# Neonatal Nutrition for Inflammatory Disorders and Necrotizing Enterocolitis

# Neonatal Nutrition for Inflammatory Disorders and Necrotizing Enterocolitis

Editor

**Misty Good**

MDPI • Basel • Beijing • Wuhan • Barcelona • Belgrade • Manchester • Tokyo • Cluj • Tianjin

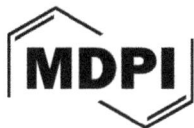

*Editor*
Misty Good
Washington University School of Medicine in St. Louis
USA


*Editorial Office*
MDPI
St. Alban-Anlage 66
4052 Basel, Switzerland


This is a reprint of articles from the Special Issue published online in the open access journal *Nutrients* (ISSN 2072-6643) (available at: https://www.mdpi.com/journal/nutrients/special_issues/Neonatal_Inflammatory_Enterocolitis).


For citation purposes, cite each article independently as indicated on the article page online and as indicated below:

LastName, A.A.; LastName, B.B.; LastName, C.C. Article Title. *Journal Name* **Year**, *Article Number*, Page Range.


**ISBN 978-3-03943-481-7 (Hbk)**
**ISBN 978-3-03943-482-4 (PDF)**


© 2020 by the authors. Articles in this book are Open Access and distributed under the Creative Commons Attribution (CC BY) license, which allows users to download, copy and build upon published articles, as long as the author and publisher are properly credited, which ensures maximum dissemination and a wider impact of our publications.
The book as a whole is distributed by MDPI under the terms and conditions of the Creative Commons license CC BY-NC-ND.

# Contents

**About the Editor** . . . . . . . . . . . . . . . . . . . . . . . . . . . . . . . . . . . . . . . . . . . . . . . . . . . . . . . . . **vii**

**Preface to "Neonatal Nutrition for Inflammatory Disorders and Necrotizing Enterocolitis"** . . **ix**

**Emma Altobelli, Paolo Matteo Angeletti, Alberto Verrotti and Reimondo Petrocelli**
The Impact of Human Milk on Necrotizing Enterocolitis: A Systematic Review and Meta-Analysis
Reprinted from: *Nutrients* **2020**, *12*, 1322, doi:10.3390/nu12051322 . . . . . . . . . . . . . . . . . . . . . **1**

**Lila S. Nolan, Olivia B. Parks and Misty Good**
A Review of the Immunomodulating Components of Maternal Breast Milk and Protection Against Necrotizing Enterocolitis
Reprinted from: *Nutrients* **2020**, *12*, 14, doi:10.3390/nu12010014 . . . . . . . . . . . . . . . . . . . **15**

**Julie D. Thai and Katherine E. Gregory**
Bioactive Factors in Human Breast Milk Attenuate Intestinal Inflammation during Early Life
Reprinted from: *Nutrients* **2020**, *12*, 581, doi:10.3390/nu12020581 . . . . . . . . . . . . . . . . . . **29**

**David Ramiro-Cortijo, Pratibha Singh, Yan Liu, Esli Medina-Morales, William Yakah, Steven D. Freedman and Camilia R. Martin**
Breast Milk Lipids and Fatty Acids in Regulating Neonatal Intestinal Development and Protecting against Intestinal Injury
Reprinted from: *Nutrients* **2020**, *12*, 534, doi:10.3390/nu12020534 . . . . . . . . . . . . . . . . . . **45**

**Kathryn Burge, Erynn Bergner, Aarthi Gunasekaran, Jeffrey Eckert and Hala Chaaban**
The Role of Glycosaminoglycans in Protection from Neonatal Necrotizing Enterocolitis: A Narrative Review
Reprinted from: *Nutrients* **2020**, *12*, 546, doi:10.3390/nu12020546 . . . . . . . . . . . . . . . . . . **63**

**Jeffrey D. Galley and Gail E. Besner**
The Therapeutic Potential of Breast Milk-Derived Extracellular Vesicles
Reprinted from: *Nutrients* **2020**, *12*, 745, doi:10.3390/nu12030745 . . . . . . . . . . . . . . . . . . **83**

**Shiloh R Lueschow, Stacy L Kern, Huiyu Gong, Justin L Grobe, Jeffrey L Segar, Susan J Carlson and Steven J McElroy**
Feeding Formula Eliminates the Necessity of Bacterial Dysbiosis and Induces Inflammation and Injury in the Paneth Cell Disruption Murine NEC Model in an Osmolality-Dependent Manner
Reprinted from: *Nutrients* **2020**, *12*, 900, doi:10.3390/nu12040900 . . . . . . . . . . . . . . . . . . **97**

**Jocelyn Ou, Cathleen M. Courtney, Allie E. Steinberger, Maria E. Tecos and Brad W. Warner**
Nutrition in Necrotizing Enterocolitis and Following Intestinal Resection
Reprinted from: *Nutrients* **2020**, *12*, 520, doi:10.3390/nu12020520 . . . . . . . . . . . . . . . . . . **117**

**Oluwabunmi Olaloye, Matthew Swatski and Liza Konnikova**
Role of Nutrition in Prevention of Neonatal Spontaneous Intestinal Perforation and Its Complications: A Systematic Review
Reprinted from: *Nutrients* **2020**, *12*, 1347, doi:10.3390/nu12051347 . . . . . . . . . . . . . . . . . . **133**

**Sierra A. Kleist and Kathryn A. Knoop**
Understanding the Elements of Maternal Protection from Systemic Bacterial Infections during Early Life
Reprinted from: *Nutrients* **2020**, *12*, 1045, doi:10.3390/nu12041045 . . . . . . . . . . . . . . . . . . **149**

**Estefanía Martín-Álvarez, Javier Diaz-Castro, Manuela Peña-Caballero, Laura Serrano-López, Jorge Moreno-Fernández, Belen Sánchez-Martínez, Francisca Martín-Peregrina, Mercedes Alonso-Moya, José Maldonado-Lozano, Jose A. Hurtado-Suazo and Julio J. Ochoa**
Oropharyngeal Colostrum Positively Modulates the Inflammatory Response in Preterm Neonates
Reprinted from: *Nutrients* **2020**, *12*, 413, doi:10.3390/nu12020413 . . . . . . . . . . . . . . . . . . . . 163

**Ting Ting Fu, Paige E. Schroder and Brenda B. Poindexter**
Macronutrient Analysis of Target-Pooled Donor Breast Milk and Corresponding Growth in Very Low Birth Weight Infants
Reprinted from: *Nutrients* **2019**, *11*, 1884, doi:10.3390/nu11081884 . . . . . . . . . . . . . . . . . . 175

**Débora Cañizo Vázquez, Sandra Salas García, Montserrat Izquierdo Renau and Isabel Iglesias-Platas**
Availability of Donor Milk for Very Preterm Infants Decreased the Risk of Necrotizing Enterocolitis without Adversely Impacting Growth or Rates of Breastfeeding
Reprinted from: *Nutrients* **2019**, *11*, 1895, doi:10.3390/nu11081895 . . . . . . . . . . . . . . . . . . 187

**Rebecca Hoban, Supriya Khatri, Aloka Patel and Sharon L. Unger**
Supplementation of Mother's Own Milk with Donor Milk in Infants with Gastroschisis or Intestinal Atresia: A Retrospective Study
Reprinted from: *Nutrients* **2020**, *12*, 589, doi:10.3390/nu12020589 . . . . . . . . . . . . . . . . . . . 201

**Jennifer Canvasser, Amy B. Hair, Jae H. Kim and Sarah N. Taylor**
Parent and Provider Perspectives on the Imprecise Label of "Human Milk Fortifier" in the NICU
Reprinted from: *Nutrients* **2020**, *12*, 720, doi:10.3390/nu12030720 . . . . . . . . . . . . . . . . . . . 211

# About the Editor

**Misty Good**, M.D., M.S. is an Assistant Professor of Pediatrics at the Washington University School of Medicine in St. Louis, Missouri. Dr. Good is a board-certified neonatologist and practices in the neonatal intensive care unit at St. Louis Children's Hospital. Dr. Good also leads a translational research program that focuses on elucidating the cellular and molecular mechanisms involved in the pathogenesis of necrotizing enterocolitis (NEC). Her laboratory is characterizing the mucosal immune responses during NEC and interrogates how these responses can be modified or prevented through dietary modifications or targeted intestinal epithelial therapies.

# Preface to "Neonatal Nutrition for Inflammatory Disorders and Necrotizing Enterocolitis"

This *Nutrients* Special Issue focuses on neonatal nutritional advances for inflammatory disorders affecting infants, such as necrotizing enterocolitis (NEC). Nutrition can significantly impact the development of certain diseases that afflict infants. This Special Issue aims to bring together the latest research on the role of nutrition in preventing or impacting neonatal disorders. Specifically, this Special Issue focuses on the role of breast milk or donor breast milk and the various components in milk that have been demonstrated to protect against NEC and other inflammatory diseases. This Special Issue provides a comprehensive composite of the advances in nutritional strategies that can modulate or prevent neonatal intestinal disorders.

**Misty Good**
*Editor*

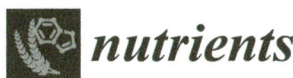 

Review

# The Impact of Human Milk on Necrotizing Enterocolitis: A Systematic Review and Meta-Analysis

**Emma Altobelli [1,*], Paolo Matteo Angeletti [1], Alberto Verrotti [2] and Reimondo Petrocelli [3]**

1. Department of Life, Health and Environmental Sciences, University of L'Aquila, 67100 L'Aquila, Italy; paolomatteoangeletti@gmail.com
2. Department of Pediatrics, University of L'Aquila, 67100 L'Aquila, Italy; alberto.verrottidipianella@univaq.it
3. Public Health Unit, ASREM, 86100 Campobasso, Italy; reimondo.petrocelli@asrem.org
* Correspondence: emma.altobelli@cc.univaq.it; Tel.: +39-0862-434666

Received: 25 March 2020; Accepted: 1 May 2020; Published: 6 May 2020

**Abstract:** Background. Premature infants receiving breastfeed have a lower incidence of NEC than those fed preterm formula. This study aimed: (1) to update a systematic review and meta-analyses to evaluate the relationship between feeding and necrotizing enterocolitis (NEC) in low weight premature infants; (2) to conduct meta-regression analyses by subgroups; (3) to describe geographical distribution of milk banks in the world. Methods. Papers included in the meta-analysis were updated as of June 2019. Relative risks were used as a measure of effect size. Random effect models were used to account for different sources of variation among studies. For milk banks, the data reviewed by the literature were integrated with the information collected from countries' institutional sites and milk bank networks. Results. Thirty-two papers were included in meta-analysis: six randomized controlled trials (RCTs) and 26 observational studies (OS). The census has found 572 milk banks around in the world. Brazil has the most active milk banks. RCTs meta-analysis indicates a risk reduction of NEC using human milk respect to formula: Relative risk (RR) = 0.62 (0.42–0.93). Seven OS compared quantities lower than human milk or higher than the 50th quantile showing a risk reduction of NEC:RR = 0.51 (0.31–0.85); 3 OS that evaluated human milk versus mixed feeding showing that human milk has a protective role on the development of NEC:RR = 0.74 (0.63–0.91). Results of subgroups analysis show that the risk reduction is statistically significant only for studies in which premature infants are given both their own and donated breastmilk. Conclusions. The possibility of preserving human milk and promoting donations guarantees an improvement in the health of newborns.

**Keywords:** human milk banks; NEC; meta-analysis; breast-feeding

## 1. Introduction

Necrotizing enterocolitis (NEC) is the most devastating intestinal disease in neonates with very-low-birth-weight (VLBW). Incidence varies in different studies. Yee et al. [1] and Fitzgibbons et al. [2] showed, in large cohort studies of VLBW infants, respectively, NEC incidence from 1.3% to 12.9% and from 3% to 12%; while more recently observational studies showed an incidence from 20.7% [3] to 16.7% [4,5].

It is universally accepted that human milk is the optimum source of nutrition for the first six months of life. The health benefits of human milk are known, not only for premature infants [6], but also for prevention of other infant diseases [7].

Premature infants receiving human milk have a lower incidence of NEC than those fed preterm formula [8]. In fact, some studies suggest that mother's milk is protective against sepsis, because it contains bioactive substances that have bactericidal and immune-modulating activities [9].

Shoji et al. support the hypothesis that breastmilk has antioxidant proprieties with a protective effect from oxidative stress [10]. In this contest, it is important to underline that not all mothers produce sufficient milk for their neonate, and donor human milk (DM) has been considered as an alternative to mother's milk (MM) [11]. Human milk inhibits the growth of *Escherichia coli*, *Staphylococcus aureus* and *Candida* sp. [12]. DM is generally pasteurized to prevent the potential risk for the transmission of pathogens from donor mothers to preterm infants. Its safety must be considered accurately because pasteurization reduces the concentration of immunological proteins in human milk [13,14]. Human milk banking is an absolute necessity, especially for premature infants. Unfortunately, human milk banks are not present in each country of the world. Infants can suffer the consequences if there are no banks. Generally, the collection and processing of human milk is established by guidelines. Globally, there is a growing interest to increase milk banks by also raising awareness campaigns to donate milk.

The aims of our study are: (i) to update a systematic review and meta-analyses of observational and RCT studies that evaluated the possible relationship between feeding (maternal, preterm formula, mixed maternal-formula) and development of necrotizing enterocolitis (NEC) in premature infants low weight; (ii) to conduct meta-regression analyses evaluating continuous and geographical variables; (iii) to describe the geographical distribution of milk banks in the world.

## 2. Materials and Methods

The papers included in the meta-analysis were sought in the MEDLINE, EMBASE, Scopus, Clinicaltrials.gov, Web of Science, and Cochrane Library databases as of June 2019. The search terms used were milk, human OR breast feeding OR milk banks OR breast milk expression OR breastfeed* OR breastfed OR breast OR HM OR fed OR feed* OR enteral nutrition AND enteral nutrition AND infant, premature OR infants, extremely premature OR infant, low birth weight OR infant, very low birth weight OR intensive care units, neonatal OR intensive care, neonatal OR premature birth AND low birthweight OR low birth weight OR VLBW OR ELBW OR Prematur* OR Preterm OR pre-term OR infant* OR newborn* OR new-born* OR baby* OR babies OR neonatal intensive care OR NICU AND enterocolitis, necrotizing. Filters: Filters: 15 years, Humans, Child: birth-18 years.

Papers were selected using the Preferred Reporting Items for Systematic Reviews and Meta-Analyses (PRISMA) flowchart (Figure 1) and the PRISMA checklist (Table S1) [15]. A manual search of possible references of interest was also performed. Only studies published in English over the previous 15 years were considered. The papers were selected by two independent reviewers (P.M.A. and A.V.); a methodologist (E.A.) resolved any disagreements. Bias was assessed using the Cochrane Collaboration tool for assessing risk of bias and the Newcastle–Ottawa scale for cohort studies (Tables S2 and S3) [16,17].

For the research of milk banks, place where HM is collected and/or treated and/or distributed, the data reviewed by the literature were integrated with the information collected from the institutional sites of the individual countries and from European and North American milk bank networks. Other information sources have been obtained from the literature using the following words: "human milk banks" AND "state name". Moreover, we used the information obtained from the institutional sites for each country [18,19]. Data on premature births were derived from WHO datasets [20]. The ratio between milk banks and premature births per 100,000 was performed.

*Statistical Analysis*

We consider NEC if patients had a Bell's score ≥2. Relative risks (RRs), with 95% CI and p-value, were used as a measure of effect size. Random effect models were used to account for different sources of variation among studies. Heterogeneity was assessed using Q statistics and $I^2$. The stability of study findings was checked with moderator analysis. Publication bias was analyzed and represented by a funnel plot, and funnel plot symmetry was assessed with Egger's test [21,22]. Publication bias was checked using the trim and fill procedure [22,23]; PROMETA 3 software (IDo Statistics-Internovi, Cesena, Italy) was used. Finally, meta-regression analyses, using a random effects model, were utilized for the following variables: publication year of article, gender, birth weight and gestational age and geographical area; for continuous variables, regression models were used; for categorical variables, an ANOVA-Q test was used. Meta-regressions were performed when the number of studies containing the variables to be analyzed was ≥3. Meta-analyses and meta-regressions were conducted according to the study design: randomized and observational studies. In the context of observational studies, a distinction was made based on the type of comparison HM vs mixed feeding, HM vs only preterm formula and mixed feeding vs only preterm formula. The articles presenting data in quantiles of consumed milk were analyzed by dichotomically dividing the patients into two groups on the basis of the presence of human milk in their diet: inferior or superior to the 50° quantile. A subgroup analysis was also conducted, excluding studies that, in the preterm formula group, had an incidence of NEC above 15%.

## 3. Results

### 3.1. Literature Search Results

Research has highlighted the presence of 307 records. In the screening phase, 271 references were excluded; therefore, 36 full texts were considered. Of these, 4 were not considered for different reasons: one paper was a meta-analysis [23], one was an RCT that reviewed early progressive feeding [24], one had another outcome regarding neurological follow-up of premature children respect to the nourishment adopted [25], one paper analyzed only children that took maternal milk or formula or donated milk the same or more than 50° quantile not allowing consistent comparisons with the other primary studies selected [26]. Finally, 32 papers were included in quantitative analysis: six clinical trials [6,27–32] and 26 observational studies [3–5,33–54].

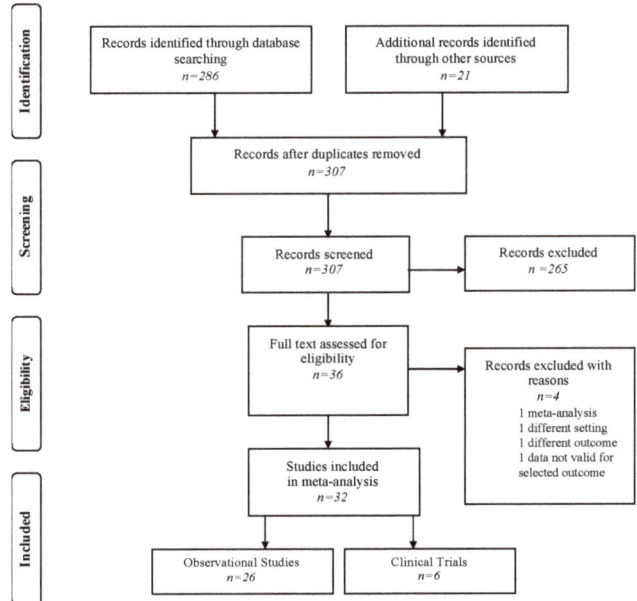

**Figure 1.** Flow-chart of search strategy.

The characteristics of the studies, compared to the type of human milk adopted, are reported in the Tables S4, S5. The characteristics concerning the population of the single studies are reported in the Table S6.

## 3.2. Meta-Analysis and Meta-Regression Results

Selected trials [6,27–31] investigated the occurrence of NEC in breastfed premature infants compared to those fed preterm formula. Their total sample size is 1626 newborns. The meta-analysis indicates that there is a clear indication of risk reduction in the use of human milk respect to formula, RR = 0.62 (0.42–0.93), and this result occurs in presence of statistical heterogeneity among primary studies analyzed ($I^2$ = 47.03, $p$ = 0.009) (Table 1, Figure S1).

The meta-regression analyses by year of publication, male gender, birth weight, gestational age and ethnicity do not show statistically significant results; in fact, it is important to underline that these variables do not influence NEC incidence (Table 2). Trim and fill analyses do not show differences among observed and estimated values and any studies were trimmed.

Eighteen observational studies [3–5,32–47] investigated the comparison between human milk vs formula for a total of 6,405 newborns. The overall result indicates that there is a reduction in the risk of NEC, RR = 0.45 (0.32–0.62, $p$ < 0.001), with statistically significant heterogeneity among primary studies analyzed ($I^2$ = 55.25, $p$ = 0.002) (Table 1, Figure S1).

The meta-regression analyses by year of publication, gender, birth weight, gestational age and ethnicity does not show statistically significant results (Table 2). The analysis by geographical area shows statistically significant differences, with risk reduction in Europe and USA, but not in Japan, probably because there is only one study with a small sample (Table 3).

Seven observational studies [49–55] compared high consumption of human milk against low consumption for a total of 2,453 newborns. The results show a risk reduction of NEC, RR = 0.51 (0.31–0.85, $p$ = 0.01), without statistically significant heterogeneity ($I^2$ = 9.21, $p$ = 0.359) (Table 1, Figure S1).

The meta-regression analyses show that there are no significant results regarding the year of publication, birth weight and ethnicity, but they show a statistically significant result with regard to male gender (Table 2).

Three studies [35–37] that evaluated breastfeeding versus mixed feeding (Table 1) show that human milk could have a protective role on the development of NEC, RR = 0.74 (0.63–0.91, $p$ = 0.003), both without statistically significant heterogeneity ($I^2$ = 0.00, $p$ = 0.407) and in the absence of publication bias (Table 1, Figure S1).

The meta-regression analyses for publication year and birth weight do not show statistically significant results (Table 2).

Finally, four studies concerned the comparison between mixed feeding and preterm formula (Table 1) [35–38]. In these it is revealed that mixed feeding is a risk factor for the development of NEC, RR = 1.37 (1.13–1.65, $p$ = 0.001), without statistically significant heterogeneity ($I^2$ = 0.00, $p$ = 0.774) and publication bias (Table 1, Figure S1).

The meta-regression analysis for year of publication shows a statistically significant result (Table 2), but not for birth weight.

Finally, trim and fill analysis do not show differences among observed and estimated values and any study were trimmed.

Table 1. Meta-analysis results.

| | Pooled Analysis | | Heterogeneity | | Publication Bias | | | |
| --- | --- | --- | --- | --- | --- | --- | --- | --- |
| | | | | | Egger's Test | | Begg's and Mazdumdar's Tests | |
| | RR (95% CI) | p-Value | I² | p-Value | T | p-Value | Z | p-Value |
| **RCT** | | | | | | | | |
| Human milk (breastfeeding and donor) vs preterm formula k = 6 [6,27–31] | 0.62 (0.42–0.93) | 0.02 | 47.03 | 0.009 | −1.82 | 0.144 | −2.44 | 0.015 |
| Human milk (breastfeeding and donor) vs preterm formula k = 4 * [27–30] | 0.57 (0.32–1.01) | 0.054 | 64.01 | 0.040 | −1.64 | 0.243 | −2.04 | 0.174 |
| **Observational studies** | | | | | | | | |
| >50° quantile of human milk of total enteral feeding k = 7 [48–54] | 0.51 (0.31–0.85) | 0.001 | 9.21 | 0.359 | −2.02 | 0.078 | −02.27 | 0.788 |
| Human milk (breastfeeding and donor) vs preterm formula k = 18 [3–5,32–47] | 0.45 (0.32–0.62) | <0.001 | 55.25 | 0.002 | −0.35 | 0.731 | 0.11 | 0.910 |
| Human milk (breastfeeding and donor) vs preterm formula k = 15 [32–47] | 0.45 (0.30–0.69) | <0.001 | 56.61 | 0.004 | −0.97 | 0.35 | 0.35 | 0.729 |
| Human milk (breastfeeding and donor) vs mixed feeding k = 3 [35–37] | 0.74 (0.63–0.91) | 0.003 | 0.00 | 0.407 | 0.11 | 0.925 | −0.68 | 0.497 |
| Mixed feeding vs preterm formula k = 4 [37,38] | 1.37 (1.13–1.65) | 0.001 | 0.00 | 0.774 | 0.23 | 0.871 | 0.00 | 1.00 |

Legend: RCT: randomized controlled trial; RR: relative risk; CI: confidence interval; k: numbers of primary studies *Excluding paper reporting NEC (necrotizing enterocolitis) incidence >15% of in preterm formula groups.

## 3.3. Human Milk Bank for Premature Birth

The census of milk banks has found in the world 572 milk banks, not evenly distributed and were reported on Table S7. Brazil holds the record for the number of active milk banks (214), followed by South Africa with 44, Italy with 37 banks and in Europe 238. Norway, Sweden, Finland, Estonia, Switzerland, Slovakia and Cuba have the largest number of milk banks per premature baby (Figure 2).

Table 2. Meta-regressions: results for continuous variables.

|  | No. of Primary Studies | Total Sample Size | Intercept (y) | Slope (x) | $p$-Value |
|---|---|---|---|---|---|
| **RCT** | | | | | |
| Human milk vs preterm formula | | | | | |
| Publication year | 6 | 1626 | −107.64 | 0.05 | 0.472 |
| Male (%) | 4 | 775 | −2.96 | 0.04 | 0.383 |
| Birth weight | 4 | 1084 | −5.21 | 0.00 | 0.068 |
| Gestational age | 5 | 1253 | −5.21 | 0.26 | 0.393 |
| Caucasians (%) | 3 | 1030 | −0.20 | −0.02 | 1.186 |
| **Observational Studies** | | | | | |
| High vs low dose | | | | | |
| Publication year | 7 | 2453 | 21.34 | −0.02 | 0.883 |
| Male (%) | 5 | 1950 | 7.84 | −0.18 | 0.039 |
| Birth weight | 3 | 835 | 2.88 | 0.0 | 0.189 |
| Caucasians (%) | 4 | 1982 | 2.22 | −0.05 | 0.064 |
| Human milk vs preterm formula | | | | | |
| Publication year | 18 | 6405 | 145.52 | −0.07 | 0.077 |
| Male (%) | 15 | 4730 | 0.16 | −0.02 | 0.682 |
| Birth weight | 14 | 5424 | 0.63 | 0.00 | 0.234 |
| Gestational age | 11 | 2875 | 1.56 | −0.08 | 0.680 |
| Caucasians (%) | 5 | 3558 | −0.18 | −0.02 | 0.096 |
| Human milk vs mixed feeding | | | | | |
| Publication year | 3 | 2071 | 190.88 | −0.09 | 0.624 |
| Birth weight | 3 | 2071 | −0.83 | 0.00 | 0.659 |
| Mixed feeding vs preterm formula | | | | | |
| Publication year | 4 | 2089 | −110.88 | −0.05 | 0.009 |
| Birth weight | 3 | 1708 | −0.75 | 0.00 | 0.491 |

Table 3. Observational studies regarding human milk vs preterm formula: meta-regression results of geographical areas.

|  | No. of Primary Studies | Total Sample Size | RR (95% CI) | $p$-Value | $I^2$ | Q | $p$-Value | Overall ANOVA Q-Test |
|---|---|---|---|---|---|---|---|---|
| Europe | 9 | 3398 | 0.53 (0.35–0.79) | 0.02 | 35.82 | 12.31 | 0.138 | 0.42, $p = 0.811$ |
| Japan | 1 | 18 | 0.81 (0.01–45.22) | 0.92 | - | - | - | |
| USA | 8 | 3876 | 0.43 (0.26–0.71) | 0.71 | 72.19 | 25.17 | 0.001 | |

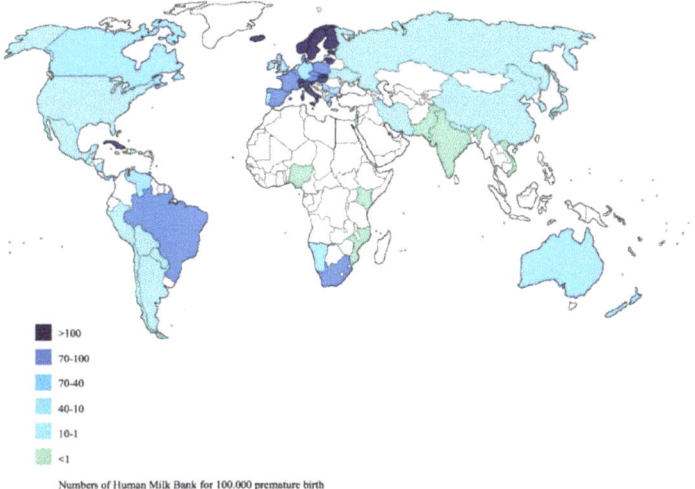

**Figure 2.** Distribution of Human Milk Bank in the world.

## 4. Discussion

Some fundamental aspects emerge from our work: the first is that human milk, breastfeed or donor, has a protective effect in the development of NEC in premature babies: in fact, it can be seen that the use of human milk is a protective factor in the development of NEC in premature babies; the second underlines that there is no homogeneous distribution of the places of the milk banks where HM is collected and/or pasteurized and/or distributed. The latter represents a limitation of the study: particularly the pasteurization, with thermal damage, reduces microbial contamination and immunological components [9]. A second limitation is that, considering the primary studies, it was not possible to extrapolate the policies relating to the implementation of the milk banks; in addition, breast milk and donated milk were considered as a single entity of comparison with breastfeeding with formula, although statistically there is no evidence for publication bias.

A third limitation consists in the fact that the countries considered are very heterogeneous, both from the socio-cultural point of view and from the point of view of organizing health systems. In addition, it should be emphasized that, even within the same state, there are differences between the north and south. Heterogeneity between countries and between north and south of the same country can present socio-cultural differences. There may be religious differences between one state and another or between one continent and another. Another fundamental difference is represented by the income.

Finally, some works [3–6,31] show a higher incidences of NEC compared to the others. This could partially justify the clinical heterogeneity of the studies, although the analysis of the risk of bias does not highlight substantial critical issues.

The United Nations Objective 3.4 for "Sustainable development is linked to the reduction of premature mortality" [55]. The guidelines of the WHO and the main American and European scientific associations indicate that, in the absence of breast milk, donated milk is the second food of choice [56]. Where breastfeeding is not possible, donated milk stored in milk banks can be used [57–60]. Our work highlighted that there is an inhomogeneous distribution of milk banks (Figure 2).

It has been estimated that 52.9% of premature births occur in Asia, 25% in sub-Saharan Africa, 7.7% in Latin America, 5.7% in Europe, 4.1 % in North Africa, 3.1 in North America and 0.5% in Oceania. This data obviously reflects differences in terms of methodological qualities between countries with high and low incomes [61]. A European study shows that the costs of hospitalization of a premature are 10,000 euros more than a not premature one [62]. Regarding milk banks, in Asia and Africa there is a lower presence (more concentrated only in some countries) both in percentage terms and in relation to the number of premature per 100,000 births. This data shows that there are inequalities in access to donated breast milk.

A liter of donated milk has been estimated 82.88 euro in Germany [63], while in the US the costs is 150 dollars [64,65].

It is important to underline that the administration of donated breast milk, as we have seen, associated with the continuous improvement of neonatal techniques, could significantly reduce the costs of hospitalization and assistance in the short term.

A study conducted in the US shows that treatment with breast feed fortifier derived from human donated milk in the prevention of NEC is cost effective with respect to breast feed fortifier derived from bovine milk [66]. This effect could be very important in the long run. It is known that breast milk improves neuro-cognitive development, potentially also reducing the costs of social and scholastic assistance linked to any deficit, even if there are no studies on the subject to date. Therefore, the establishment of a milk bank does not appear to be anti-economical, but rather as a precise choice in maternal and child health policies aimed at reducing social inequalities. Online sales of breast milk are also described, but being out of the milk bank circuit, do not have the same quality standard [67]. Within the advanced countries there are differences in the distribution of milk banks: for example, in Italy there is a difference between the north and south, being more widespread in the north of the country with a higher income to the detriment of the southern areas with a lower income [68]. At the same time, the scarcity of the resource imposes choices with respect to whom should administer this good.

Our results show that feeding with breast milk reduces the risk of NEC. In particular, it is noted that in studies that compared the low versus high consumption of their own breast milk, there is a significant reduction in the risk of NEC. This information is also confirmed in observational studies and in clinical trials in which human milk (donated or own) is compared with formulas: in both cases there is a risk reduction. In addition, subgroup analysis is particularly interesting. It shows that the risk reduction is statistically significant only for studies in which premature are given both their own and donated breastmilk. It should be emphasized that heterogeneity is statistically significant in the absence of publication bias. The nature of these results could be explained by the difference between maternal milk and donated maternal milk, which undergoes pasteurization processes to eliminate possible pathogens. In fact, in a recent study a difference of macronutrients and proteins is highlighted: the donated milk would have less grams of protein per deciliter (1.42 vs. 1.52) and less fat content per deciliter (3.41 vs. 3.79), therefore a lower energy content (63.80 vs. 67.29) [58]. However, the pasteurization of breast milk appears to be a hygiene practice of fundamental importance in order to eliminate the bacterial and viral load, despite sacrificing some beneficial components in breast milk [58,59]. Alternative methods to pasteurization are being studied to preserve all the qualities of breast milk [58].

The variables investigated with meta-regression analysis do not provide explanations on the factors that may affect the risk of NEC, with the exception of publication year and male gender. In the first case, this result could be justified by an overall improvement in the health care of premature neonates, as highlighted also in the most recently published papers [28]. In the second, the result could be influenced by selection methods of the patients, not being known in the literature a greater predisposition of male gender on the incidence of prematurity.

Furthermore, it is important to remember that the use of the random effects model, also for meta-regressions, allows to ascertain the possible epidemiological link between the observed effect and the variables investigated; this aspect is strengthened in the absence of statistically significant publication bias.

## 5. Conclusions

In conclusion, our study shows a clear benefit of breastfeeding or, in its absence, with donated milk and highlights a heterogeneity in the distribution of milk banks between countries and within the same country. Particularly in Africa, the Middle East and Asia, where Muslim populations are dominant. In addition, our results underline the relationship between feeding and development of NEC [69].

It therefore highlights the potential benefit of accessing a resource, breast milk, appropriately stored at the milk banks. In addition, this breastfeeding should also be encouraged in order to reduce the impact of other pathologies related to lactation [23]. Failure to access socio-health infrastructures such as milk banks could create inequalities for the prevention of a high mortality disease. Further investigations, which go beyond the objectives of this meta-analysis, should be addressed on the link between NEC and pasteurized or unpasteurized human milk.

Finally, almost all primary studies have been conducted in Europe and the United States. The possibility of preserving breast milk and promoting donations (implicitly also supporting control over maternal health conditions, promoting virtuous behavior) guarantees an improvement in the health of newborns. Of particular interest would be to evaluate the incidence of NEC in Arab countries, where breastfeeding is abandoned early and the donation of breast milk is not particularly successful for religious reasons.

International cooperation and the authorities of the single countries should provide some targeted interventions for the realization of milk banks that, in the last analysis, represent a fortress of health and social justice. In particular, the use of donor milk is widely endorsed.

**Supplementary Materials:** The following are available online at http://www.mdpi.com/2072-6643/12/5/1322/s1, Table S1: Prisma Checklist, Table S2: Trial bias assessment according to Cochrane Collaboration, Table S3 Observational Studies bias assessment according to New Castle-Ottawa scale, Table S4: Nutritional Pattern of Interventional Studies, Table S5: Nutritional Pattern of Observational Studies, Table S6: Characteristics of included studies, Table S7: Human Milk Banks in the world. Figure S1: Meta-analysis: results from RCT and observational studies. Forest plot for selected outcomes.

**Author Contributions:** E.A.: Guarantor of the article, study concept and design, literature search, data analysis, and manuscript writing. P.M.A.: literature search, data abstraction, participant manuscript writing. A.V.: literature search. R.P.: literature search. All authors have read and agreed to the published version of the manuscript.

**Funding:** This research received no external funding.

**Acknowledgments:** We have not received funds in support of research work or for covering the costs to public in open access.

**Conflicts of Interest:** The authors declare no conflict of interest. The founding sponsors had no role in the design of the study; in the collection, analyses, or interpretation of data; in the writing of the manuscript, and in the decision to publish the results.

## References

1. Yee, W.H.; Soraisham, A.S.; Shah, V.S.; Aziz, K.; Yoon, W.; Lee, S.K. Canadian neonatal network incidence and timing of presentation of necrotizing enterocolitis in preterm infants. *Pediatrics* **2012**, *129*, e298–e304. [CrossRef] [PubMed]
2. Fitzgibbons, S.C.; Ching, Y.; Yu, D.; Carpenter, J.; Kenny, M.; Weldon, C.; Lillehei, C.; Valim, C.; Horbar, J.D.; Jaksic, T. Mortality of necrotizing enterocolitis expressed by birth weight categories. *J. Pediatr. Surg.* **2009**, *44*, 1072–1075. [CrossRef] [PubMed]
3. Verd, S.; Porta, R.; Botet, F.; Gutiérrez, A.; Ginovart, G.; Barbero, A.H.; Ciurana, A.; Plata, I.I. Hospital outcomes of extremely low birth weight infants after introduction of donor milk to supplement mother's milk. *Breastfeed. Med.* **2015**, *10*, 150–155. [CrossRef] [PubMed]
4. Huston, R.K.; Markell, A.M.; McCulley, E.A.; Pathak, M.; Rogers, S.P.; Sweeney, S.L.; Dolphin, N.G.; Gardiner, S.K. Decreasing necrotizing enterocolitis and gastrointestinal bleeding in the neonatal intensive care unit: The role of donor human milk and exclusive human milk diets in infants ≤1500 g birth weight. *Infant. Child Adolesc. Nutr.* **2014**, *6*, 86–93. [CrossRef]

5. Hair, A.B.; Rechtman, D.J.; Lee, M.L.; Niklas, V. Beyond necrotizing enterocolitis: Other clinical advantages of an exclusive human milk diet. *Breastfeed. Med.* **2018**, *13*, 408–411. [CrossRef]
6. Cristofalo, E.A.; Schanler, R.J.; Blanco, C.L.; Sullivan, S.; Trawoeger, R.; Kiechl-Kohlendorfer, U.; Dudell, G.; Rechtman, D.J.; Lee, M.L.; Lucas, A.; et al. Randomized trial of exclusive human milk versus preterm formula diets in extremely premature infants. *J. Pediatr.* **2013**, *163*, 1592–1595. [CrossRef]
7. Altobelli, E.; Petrocelli, R.; Verrotti, A.; Chiarelli, F.; Marziliano, C. Genetic and environmental factors affect the onset of type 1 diabetes mellitus. *Pediatr. Diabetes* **2016**, *17*, 559–566. [CrossRef]
8. Schanler, R.J.; Shulman, R.J.; Lau, C. Feeding strategies for premature infants: Beneficial outcomes of feeding fortified human milk versus preterm formula. *Pediatrics* **1999**, *103*, 1150–1157. [CrossRef]
9. Van Gysel, M.; Cossey, V.; Fieuws, S.; Schuermans, A. Impact of pasteurization on the antibacterial properties of human milk. *Eur. J. Pediatr.* **2012**, *171*, 1231–1237. [CrossRef]
10. Shoji, H.; Shimizu, T.; Shinohara, K.; Oguchi, S.; Shiga, S.; Yamashiro, Y. Suppressive effects of breast milk on oxidative DNA damage in very low birthweight infants. *Arch. Dis. Child Fetal. Neonatal. Edit.* **2004**, *89*, F136–F138. [CrossRef]
11. Hylander, M.A.; Strobino, D.M.; Dhanireddy, R. Human milk feedings and infection among very low birth weight infants. *Pediatrics* **1998**, *102*, e38. [CrossRef] [PubMed]
12. Dan, L.; Liu, S.; Shang, S.; Zhang, H.; Zhang, R.; Li, N. Expression of recombinant human lysozyme in bacterial artificial chromosome transgenic mice promotes the growth of Bifidobacterium and inhibits the growth of *Salmonella* in the intestine. *J. Biotechnol.* **2018**. [CrossRef] [PubMed]
13. Picaud, J.C. Buffin human milk-treatment and quality of banked human milk. *R Clin Perinatol.* **2017**, *44*, 95–119. [CrossRef] [PubMed]
14. Peila, C.; Moro, G.E.; Bertino, E.; Cavallarin, L.; Giribaldi, M.; Giuliani, F.; Cresi, F.; Coscia, A. The effect of holder pasteurization on nutrients and biologically-active components in donor human milk: A review. *Nutrients* **2016**, *2*, 477. [CrossRef]
15. Moher, D.; Altman, D.G.; Liberati, A.; Tetzlaff, J. PRISMA statement. *Epidemiology* **2011**, *22*, 128. [CrossRef]
16. Higgins, J.P.T.; Green, S.; Altman, D.G. Assessing risk of bias in included studies published online. In *Cochrane Handbook for Systematic Reviews of Interventions*; Wiley: Hoboken, NJ, USA, 2008; Chapter 8.
17. Wells, G.A.; Shea, B.; O'Connell, D.; Peterson, J.; Welch, V.; Losos, M.; Tugwell, P. The Newcastle-Ottawa Scale (NOS) for Assessing the Quality of Non Randomised Studies in Meta-Analyses. 2001. Available online: http://www.ohri.ca/programs/clinical_epidemiology/oxford.asp (accessed on 10 November 2019).
18. European Milk Bank Association. Available online: https://europeanmilkbanking.com/ (accessed on 10 November 2019).
19. Human Milk Banking Association North America. Available online: https://www.hmbana.org/ (accessed on 10 November 2019).
20. WHO. Preterm Birth. Available online: http://ptb.srhr.org/ (accessed on 10 November 2019).
21. Rothstein, H.R.; Sutton, A.J.; Borenstein, M. *Publication Bias in Meta-Analysis*; Wiley: Chichester, UK, 2005.
22. Fragkos, K.C.; Tsagris, M.; Frangos, C.C. Publication bias in meta-analysis: Confidence intervals for Rosenthal's fail-safe number. *Int. Sch. Res. Not.* **2014**, *2014*, 825383. [CrossRef]
23. Miller, J.; Tonkin, E.; Damarell, R.A.; McPhee, A.J.; Suganuma, M.; Suganuma, H.; Middleton, P.F.; Makrides, M.; Collins, C.T. A systematic review and meta-analysis of human milk feeding and morbidity in very low birth weight infants. *Nutrients* **2018**, *10*, 707. [CrossRef]
24. Salas, A.A.; Li, P.; Parks, K.; Lal, C.V.; Martin, C.R.; Carlo, W.A. Early progressive feeding in extremely preterm infants: A randomized trial. *Am. J. Clin. Nutr.* **2018**, *107*, 365–370. [CrossRef]
25. Vohr, B.R.; Poindexter, B.B.; Dusick, A.M.; McKinley, L.T.; Higgins, R.D.; Langer, J.C.; Poole, W.K. National institute of child health and human development national research network. Persistent beneficial effects of breast milk ingested in the neonatal intensive care unit on outcomes of extremely low birth weight infants at 30 months of age. *Pediatrics* **2007**, *120*, e953. [CrossRef]
26. Sisk, P.M.; Lovelady, C.A.; Dillard, R.G.; Gruber, K.J.; O'Shea, T.M. Early human milk feeding is associated with a lower risk of necrotizing enterocolitis in very low birth weight infants. *J. Perinatol.* **2007**, *27*, 428–433. [CrossRef]
27. Sisk, P.M.; Lambeth, T.M.; Rojas, M.A.; Lightbourne, T.; Barahona, M.; Anthony, E.; Auringer, S.T. Necrotizing enterocolitis and growth in preterm infants fed predominantly maternal milk, pasteurized donor milk, or preterm formula: A retrospective study. *Am. J. Perinatol.* **2017**, *34*, 676–683. [PubMed]

28. Schanler, R.J.; Lau, C.; Hurst, N.M.; Smith, E.O. Randomized trial of donor human milk versus preterm formula as substitutes for mothers' own milk in the feeding of extremely premature infants. *Pediatrics* **2005**, *116*, 400–406. [CrossRef] [PubMed]
29. Manzoni, P.; Stolfi, I.; Pedicino, R.; Vagnarelli, F.; Mosca, F.; Pugni, L.; Bollani, L.; Pozzi, M.; Gomez, K.; Tzialla, C.; et al. Human milk feeding prevents retinopathy of prematurity (ROP) in preterm VLBW neonates. *Early Hum. Dev.* **2013**, *89*, S64–S68. [CrossRef]
30. O'Connor, D.L.; Gibbins, S.; Kiss, A.; Bando, N.; Brennan-Donnan, J.; Ng, E.; Campbell, D.M.; Vaz, S.; Fusch, C.; Asztalos, E.; et al. Effect of supplemental donor human milk compared with preterm formula on neurodevelopment of very low-birth-weight infants at 18 months: A randomized clinical trial. *JAMA* **2016**, *316*, 1897–1905. [CrossRef]
31. Corpeleijn, W.E.; de Waard, M.; Christmann, V.; van Goudoever, J.B.; Jansen-van der Weide, M.C.; Kooi, E.M.; Koper, J.F.; Kouwenhoven, S.M.; Lafeber, H.N.; Mank, E.; et al. Effect of donor milk on severe infections and mortality in very low-birth-weight infants: The early nutrition study randomized clinical trial. *JAMA Pediatr.* **2016**, *170*, 654–661. [CrossRef]
32. Sullivan, S.; Schanler, R.J.; Kim, J.H.; Patel, A.L.; Trawöger, R.; Kiechl-Kohlendorfer, U.; Chan, G.M.; Blanco, C.L.; Abrams, S.; Cotton, C.M.; et al. An exclusively human milk-based diet is associated with a lower rate of necrotizing enterocolitis than a diet of human milk and bovine milk-based products. *J. Pediatr.* **2010**, *156*, 562–567. [CrossRef]
33. Bishop, C.E.; Vasquez, M.; Petershack, J.A.; Blanco, C.L. Pasteurized donor human milk for VLBW infants: The effect on necrotizing enterocolitis and related factors. *J. Neonatal Perinat. Med.* **2010**, *3*, 87–93. [CrossRef]
34. Chowning, R.; Radmacher, P.; Lewis, S.; Serke, L.; Pettit, N.; Adamkin, D.H. A retrospective analysis of the effect of human milk on prevention of necrotizing enterocolitis and postnatal growth. *J. Perinat.* **2016**, *36*, 221–224. [CrossRef]
35. Manea, A.; Boia, M.; Iacob, D.; Dima, M.; Iacob, R.E. Benefits of early enteral nutrition in extremely low birth weight infants. *Singap. Med. J.* **2016**, *57*, 616–618. [CrossRef]
36. German Neonatal Network (GNN); Spiegler, J.; Preuß, M.; Gebauer, C.; Bendiks, M.; Herting, E.; Göpel, W. Does breastmilk influence the development of bronchopulmonary dysplasia? *J. Pediatr.* **2016**, *169*, 76–80.
37. Berkhout, D.J.C.; Klaassen, P.; Niemarkt, H.J.; de Boode, W.P.; Cossey, V.; van Goudoever, J.B.; Hulzebos, C.V.; Andriessen, P.; van Kaam, A.H.; Kramer, B.W.; et al. Risk factors for necrotizing enterocolitis: A prospective multicenter case-control study. *Neonatology* **2018**, *114*, 277–284. [CrossRef] [PubMed]
38. Zamrik, S.; Giachero, F.; Heldmann, M.; Hensel, K.O.; Wirth, S.; Jenke, A.C. Impact of an in-house pediatric surgery unit and human milk centered enteral nutrition on necrotizing enterocolitis. *Biomed. Res. Int.* **2018**, *2018*, 5042707. [CrossRef] [PubMed]
39. Corpeleijn, W.E.; Kouwenhoven, S.M.; Paap, M.C.; van Vliet, I.; Scheerder, I.; Muizer, Y.; Helder, O.K.; van Goudoever, J.B.; Vermeulen, M.J. Intake of own mother's milk during the first days of life is associated with decreased morbidity and mortality in very low birth weight infants during the first 60 days of life. *Neonatology* **2012**, *102*, 276–281. [CrossRef] [PubMed]
40. Kreissl, A.; Sauerzapf, E.; Repa, A.; Binder, C.; Thanhaeuser, M.; Jilma, B.; Ristl, R.; Berger, A.; Haiden, N. Starting enteral nutrition with preterm single donor milk instead of formula affects time to full enteral feeding in very low birth weight infants. *Acta Paediatr.* **2017**, *106*, 1460–1467. [CrossRef] [PubMed]
41. Herrmann, K.; Carroll, K. An exclusively human milk diet reduces necrotizing enterocolitis. *Breastfeed. Med.* **2014**, *9*, 184–190. [CrossRef] [PubMed]
42. Alshaikh, B.; Kostecky, L.; Blachly, N.; Yee, W. Effect of a quality improvement project to use exclusive mother's own milk on rate of necrotizing enterocolitis in preterm infants. *Breastfeed. Med.* **2015**, *10*, 355–361. [CrossRef]
43. Montjaux-Regis, N.; Cristini, C.; Arnaud, C.; Glorieux, I.; Vanpee, M.; Casper, C. Improved growth of preterm infants receiving mother's own raw milk compared with pasteurized donor milk. *Acta Paediatr.* **2011**, *100*, 1548–1554. [CrossRef]
44. Maayan-Metzger, A.; Avivi, S.; Schushan-Eisen, I.; Kuint, J. Human milk versus formula feeding among preterm infants: Short-term outcomes. *Am. J. Perinatol.* **2012**, *29*, 121–126. [CrossRef]
45. Colacci, M.; Murthy, K.; Deregnier, R.A.O.; Khan, J.Y.; Robinson, D.T. Growth and development in extremely low birth weight infants after the introduction of exclusive human milk feedings. *Am. J. Perinatol.* **2017**, *34*, 130–137. [CrossRef]

46. Tanaka, K.; Kon, N.; Ohkawa, N.; Yoshikawa, N.; Shimizu, T. Does breastfeeding in the neonatal period influence the cognitive function of very-low-birth-weight infants at 5 years of age? *Brain Dev.* **2009**, *31*, 288–293. [CrossRef]
47. Ginovart, G.; Gich, I.; Verd, S. Human milk feeding protects very low-birth-weight infants from retinopathy of prematurity: A pre–post cohort analysis. *J. Matern. Fetal. Neonatal. Med.* **2016**, *29*, 3790–3795. [CrossRef] [PubMed]
48. Giuliani, F.; Prandi, G.; Coscia, A.; Cresi, F.; Di Nicola, P.; Raia, M.; Sabatino, G.; Occhi, L.; Bertino, E. Donor human milk versus mother's own milk in preterm VLBWIs: A case control study. *J. Biol. Regul. Homeost. Agents.* **2012**, *26*, 19–24. [PubMed]
49. Vohr, B.R.; Poindexter, B.B.; Dusick, A.M.; McKinley, L.T.; Wright, L.L.; Langer, J.C.; Poole, W.K. Beneficial effects of breast milk in the neonatal intensive care unit on the developmental outcome of extremely low birth weight infants at 18 months of age. *Pediatrics* **2006**, *118*, e115–e123. [CrossRef] [PubMed]
50. Parker, L.A.; Krueger, C.; Sullivan, S.; Kelechi, T.; Mueller, M. Effect of breast milk on hospital costs and length of stay among very low-birth-weight infants in the NICU. *Adv. Neonatal. Care* **2012**, *12*, 254–259. [CrossRef] [PubMed]
51. Jacobi-Polishook, T.; Collins, C.T.; Sullivan, T.R.; Simmer, K.; Gillman, M.W.; Gibson, R.A.; Makrides, M.; Belfort, M.B. Human milk intake in preterm infants and neurodevelopment at 18 months corrected age. *Pediatr. Res.* **2016**, *80*, 486–492. [CrossRef] [PubMed]
52. Furman, L.; Taylor, G.; Minich, N.; Hack, M. The effect of maternal milk on neonatal morbidity of very low-birth-weight infants. *Arch. Pediatr. Adolesc. Med.* **2003**, *157*, 66–71. [CrossRef]
53. Colaizy, T.T.; Carlson, S.; Saftlas, A.F.; Morriss, F.H., Jr. Growth in VLBW infants fed predominantly fortified maternal and donor human milk diets: A retrospective cohort study. *BMC Pediatr.* **2012**, *12*, 124. [CrossRef]
54. O'Connor, D.L.; Jacobs, J.; Hall, R.; Adamkin, D.; Auestad, N.; Castillo, M.; Connor, W.E.; Connor, S.L.; Fitzgerald, K.; Groh-Wargo, S.; et al. Growth and development of premature infants fed predominantly human milk, predominantly premature infant formula, or a combination of human milk and premature formula. *J. Pediatr. Gastroenterol. Nutr.* **2003**, *37*, 437–446. [CrossRef]
55. WHO. The 2030 Agenda for Sustainable Development. Available online: https://sustainabledevelopment.un.org/sdgs (accessed on 10 November 2019).
56. WHO. Recommended definitions, terminology and format for statistical tables related to the perinatal period and use of a new certificate for cause of perinatal deaths. Modifications recommended by FIGO as amended October 14, 1976. *Acta Obstet. Gynecol. Scand.* **1977**, *56*, 247–253.
57. Weaver, G.; Bertino, E.; Gebauer, C.; Grovslien, A.; Mileusnic-Milenovic, R.; Arslanoglu, S.; Barnett, D.; Boquien, C.Y.; Buffin, R.; Gaya, A.; et al. Recommendations for the establishment and operation of human milk banks in Europe: A consensus statement from the European milk bank association (EMBA). *Front. Pediatr.* **2019**, *7*, 53. [CrossRef]
58. De Halleux, V.; Pieltain, C.; Senterre, T.; Rigo, J. Use of donor milk in the neonatal intensive care unit. *Semin. Fetal. Neonatal. Med.* **2017**, *22*, 23–29. [CrossRef] [PubMed]
59. Moro, G.E.; Billeaud, C.; Rachel, B.; Calvo, J.; Cavallarin, L.; Christen, L.; Escuder-Vieco, D.; Gaya, A.; Lembo, D.; Wesolowska, A.; et al. Processing of donor human milk: Update and recommendations from the European milk bank association (EMBA). *Front. Pediatr.* **2019**, *7*, 4. [CrossRef] [PubMed]
60. Asztalos, E.V. Supporting mothers of very preterm infants and breast milk production: A review of the role of galactogogues. *Nutrients* **2018**, *12*, 600. [CrossRef] [PubMed]
61. Chawanpaiboon, S.; Vogel, J.P.; Moller, A.B.; Lumbiganon, P.; Petzold, M.; Hogan, D.; Landoulsi, S.; Jampathong, N.; Kongwattanakul, K.; Laopaiboon, M.; et al. Global, regional, and national estimates of levels of preterm birth in 2014: A systematic review and modelling analysis. *Lancet Glob. Health* **2019**, *7*, e37–e46. [CrossRef]
62. Jacob, J.; Lehne, M.; Mischker, A.; Klinger, N.; Zickermann, C.; Walker, J. Cost effects of preterm birth: A comparison of health care costs associated with early preterm, late preterm, and full-term birth in the first 3 years after birth. *Eur. J. Health Econ.* **2017**, *18*, 1041–1046. [CrossRef]
63. Fengler, J.; Heckmann, M.; Lange, A.; Kramer, A.; Flessa, S. Cost analysis showed that feeding preterm infants with donor human milk was significantly more expensive than mother's milk or formula. *Acta Paediatr.* **2019**, *108*, 1978–1984. [CrossRef]
64. Spatz, D.L.; Robinson, A.C.; Froh, E.B. Cost and use of pasteurized donor human milk at a children's hospital. *J. Obstet. Gynecol. Neonatal. Nurs.* **2018**, *47*, 583–588. [CrossRef]

65. Johnson, T.J.; Patel, A.L.; Bigger, H.R.; Engstrom, J.L.; Meier, P.P. Cost savings of human milk as a strategy to reduce the incidence of necrotizing enterocolitis in very low birth weight infants. *Neonatology* **2015**, *107*, 271–276. [CrossRef]
66. Ganapathy, V.; Hay, J.W.; Kim, J.H. Costs of necrotizing enterocolitis and cost-effectiveness of exclusively human milk-based products in feeding extremely premature infants. *Breastfeed. Med.* **2012**, *7*, 29–37. [CrossRef]
67. St-Onge, M.; Chaudhry, S.; Koren, G. Donated breast milk stored in banks versus breast milk purchased online. *Can. Fam. Physician.* **2015**, *61*, 143–146.
68. De Nisi, G.; Moro, G.E.; Arslanoglu, S.; Ambruzzi, A.M.; Biasini, A.; Profeti, C.; Tonetto, P.; Bertino, E. Members of the Italian association of donor human milk banks (associazione Italiana banche del latte umano donato). Survey of Italian human milk banks. *J. Hum. Lact.* **2015**, *31*, 294–300. [CrossRef] [PubMed]
69. Rigourd, V.; Nicloux, M.; Giuseppi, A.; Brunet, S.; Vaiman, D.; TerkiHassaine, R.; Jébali, S.; Kanaan, Z.; Ayachi, A. Breast milk donation in the muslim population: Why it is possible. *Am. J. Pediatr.* **2018**, *4*, 12–14. [CrossRef]

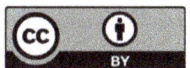

© 2020 by the authors. Licensee MDPI, Basel, Switzerland. This article is an open access article distributed under the terms and conditions of the Creative Commons Attribution (CC BY) license (http://creativecommons.org/licenses/by/4.0/).

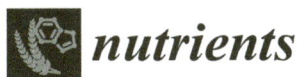 

*Review*

# A Review of the Immunomodulating Components of Maternal Breast Milk and Protection Against Necrotizing Enterocolitis

Lila S. Nolan [1], Olivia B. Parks [2] and Misty Good [1,*]

[1] Department of Pediatrics, Division of Newborn Medicine, Washington University School of Medicine, St. Louis, MO 63110, USA; lilanolan@wustl.edu
[2] University of Pittsburgh School of Medicine, Medical Scientist Training Program, Pittsburgh, PA 15213, USA; Parks.Olivia@medstudent.pitt.edu
* Correspondence: mistygood@wustl.edu; Tel.: +314-286-1329

Received: 12 November 2019; Accepted: 17 December 2019; Published: 19 December 2019

**Abstract:** Breast milk contains immunomodulating components that are beneficial to newborns during maturation of their immune system. Human breast milk composition is influenced by an infant's gestational and chronological age, lactation stage, and the mother and infant's health status. Major immunologic components in human milk, such as secretory immunoglobulin A (IgA) and growth factors, have a known role in regulating gut barrier integrity and microbial colonization, which therefore protect against the development of a life-threatening gastrointestinal illness affecting newborn infants called necrotizing enterocolitis (NEC). Breast milk is a known protective factor in the prevention of NEC when compared with feeding with commercial formula. Breast milk supplements infants with human milk oligosaccharides, leukocytes, cytokines, nitric oxide, and growth factors that attenuate inflammatory responses and provide immunological defenses to reduce the incidence of NEC. This article aims to review the variety of immunomodulating components in breast milk that protect the infant from the development of NEC.

**Keywords:** breast milk; necrotizing enterocolitis; prematurity; immunity; newborn; inflammation

## 1. Introduction

Necrotizing enterocolitis (NEC) is a severe gastrointestinal disease in preterm infants with associated mortality as high as 50% in cases that require surgical intervention [1]. NEC occurs in 1–5% of patients admitted to a neonatal intensive care unit (NICU), and increased incidence and fatality occurs in infants with prematurity and low birth weight [2]. The etiology of NEC is complex, and pathogenesis is attributed to inflammation of the neonatal gastrointestinal tract by triggers such as commercial formula feeds, intestinal dysbiosis, and immaturity of gut mucosal immunity. Treatment of NEC requires withholding enteral feeds and potent antimicrobial agents, and these infants are at risk of adverse long term outcomes. Identification of factors that contribute to the prevention of NEC remains a high priority in neonatal research. There is a consensus regarding the protective nature of breast milk in the prevention of NEC development. Human breast milk, in contrast to commercial formulas, contains soluble and cellular components that provide infants with passive immunity to their gastrointestinal tract. These antimicrobial and bioactive factors are multi-functional and anti-inflammatory, with an established protective role against the development of NEC. An early prospective study of 926 infants showed that exclusively formula-fed preterm infants were six to ten times more likely to acquire NEC as compared to preterm infants nourished with human milk alone [3]. Furthermore, an analysis of 243 infants in a randomized trial showed that preterm infants less than 30 weeks' gestation who received maternal milk had reduced incidence of late-onset sepsis or NEC as compared with preterm infants who received donor breast milk or commercial formula [4]. Sullivan and colleagues demonstrated in a randomized, controlled, multicenter trial that extremely premature infants who received only human milk, including human milk-derived fortification, had decreased rates of NEC compared to those infants exposed to bovine milk-derived products with a number needed to treat of 10 infants to prevent one NEC case [5].

Breast milk composition is complex, dynamic, and influenced by a variety of maternal factors. Immunoglobulins, antimicrobial peptides, growth factors, human milk oligosaccharides, cytokines, L-glutamine, and nitric oxide in breast milk maintain roles in the enhancement of the neonatal intestinal barrier function and the reduction of NEC. This article aims to review the protective role of breast milk and its components against NEC, as shown in Figure 1.

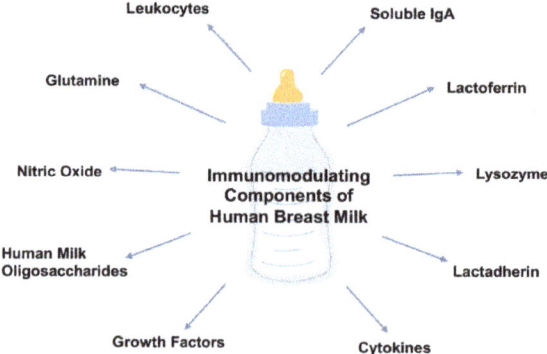

**Figure 1.** Overview of the immunomodulatory components of maternal breast milk.

## 2. Breast Milk and the Host-Microbial Relationship

### 2.1. Maternal Soluble IgA

Bioactive components of maternal milk, particularly immunoglobulin A (IgA), have known influential effects on the neonatal microbiota. IgA is the most plentiful antibody in human milk and comprises a significant portion of total protein content in colostrum [6]. IgA produced by the maternal mammary glands undergoes proteolytic cleavage to release secretory IgA (sIgA), permitting transport into human milk [7]. Breast milk sIgA provides critical antimicrobial defense to the neonatal gastrointestinal tract through inhibition of pathogen attachment to mucosal surfaces, neutralization of microbial toxins, and provision of passive immunity. IgM and IgG are of lesser abundance in human milk but also have known immune-surveillance properties.

The sIgA levels in breast milk decrease over time during the postpartum period [8]. Recent studies have identified no difference in breast milk sIgA concentration of preterm versus term breast milk [6,8], although Mehta and Petrova identified that preterm milk contains a higher concentration of sIgA in the first six to eight days of lactation [9]. Breast milk sIgA is a critical component, as it promotes colonization of commensal microbiota, decreasing the activity of pattern recognition receptors and subsequent downstream inflammation within the intestinal epithelium [10]. A humoral response with increased levels of sIgA in mature breast milk has been shown to occur in response to an infection in the mother or infant [11]. Gopalakrishna and colleagues studied the role that sIgA in breast milk plays in the pathogenesis of NEC [12]. They determined the proportion of IgA-associated intestinal bacteria and discovered that premature infants with an exclusive formula-fed diet contained very low levels of IgA-associated intestinal bacteria. Furthermore, infants with NEC had higher levels of IgA-unbound Enterobacteriaceae when compared with healthy age-matched controls. This suggests that insufficient concentrations of IgA and decreased IgA-bound bacteria in the intestine may be causative factors of insufficient microbiome diversity and increased risk of NEC development [12]. In a neonatal mouse model of NEC, pups reared by IgA-deficient mothers showed susceptibility to intestinal disease despite receiving maternal milk, suggesting that maternal IgA can define the host-microbiota relationship and underscoring that the IgA in milk plays an important role in the susceptibility to NEC [12].

## 2.2. Lactoferrin

Lactoferrin is an abundant peptide in human milk and has known roles in host defense and antimicrobial properties. When lactoferrin encounters proteolysis in acidic conditions, such as in the stomach, lactoferricin is produced. Lactoferricin has both strong antibacterial and some antiviral activity with immunomodulatory capabilities [13]. In particular, human lactoferricin has a potent ability to neutralize endotoxin activity, prevent activation of mononuclear cells, and ultimately prevent the secretion of cytokines, such as interleukin (IL)-1β, IL-6, tumor necrosis factor (TNF)-α, and IL-8, that contribute to inflammation [13,14]. Togawa and colleagues demonstrated that the administration of enteral lactoferrin in rats attenuated colonic inflammation after induction of colitis [15]. Many studies have subsequently evaluated the modulatory role of lactoferrin in antimicrobial and immunological defenses in infants. A Cochrane Review of six, small, randomized control trials (RCT) that provided lactoferrin supplementation to enteral feeds found decreased late-onset bacterial and fungal sepsis in preterm infants, although the evidence was identified as low in quality [16]. A systematic review and meta-analysis reviewed nine RCTs and showed that prophylactic lactoferrin significantly reduced the incidence of late-onset sepsis and NEC (Bell's stage II or greater) [17]. Most recently, a large randomized control trial of 2203 infants contrasted these prior findings, demonstrating that enteral supplementation with bovine lactoferrin did not reduce NEC or the incidence of infection or mortality [18].

## 2.3. Lysozyme

Lysozyme, as an immune-active enzyme in colostrum and breast milk, has many bactericidal effects. In synergy with lactoferrin, lysozyme can bind to lipopolysaccharide (LPS) on outer bacterial membranes, which provides lysozyme access to degrade internal proteoglycan matrices of bacterial membranes. Studies of breast milk composition have shown that premature breast milk as compared to term breast milk has higher lysozyme content [6,9], although other studies have found no difference [8]. In the gastrointestinal tract, Paneth cells within the crypts of Lieberkühn produce a variety of antimicrobial peptides, including lysozyme, which are secreted in response to enteric pathogens [19]. Of relevance to NEC, in the small intestinal biopsies of premature infants with NEC, there were decreased concentrations of Paneth cells compared to controls [20]. The role of lysozyme has been studied in a mouse model of NEC utilizing Paneth cell ablation. This model consists of 14-day-old pups treated with dithizone, a heavy metal chelator, followed by luminal infection with *Klebsiella* [21]. The pups in this experimental group developed a NEC-like injury, suggesting the significance of lysozyme and antimicrobial protection provided by Paneth cells can regulate the inflammatory response in NEC [21]. A subsequent study using an experimental murine NEC model demonstrated that Paneth cell deficiency induces a disruption in the intestinal microbiome, and in particular, the development of an Enterobacteriaceae bloom, which has been shown to precede NEC in humans [22]. These results signify the potential significance of breast milk lysozyme in protecting breast fed infants from the intestinal inflammatory insult seen in NEC.

## 2.4. Lactadherin

Lactadherin (milk fat globule-epidermal growth factor (EGF) factor VIII) is a human milk glycoprotein that contributes to apoptotic cell phagocytosis [23]. A deficiency of lactadherin has been strongly associated with inflammatory and autoimmune diseases and has been shown to maintain homeostasis of the intestinal epithelium through the migration of epithelial cells. In a model of seven-week-old mice, treatment with recombinant lactadherin resulted in protection from colitis, as demonstrated by downregulation of pro-inflammatory cytokines and improved histological scores [23]. Additionally, in a neonatal rat model of NEC-like intestinal injury, supplementation with recombinant human lactadherin attenuated the disruption of cellular tight junctions [24].

## 2.5. Epidermal Growth Factor

The growth factors in breast milk serve a protective role in helping to facilitate the intestinal mucosal barrier maturation. Maternal milk and colostrum contain epidermal growth factor (EGF) and are the predominant sources of intestinal EGF during the postnatal phase. The roles of EGF in the development of the intestine, as well as the response and repair of the intestine during intestinal injury or infection, have been reported [25]. EGF levels are decreased in the saliva and serum of premature infants with NEC when compared to infants without NEC. In a study of salivary EGF, infants with NEC had lower salivary EGF in the first week after birth and greater increases from week of life one to two as compared to infants without NEC, suggesting that NEC development may be attributed to overall lower EGF concentrations in the at-risk neonate [26]. EGF also has proposed effects on goblet cells and the production of mucin in the intestinal epithelium. Clark and colleagues showed that treatment with EGF resulted in an increased number of goblet cells and increased the production of mucin in the small intestine [27].

NEC has been associated with impaired intestinal barrier function and epithelial cell apoptosis. The in vivo treatment with enteral EGF has shown to regulate the expression of tight junction proteins, occludin and claudin-3 as well as normalize their expression at the site of NEC injury, helping to maintain the gut barrier [27]. Additionally, enteral EGF administration can increase expression of the anti-apoptotic protein, Bcl-2, and decrease levels of the pro-apoptotic protein, Bax. The role of EGF in balancing apoptosis regulators provides implications of an opportunity for future therapeutic strategies to protect the intestinal barrier from injury in NEC [28,29].

## 2.6. Heparin-Binding Epidermal Growth Factor

The developing fetus and the breast fed newborn are continually exposed to Heparin-binding epidermal growth factor (HB-EGF), which is present in both amniotic fluid and breast milk, suggesting its possible role in gastrointestinal epithelium development both in utero and during the neonatal period [30]. As a member of the EGF family, HB-EGF binds to the EGF receptor (EGFR) and has known mitogenic effects. HB-EGF is expressed in response to hypoxia, tissue damage, and oxidative stress, including in the intestine, and has a pivotal role in tissue regeneration and repair [31,32]. In seeking to evaluate the role of exogenous HB-EGF in the context of NEC, Dvorak and colleagues demonstrated that either the oral administration of HB-EGF or EGF significantly reduced NEC in a premature rat model through increased production of MUC2, a secretory mucin [33]. However, the concurrent administration of both growth factors did not confer better protection and physiologic doses of EGF provided better protection [33]. In another study, enteral administration of HB-EGF to neonatal rat pups decreased the incidence and severity of NEC and reduced intestinal permeability as demonstrated by a low serum concentration of enterally-administered fluorescein isothiocyanate-dextran [32]. The results of these studies suggest a potential role of HB-EGF in the attenuation of intestinal injury during NEC.

## 2.7. Transforming Growth Factor-β2

Human milk contains high concentrations of the transforming growth factor-β isoform, transforming growth factor-β2 (TGF-β2), which has immunomodulatory effects on intestinal maturation, immunoglobulin production, and a suppressive effect on T cells [34]. Breast milk with higher concentrations of TGF-β2 is associated with a higher diversity of intestinal microbial composition in the neonate, a factor that is known to lower the risk of adult immunological diseases [34]. Of note, preterm human milk has been shown to have reduced TGF-β bioactivity [35]. Maheshwari and colleagues analyzed TGF-β2 expression in premature infant intestinal tissue samples and observed lower TGF-β2 expression and bioactivity in patients with NEC as compared with controls [36]. In a murine experimental model of NEC, enterally administered recombinant TGF-β2 showed protective effects against NEC-like mucosal injury [36]. The addition of recombinant TGF-β2 to milk has been investigated as a preventative strategy to boost the anti-inflammatory properties of milk and prevent the development of NEC. However, it was discovered that in human preterm milk, TGF-β2 is sequestered by chondroitin sulfate proteoglycans, which therefore inhibits its biological activity [35]. Consequently, the digestion of human preterm milk with chondroitinase resulted in the activation of endogenous TGF-β2 and also restored the bioactivity of recombinant TGF-β2 [35]. These findings suggest chondroitinase digestion of preterm milk may be an option for preventing NEC by enhancing the anti-inflammatory properties of the milk.

*2.8. Prebiotics and Oligosaccharides*

Human milk oligosaccharides (HMOs) are complex sugars present in high abundance in breast milk. HMOs serve as prebiotics and metabolic substrates with targeted antimicrobial activity, allowing beneficial bacteria to thrive while suppressing those which are potentially harmful [37,38]. In an in vitro epithelial model of the crypt-villus axis, treatment with HMOs resulted in reduced intestinal cell proliferation, but promoted epithelial cell differentiation, indicating a potential role in intestinal maturation [39].

HMOs ingested from breast milk undergo only minimal degradation in the infant's acidic stomach and by the pancreatic and brush border enzymes in order to reach the distal small intestine and colon [37,38]. Preclinical animal studies as well as human studies in mother–infant dyads support the contributions of HMOs in reduction of the development of NEC. In a cohort study comprised of 200 mother–infant dyads, the composition of HMOs in breast milk was analyzed [40]. One specific HMO, disialyllacto-N-tetraose (DSLNT) was identified to be present in significantly lower concentrations in those infants who developed NEC [40]. Measurement of DSLNT levels in maternal milk may therefore provide additional insight into why some breast fed infants are still at risk of NEC.

Enteral administration with supplemental HMOs have been studied as potential therapeutics in reducing the risk of NEC [41,42]. For example, in a neonatal rat model of NEC, animals were fed with DSLNT-containing formula, which resulted in reduced severity of NEC based on pathology scores and improved survival [43]. The same study showed that galacto-oligosaccharides, an infant formula additive, similar although structurally different from HMOs, demonstrated no effect on NEC severity or survival in neonatal rats [43]. In a preterm pig model of NEC, receiving supplemental feeds with a mixture of HMOs have not shown a significant difference in NEC severity, gut microbial colonization, or intestinal permeability [42]. However, in a neonatal mouse model of NEC, enteral administration of another HMO found in breast milk, 2'fucosyllactose (HMO-2'FL), resulted in the preservation of mesenteric perfusion and restored the expression of endothelial nitric oxide synthase (eNOS), a vasodilatory molecule necessary for intestinal perfusion [44]. The results of these studies suggest key roles of HMO-2'FL and DSLNT as protective components of breast milk in the prevention of NEC development.

*2.9. Glutamine*

Free amino acids comprise 3–5% of the total amino acids in human milk [45]. In a longitudinal analysis of breast milk from healthy mothers of term infants, glutamine and glutamic acid were among the most plentiful free amino acids in the first three months of lactation [45]. Levels of glutamine increased significantly during the first to the third month of lactation [45,46]. In addition, breast milk, which contains higher concentrations of glutamine, amongst other free amino acids, is associated with more rapid weight gain [46] and increased length [47] in the infant. Glutamine also holds a relevant role in maintaining gut barrier integrity. For example, glutamine augments the effects of growth factors and influences cell signaling pathways involved in intestinal cell proliferation and differentiation, as well as the expression of tight junctions [48,49]. Glutamine has also exhibited anti-apoptotic properties in intestinal cells, attributed to its role in the production of glutathione [48,49].

Neonates deficient in circulating amino acids such as glutamine and arginine, are associated with a higher risk of NEC development [50]. In a neonatal rat model of NEC, pups receiving exogenous administration of glutamine had reduced pathology injury scores and reduced ileal mRNA expression of the innate immune receptors, Toll-like receptor (TLR)-2 and TLR-4 [51]. As TLR-2 and TLR-4 have established roles in inducing synthesis of inflammatory mediators and increasing apoptosis in NEC [52–54], their reduced expression by glutamine supplementation suggests a mechanism by which it mediates protection. In a small study that evaluated the outcomes of arginine and glutamine supplementation in 25 preterm neonates of less than 34 weeks' gestation, there were no infants that developed NEC in the glutamine group and no difference in the NEC incidence in the arginine group [55]. However, large RCTs of infants diagnosed with severe gastrointestinal disease, including NEC, spontaneous intestinal perforation, and intestinal structural anomalies, did not show a decreased risk of death or severe infections while receiving enteral glutamine [56]. Additional large RCTs evaluating glutamine supplementation in preterm infants did not show a benefit in decreasing the risk of death, intestinal disease, or long term developmental outcomes [57]. Therefore, despite the significant levels of glutamine in human breast milk, there is insufficient evidence for exogenous supplementation of glutamine as a preventative strategy for NEC at this time.

## 3. Breast Milk and Immune Homeostasis

### 3.1. Cellular Mechanisms

There are two primary pathways for maternal cellular transfer to the infant—placental transmission and oral transmission through breastfeeding [58]. Breast milk leukocytes, including macrophages and neutrophils, survive passage through the neonatal gastrointestinal tract and translocate to blood, lymph nodes, spleen, and liver [11,58,59]. Understanding the physiological significance of the transfer of human milk cells to neonates can provide insight into the protective properties of breast milk on the infant recipient.

The progression through maturational stages of lactation involves alterations in breast milk leukocyte composition and concentration. In an analysis of $CD45^+$ leukocytes in breast milk, colostrum contained the highest number of leukocytes compared with transitional milk (8–12 days postpartum) and mature milk (26–30 days postpartum) [60]. The infant's gestational age at birth is also associated with changing concentrations of certain types of breast milk leukocytes. Colostrum contains lower levels of non-cytotoxic T cells and B lymphocytes with increased gestational age whereas mature milk of preterm mothers contains lower cytotoxic T cell and natural killer (NK) cell levels when compared to term milk [60]. In seeking to understand the impact of maternal milk leukocytes on the breastfeeding infant, Cabinian and colleagues used a murine model to examine the transport and survival of maternal breast milk leukocytes, primarily T cells, to the gastrointestinal Peyer's patches of the suckling pup [61]. The observed transfer of cells to the Peyer's patches implicates the role of breast milk leukocytes in neonatal intestinal development and localized immunological maturation. The overall relevance of the differences in human milk cellular content and transfer on the development of NEC requires further study.

Additionally, maternal and infant bacterial infections influenced concentrations of breast milk leukocytes and cytokines, notably macrophages and TNF-α levels [11,62]. Maternal infection can induce a significant leukocyte surge that ranges from 0.7% to 93.6% of total cells in breast milk [11]. A smaller increase in breast milk leukocytes has been observed when the breastfeeding infant develops an infection [11]. Riskin and colleagues identified that macrophages, as well as neutrophils, comprise the majority of breast milk leukocytes in mothers with a sick infant [62]. The increase in breast milk leukocytes in response to an inflammatory process in the mother/infant dyad suggests a dynamic interaction between maternal and infant immune systems and further supports the benefits of breast milk.

## 3.2. Cytokines

Preterm infants, when compared with their term counterparts, exhibit immune immaturity, which includes lower production of cytokines and other immunological proteins during challenge with an inflammatory insult [59]. The presence of cytokines in breast milk provides passive protection and immune modulation in the infant recipient and results in absorption into the systemic circulation. In particular, these cytokines include IL-1, IL-2, IL-6, IL-8, IL-10, interferon (IFN)-γ, and TNF-α (Table 1). Breast milk produced by mothers of full-term infants contains high levels of IL-2, IL-8, and IL-10, with levels decreasing drastically by day 21 of lactation. In contrast, mothers of preterm infants have significantly lower levels of cytokines in the colostrum when compared to mothers of full-term infants [63].

**Table 1.** Cytokines present in human breast milk and physiologic relevance to the infant.

| Cytokine | Composition in Human Milk and Significance | References |
|---|---|---|
| Interleukin (IL)-1 | - Human milk IL-1β attenuates the activation of pro-inflammatory IL-8 and suppresses pro-inflammatory responses of nuclear factor kappa beta (NF-kB) signaling. | [53,64] |
| IL-2 | - Highest in concentration in colostrum and reduced in later stages of lactation.<br>- Recruits T cells to stimulate an antigen-specific immune response. | [63,65,66] |
| IL-6 | - Detected in higher levels in term breast milk.<br>- Pro-inflammatory properties and is present in the acute phase of infection.<br>- Colostrum may contain anti-IL-6 antibodies that cause decreased immunoglobulin A (IgA) production by breast milk leukocytes. | [63,67,68] |
| IL-8 | - Decreased levels of detection in later stages of lactation.<br>- Provides chemotactic response of neutrophils.<br>- Recombinant IL-8 may improve the viability of intestinal cells when exposed to injury. | [63,69,70] |
| IL-10 | - Maintains anti-inflammatory mechanisms involving limiting the $T_h1$ response, inhibiting production of inflammatory cytokines, and promoting immunoglobulin synthesis. | [71–75] |
| IFN-γ | - Detected in decreasing levels with later stages of lactation.<br>- Increases activation of intestinal macrophages and is present in higher concentrations in the ileum of infants with necrotizing enterocolitis (NEC).<br>- Pro-inflammatory mechanism of action may provide an infant with defense against inflammation and infection. | [76–79] |
| TNF-α | - Detected in decreased levels in colostrum of preterm milk.<br>- Present in breast milk in association with its soluble receptor, reducing its pro-inflammatory activity. | [63,80,81] |

High levels IL-1RA, an IL-1 receptor, have been detected in breast milk [64]. IL-1β is a member of the IL-1 family and is known to induce an endogenous innate inflammatory response in enterocytes, upregulate expression of pro-inflammatory IL-8, and stimulate the nuclear factor kappa beta (NF-kB) pathway. However, human milk has demonstrated the ability to attenuate the IL-1β-dependent activation of IL-8 [64]. The protective effects of breast milk on suppressing this NF-kB-mediated pro-inflammatory immune response has been shown in intestinal epithelial cells both in vitro and in vivo, providing evidence of a mechanism mediating protection against NEC development [53,64].

Neonates have a known deficiency in the production of IL-2, which is a necessary cytokine in the recruitment of T cells required to produce an antigen-specific immune response [65,66]. Human milk, therefore, provides an ideal source of IL-2 for the newborn. Levels of aqueous IL-2 in human milk are of highest concentration in colostrum with reduced levels in later stages of lactation [63,65]. The presence of IL-2 in breast milk, which is absorbed by the gastrointestinal tract of the infant, may enter the systemic circulation to influence the maturing immune system.

IL-6 is a pro-inflammatory cytokine in the acute phase of the inflammatory response [59]. Multiple studies have observed high levels of IL-6 in colostrum [63,67,68]. An early analysis of IL-6 in breast milk showed that the presence of an anti-IL-6 antibody in colostrum caused decreased production of IgA by mononuclear leukocytes, suggesting a relationship between IL-6 and IgA production in breast milk [67]. Ustundag and colleagues noted higher levels of breast milk IL-6 at two weeks postpartum in mothers of term infants when compared to milk from mothers of preterm infants [63]. The prevalence of IL-6 in breast milk with uptake by the infant recipient may have a significant biologic role in neonatal immune homeostasis.

IL-8 expression by macrophages, endothelial cells, and epithelial cells provides chemotactic activity for a neutrophil-dependent response to acute inflammation, such as in sepsis and NEC. A decline in IL-8 levels in breast milk occurs with the advancement in lactational stage [69,70]. Although one study found no difference in breast milk IL-8 expression in mothers of infants of different gestational ages [63], others have identified higher IL-8 levels in the breast milk of mothers of preterm infants [69]. Maheshwari and colleagues showed that fetal and adult human intestinal cells treated with recombinant IL-8 in vitro had increased cell proliferation and differentiation [69]. Additionally, intestinal cells exposed to injury in vitro demonstrated increased viability when treated with recombinant IL-8 [69]. Thus, the dynamic effects of IL-8 on the developing intestine suggests its physiologic role in intestinal development as a component of human breast milk.

The anti-inflammatory properties of IL-10 attenuate the immune response to an infection and maintain tissue homeostasis by inhibition of the activity of $T_h1$ effector cells, NK cells, and macrophages [71,72]. IL-10 can inhibit the production of inflammatory IL-1, IL-6, IL-8, and TNF-$\alpha$ [72,73]. One study found IL-10 in the aqueous and non-aqueous phases of human milk, with concentrations found to be highest within the first 24 hours of lactation [72]. IL-10 in breast milk affects the infant by attracting $CD8^+$ T lymphocytes [72,74] and promoting immunoglobulin synthesis by B cells [72,75].

IFN-$\gamma$ is a pro-inflammatory cytokine found in human milk in low concentrations with decreasing levels in the months following birth [76]. IFN-$\gamma$ is secreted by activated T cells and NK cells and enhances intestinal macrophage activation [76]. IFN-$\gamma$ is involved in the signaling pathways that increase intestinal epithelial barrier permeability [77] and is also detected in higher concentrations in the ileum of patients with NEC [78]. As infants have a reduced ability to produce IFN-$\gamma$ due to an immature immune system [79], breast milk may provide the infant with IFN-$\gamma$ and other pro-inflammatory cytokines needed to produce a host defense response against inflammation or infection.

Neonates are deficient in the production of the pro-inflammatory cytokine TNF-$\alpha$ and its receptors, TNF-$\alpha$ receptor I and II, increasing susceptibility to infection due to immune cell dysregulation. TNF-$\alpha$ is produced by a variety of immune cell types, including granulocytes and $CD4^+$ lymphocytes. TNF-$\alpha$, as an endogenous pyrogen, contributes to systemic inflammation and immune cell regulation. One study quantified the amount of detectable TNF-$\alpha$ in breast milk and colostrum and identified the majority of TNF-$\alpha$ to be in association with its soluble receptor [80]. The low amount of unbound TNF-$\alpha$ in breast milk was theorized to decrease TNF-$\alpha$ pro-inflammatory bioactivity [80]. Two additional studies have identified a significantly decreased amount of TNF-$\alpha$ in colostrum of mothers who delivered very preterm (less than 30 weeks' gestation) when compared to term and preterm groups, suggesting one reason why preterm infants have increased susceptibility to infection and impaired immunity [63,81].

Overall, the evidence suggests that infants, particularly those born preterm, have insufficient ability to mount an adequate immunological defense due to reduced production of a variety of cytokines. Breast milk can therefore supplement infants with maternal cytokines that may provide immune benefits in the protection against neonatal inflammatory diseases such as NEC.

*3.3. Nitric Oxide*

Nitric oxide (NO) is a soluble molecule produced by isoforms of NO synthase (NOS) and serves as a potent vasodilator and neurotransmitter at low, physiologic levels [82,83]. Infants derive NO from dietary sodium nitrite, which is then converted to NO within the gastrointestinal tract by commensal microbes [82,83]. NO is present in breast milk, as shown in an analysis of healthy lactating mothers evaluating the concentration of breast milk nitric oxide concentration on postpartum days one through five [84]. Exclusively breastfeeding mothers had significantly higher nitric oxide concentrations in their milk, compared with milk expressed from mothers who decided to exclusively formula-feed their infant [84]. It was theorized that infant suckling activates NOS within the mammary gland with subsequent secretion of NO into breast milk, which then confers protection to the intestine of the infant through regulation of intestinal blood flow and maintenance of vascular tone [84].

The upregulation of inducible NOS (iNOS) in response to the release of cytokines and growth factors has been implicated in NEC pathogenesis [82,85]. During inflammation, high levels of NO, and its derivative peroxynitrite, contribute to epithelial damage and the disruption of the integrity of the intestinal barrier [82]. To study abnormal NOS signaling in NEC, Yazji and colleagues used a murine model of NEC and selectively deleted endothelial TLR-4 expression, which subsequently resulted in impaired microvascular intestinal perfusion, increased severity of NEC, and reduced endothelial NOS (eNOS) expression [86]. Additionally, as compared with commercial formula, breast milk was identified to have higher levels of sodium nitrate, which serves as a precursor for nitrite and nitric oxide. Enteral administration of exogenous sodium nitrate was associated with decreased severity of NEC and improved intestinal perfusion [86]. Overall, these results suggest the protective role of breast milk in augmenting physiologic nitrate-nitrite-NO signaling to improve intestinal vascular perfusion and protect against intestinal barrier disruption in NEC.

## 4. Summary

Human breast milk contains a dynamic diversity of bioactive components needed for infant growth, immune homeostasis, and intestinal maturation. The composition of human milk varies with the stage of lactation, gestational age of the infant, the health of the mother/infant dyad, and the nutritional status of the mother. The dietary intake of the breastfeeding mother has been shown to influence the variability of human milk concentrations of fat-soluble and water-soluble vitamins and other nutrients. These nutrients, including immunoglobulins, growth factors, cytokines, and immune cells, have been demonstrated to transfer from the mother to the neonate through breast milk [87,88]. The ability of these components to regulate intestinal cell proliferation and differentiation as well as influence gut microbial colonization emphasizes the protective role of breast milk in infant metabolism and neurodevelopment, intestinal microbial homeostasis, and protection against NEC [87,88]. The growing field of research studying the outcomes related to breastfeeding reinforces the immunological value of breast milk on infant nutrition and protection from inflammatory disorders such as NEC.

**Author Contributions:** L.S.N., O.B.P. and M.G. contributed to the writing—Original draft preparation, review and editing of the initial version manuscript. L.S.N. and M.G. edited and revised the manuscript. L.S.N., O.B.P. and M.G. approved the final version of the manuscript. All authors have read and agreed to the published version of the manuscript.

**Acknowledgments:** MG is supported by R01DK118568 from the National Institutes of Health, March of Dimes Foundation Grant No. 5-FY17-79, the St. Louis Children's Hospital Foundation, the Children's Discovery Institute of Washington University and St. Louis Children's Hospital, and the Department of Pediatrics at Washington University School of Medicine, St. Louis. MG has previously received sponsored research agreement funding from Astarte Medical Partners, and participated in a neonatal microbiome advisory board for Abbott Laboratories. None of the above sources had any role in this study.

**Conflicts of Interest:** The authors declare no conflicts of interest. The funders had no role in the writing of this manuscript.

## References

1. Neu, J.; Walker, W.A. Necrotizing enterocolitis. *N. Engl. J. Med.* **2011**, *364*, 255–264. [CrossRef] [PubMed]
2. Lin, P.W.; Stoll, B.J. Necrotising enterocolitis. *Lancet* **2006**, *368*, 1271–1283. [CrossRef]
3. Lucas, A.; Cole, T.J. Breast milk and neonatal necrotising enterocolitis. *Lancet* **1990**, *336*, 1519–1523. [CrossRef]
4. Schanler, R.J. Randomized trial of donor human milk versus preterm formula as substitutes for mothers' own milk in the feeding of extremely premature infants. *Pediatrics* **2005**, *116*, 400–406. [CrossRef]
5. Sullivan, S.; Schanler, R.J.; Kim, J.H.; Patel, A.L.; Trawöger, R.; Kiechl-Kohlendorfer, U.; Chan, G.M.; Blanco, C.L.; Abrams, S.; Cotten, C.M.; et al. An exclusively human milk-based diet is associated with a lower rate of necrotizing enterocolitis than a diet of human milk and bovine milk-based products. *J. Pediatr.* **2010**, *156*, 562–567.e1. [CrossRef]
6. Trend, S.; Strunk, T.; Lloyd, M.L.; Kok, C.H.; Metcalfe, J.; Geddes, D.T.; Lai, C.T.; Richmond, P.; Doherty, D.A.; Simmer, K.; et al. Levels of innate immune factors in preterm and term mothers' breast milk during the 1st month postpartum. *Br. J. Nutr.* **2016**, *115*, 1178–1193. [CrossRef]
7. Rogier, E.W.; Frantz, A.L.; Bruno, M.E.C.; Wedlund, L.; Cohen, D.A.; Stromberg, A.J.; Kaetzel, C.S. Secretory antibodies in breast milk promote long-term intestinal homeostasis by regulating the gut microbiota and host gene expression. *Proc. Natl. Acad. Sci. USA* **2014**, *111*, 3074–3079. [CrossRef]
8. Hsu, Y.C.; Chen, C.H.; Lin, M.C.; Tsai, C.R.; Liang, J.T.; Wang, T.M. Changes in preterm breast milk nutrient content in the first month. *Pediatr. Neonatol.* **2014**, *55*, 449–454. [CrossRef]
9. Mehta, R.; Petrova, A. Biologically active breast milk proteins in association with very preterm delivery and stage of lactation. *J. Perinatol.* **2011**, *31*, 58–62. [CrossRef]
10. Rogier, E.W.; Frantz, A.L.; Bruno, M.E.C.; Kaetzel, C.S. Secretory IgA is concentrated in the outer layer of colonic mucus along with gut bacteria. *Pathogens* **2014**, *3*, 390–403. [CrossRef]
11. Hassiotou, F.; Hepworth, A.R.; Metzger, P.; Tat Lai, C.; Trengove, N.; Hartmann, P.E.; Filgueira, L. Maternal and infant infections stimulate a rapid leukocyte response in breastmilk. *Clin. Transl. Immunol.* **2013**, *2*, e3. [CrossRef] [PubMed]
12. Gopalakrishna, K.P.; Macadangdang, B.R.; Rogers, M.B.; Tometich, J.T.; Firek, B.A.; Baker, R.; Ji, J.; Burr, A.H.P.; Ma, C.; Good, M.; et al. Maternal IgA protects against the development of necrotizing enterocolitis in preterm infants. *Nat. Med.* **2019**, *25*, 1110–1115. [CrossRef]
13. Gifford, J.L.; Hunter, H.N.; Vogel, H.J. Lactoferricin: A lactoferrin-derived peptide with antimicrobial, antiviral, antitumor and immunological properties. *Cell. Mol. Life Sci.* **2005**, *62*, 2588–2598. [CrossRef] [PubMed]
14. Palmeira, P.; Carneiro-Sampaio, M. Immunology of breast milk. *Rev. Assoc. Med. Bras.* **2016**, *62*, 584–593. [CrossRef]
15. Togawa, J.I.; Nagase, H.; Tanaka, K.; Inamori, M.; Nakajima, A.; Ueno, N.; Saito, T.; Sekihara, H. Oral administration of lactoferrin reduces colitis in rats via modulation of the immune system and correction of cytokine imbalance. *J. Gastroenterol. Hepatol.* **2002**, *17*, 1291–1298. [CrossRef]
16. Pammi, M.; Suresh, G. Enteral lactoferrin supplementation for prevention of sepsis and necrotizing enterocolitis in preterm infants. *Cochrane Database Syst. Rev.* **2017**, *2017*, CD007137. [CrossRef]
17. He, Y.; Cao, L.; Yu, J. Prophylactic lactoferrin for preventing late-onset sepsis and necrotizing enterocolitis in preterm infants. *Medicine (Baltimore)* **2018**, *97*, e11976. [CrossRef]
18. Griffiths, J.; Jenkins, P.; Vargova, M.; Bowler, U.; Juszczak, E.; King, A.; Linsell, L.; Murray, D.; Partlett, C.; Patel, M.; et al. Enteral lactoferrin to prevent infection for very preterm infants: The ELFIN RCT. *Health Technol. Assess.* **2018**, *22*, 1–60. [CrossRef]
19. Mara, M.A.; Good, M.; Weitkamp, J.-H. Innate and adaptive immunity in necrotizing enterocolitis. *Semin. Fetal Neonatal Med.* **2018**, *23*, 394–399. [CrossRef]

20. McElroy, S.J.; Prince, L.S.; Weitkamp, J.-H.; Reese, J.; Slaughter, J.C.; Polk, D.B. Tumor necrosis factor receptor 1-dependent depletion of mucus in immature small intestine: A potential role in neonatal necrotizing enterocolitis. *Am. J. Physiol. Gastrointest. Liver Physiol.* **2011**, *301*, G656–G666. [CrossRef]
21. Zhang, C.; Sherman, M.P.; Prince, L.S.; Bader, D.; Weitkamp, J.-H.; Slaughter, J.C.; McElroy, S.J. Paneth cell ablation in the presence of Klebsiella pneumoniae induces necrotizing enterocolitis (NEC)-like injury in the small intestine of immature mice. *Dis. Model. Mech.* **2012**, *5*, 522–532. [CrossRef] [PubMed]
22. Lueschow, S.R.; Stumphy, J.; Gong, H.; Kern, S.L.; Elgin, T.G.; Underwood, M.A.; Kalanetra, K.M.; Mills, D.A.; Wong, M.H.; Meyerholz, D.K.; et al. Loss of murine Paneth cell function alters the immature intestinal microbiome and mimics changes seen in neonatal necrotizing enterocolitis. *PLoS ONE* **2018**, *13*, e0204967. [CrossRef] [PubMed]
23. Aziz, M.M.; Ishihara, S.; Mishima, Y.; Oshima, N.; Moriyama, I.; Yuki, T.; Kadowaki, Y.; Rumi, M.A.K.; Amano, Y.; Kinoshita, Y. MFG-E8 attenuates intestinal inflammation in murine experimental colitis by modulating osteopontin-dependent alphavbeta3 integrin signaling. *J. Immunol.* **2009**, *182*, 7222–7232. [CrossRef] [PubMed]
24. Shen, H.; Lei, Y.; He, X.; Liu, D.; He, Z. Role of lactadherin in intestinal barrier integrity in experimental neonatal necrotizing enterocolitis. *J. Cell. Biochem.* **2019**, *120*, 19509–19517. [CrossRef]
25. Nair, R.R.; Warner, B.B.; Warner, B.W. Role of epidermal growth factor and other growth factors in the prevention of necrotizing enterocolitis. *Semin. Perinatol.* **2008**, *32*, 107–113. [CrossRef]
26. Warner, B.B.; Ryan, A.L.; Seeger, K.; Leonard, A.C.; Erwin, C.R.; Warner, B.W. Ontogeny of salivary epidermal growth factor and necrotizing enterocolitis. *J. Pediatr.* **2007**, *150*, 358–363. [CrossRef]
27. Clark, J.A.; Doelle, S.M.; Halpern, M.D.; Saunders, T.A.; Holubec, H.; Dvorak, K.; Boitano, S.A.; Dvorak, B. Intestinal barrier failure during experimental necrotizing enterocolitis: Protective effect of EGF treatment. *Am. J. Physiol. Liver Physiol.* **2006**, *291*, G938–G949. [CrossRef]
28. Knott, A.W.; Juno, R.J.; Jarboe, M.D.; Zhang, Y.; Profitt, S.A.; Thoerner, J.C.; Erwin, C.R.; Warner, B.W. EGF receptor signaling affects bcl-2 family gene expression and apoptosis after massive small bowel resection. *J. Pediatr. Surg.* **2003**, *38*, 875–880. [CrossRef]
29. Clark, J.A.; Lane, R.H.; Maclennan, N.K.; Holubec, H.; Dvorakova, K.; Halpern, M.D.; Williams, C.S.; Payne, C.M.; Dvorak, B. Epidermal growth factor reduces intestinal apoptosis in an experimental model of necrotizing enterocolitis. *Am. J. Physiol. Gastrointest. Liver Physiol.* **2005**, *288*, G755–G762. [CrossRef]
30. Michalsky, M.P.; Lara-Marquez, M.; Chun, L.; Besner, G.E. Heparin-binding EGF-like growth factor is present in human amniotic fluid and breast milk. *J. Pediatr. Surg.* **2002**, *37*, 1–6. [CrossRef]
31. Yang, J.; Su, Y.; Zhou, Y.; Besner, G.E. Heparin-binding EGF-like growth factor (HB-EGF) therapy for intestinal injury: Application and future prospects. *Pathophysiology* **2014**, *21*, 95–104. [CrossRef] [PubMed]
32. Feng, J.; El-Assal, O.N.; Besner, G.E. Heparin-binding EGF-like growth factor (HB-EGF) and necrotizing enterocolitis. *Semin. Pediatr. Surg.* **2005**, *14*, 167–174. [CrossRef] [PubMed]
33. Dvorak, B.; Khailova, L.; Clark, J.A.; Hosseini, D.M.; Arganbright, K.M.; Reynolds, C.A.; Halpern, M.D. Comparison of epidermal growth factor and heparin-binding epidermal growth factor-like growth factor for prevention of experimental necrotizing enterocolitis. *J. Pediatr. Gastroenterol. Nutr.* **2008**, *47*, 11–18. [CrossRef] [PubMed]
34. Sitarik, A.R.; Bobbitt, K.R.; Havstad, S.L.; Fujimura, K.E.; Levin, A.M.; Zoratti, E.M.; Kim, H.; Woodcroft, K.J.; Wegienka, G.; Ownby, D.R.; et al. Breast milk transforming growth factor β is associated with neonatal gut microbial composition. *J. Pediatr. Gastroenterol. Nutr.* **2017**, *65*, e60–e67. [CrossRef]
35. Namachivayam, K.; Coffing, H.P.; Sankaranarayanan, N.V.; Jin, Y.; MohanKumar, K.; Frost, B.L.; Blanco, C.L.; Patel, A.L.; Meier, P.P.; Garzon, S.A.; et al. Transforming growth factor-β2 is sequestered in preterm human milk by chondroitin sulfate proteoglycans. *Am. J. Physiol. Gastrointest. Liver Physiol.* **2015**, *309*, G171–G180. [CrossRef]
36. Maheshwari, A.; Kelly, D.R.; Nicola, T.; Ambalavanan, N.; Jain, S.K.; Murphy-Ullrich, J.; Athar, M.; Shimamura, M.; Bhandari, V.; Aprahamian, C.; et al. TGF-β2 suppresses macrophage cytokine production and mucosal inflammatory responses in the developing intestine. *Gastroenterology* **2011**, *140*, 242–253. [CrossRef]
37. Bode, L. Human milk oligosaccharides in the prevention of necrotizing enterocolitis: A journey from in vitro and in vivo models to mother-infant cohort studies. *Front. Pediatr.* **2018**, *6*, 385. [CrossRef]

38. Moukarzel, S.; Bode, L. Human milk oligosaccharides and the preterm infant: A journey in sickness and in health. *Clin. Perinatol.* **2017**, *44*, 193–207. [CrossRef]
39. Holscher, H.D.; Bode, L.; Tappenden, K.A. Human milk oligosaccharides influence intestinal epithelial cell maturation in vitro. *J. Pediatr. Gastroenterol. Nutr.* **2017**, *64*, 296–301. [CrossRef]
40. Autran, C.A.; Kellman, B.P.; Kim, J.H.; Asztalos, E.; Blood, A.B.; Spence, E.C.H.; Patel, A.L.; Hou, J.; Lewis, N.E.; Bode, L. Human milk oligosaccharide composition predicts risk of necrotising enterocolitis in preterm infants. *Gut* **2018**, *67*, 1064–1070. [CrossRef]
41. Rudloff, S.; Kuntz, S.; Ostenfeldt Rasmussen, S.; Roggenbuck, M.; Sprenger, N.; Kunz, C.; Sangild, P.T.; Brandt Bering, S. Metabolism of milk oligosaccharides in preterm pigs sensitive to necrotizing enterocolitis. *Front. Nutr.* **2019**, *6*, 23. [CrossRef] [PubMed]
42. Rasmussen, S.O.; Martin, L.; Østergaard, M.V.; Rudloff, S.; Roggenbuck, M.; Nguyen, D.N.; Sangild, P.T.; Bering, S.B. Human milk oligosaccharide effects on intestinal function and inflammation after preterm birth in pigs. *J. Nutr. Biochem.* **2017**, *40*, 141–154. [CrossRef] [PubMed]
43. Jantscher-Krenn, E.; Zherebtsov, M.; Nissan, C.; Goth, K.; Guner, Y.S.; Naidu, N.; Choudhury, B.; Grishin, A.V.; Ford, H.R.; Bode, L. The human milk oligosaccharide disialyllacto-N-tetraose prevents necrotising enterocolitis in neonatal rats. *Gut* **2012**, *61*, 1417–1425. [CrossRef] [PubMed]
44. Good, M.; Sodhi, C.P.; Yamaguchi, Y.; Jia, H.; Lu, P.; Fulton, W.B.; Martin, L.Y.; Prindle, T.; Nino, D.F.; Zhou, Q.; et al. The human milk oligosaccharide 2'-fucosyllactose attenuates the severity of experimental necrotising enterocolitis by enhancing mesenteric perfusion in the neonatal intestine. *Br. J. Nutr.* **2016**, *116*, 1175–1187. [CrossRef]
45. Agostoni, C.; Carratù, B.; Boniglia, C.; Lammardo, A.M.; Riva, E.; Sanzini, E. Free glutamine and glutamic acid increase in human milk through a three-month lactation period. *J. Pediatr. Gastroenterol. Nutr.* **2000**, *31*, 508–512. [CrossRef]
46. Baldeón, M.E.; Zertuche, F.; Flores, N.; Fornasini, M. Free amino acid content in human milk is associated with infant gender and weight gain during the first four months of lactation. *Nutrients* **2019**, *11*, 2239. [CrossRef]
47. Larnkjær, A.; Bruun, S.; Pedersen, D.; Zachariassen, G.; Barkholt, V.; Agostoni, C.; Mlgaard, C.; Husby, S.; Michaelsen, K.F. Free amino acids in human milk and associations with maternal anthropometry and infant growth. *J. Pediatr. Gastroenterol. Nutr.* **2016**, *63*, 374–378. [CrossRef]
48. Kim, M.-H.; Kim, H. The roles of glutamine in the intestine and its implication in intestinal diseases. *Int. J. Mol. Sci.* **2017**, *18*, 1051. [CrossRef]
49. Wang, B.; Wu, G.; Zhou, Z.; Dai, Z.; Sun, Y.; Ji, Y.; Li, W.; Wang, W.; Liu, C.; Han, F.; et al. Glutamine and intestinal barrier function. *Amino Acids* **2015**, *47*, 2143–2154. [CrossRef]
50. Becker, R.M.; Wu, G.; Galanko, J.A.; Chen, W.; Maynor, A.R.; Bose, C.L.; Rhoads, J.M. Reduced serum amino acid concentrations in infants with necrotizing enterocolitis. *J. Pediatr.* **2000**, *137*, 785–793. [CrossRef]
51. Zhou, W.; Li, W.; Zheng, X.-H.; Rong, X.; Huang, L.-G. Glutamine downregulates TLR-2 and TLR-4 expression and protects intestinal tract in preterm neonatal rats with necrotizing enterocolitis. *J. Pediatr. Surg.* **2014**, *49*, 1057–1063. [CrossRef] [PubMed]
52. Sodhi, C.P.; Neal, M.D.; Siggers, R.; Sho, S.; Ma, C.; Branca, M.F.; Prindle, T.; Russo, A.M.; Afrazi, A.; Good, M.; et al. Intestinal epithelial Toll-like receptor 4 regulates goblet cell development and is required for necrotizing enterocolitis in mice. *Gastroenterology* **2012**, *143*, 708–718.e5. [CrossRef] [PubMed]
53. Good, M.; Sodhi, C.P.; Egan, C.E.; Afrazi, A.; Jia, H.; Yamaguchi, Y.; Lu, P.; Branca, M.F.; Ma, C.; Prindle, T.; et al. Breast milk protects against the development of necrotizing enterocolitis through inhibition of Toll-like receptor 4 in the intestinal epithelium via activation of the epidermal growth factor receptor. *Mucosal Immunol.* **2015**, *8*, 1166–1179. [CrossRef] [PubMed]
54. Sodhi, C.P.; Shi, X.-H.; Richardson, W.M.; Grant, Z.S.; Shapiro, R.A.; Prindle, T.; Branca, M.; Russo, A.; Gribar, S.C.; Ma, C.; et al. Toll-like receptor-4 inhibits enterocyte proliferation via impaired beta-catenin signaling in necrotizing enterocolitis. *Gastroenterology* **2010**, *138*, 185–196. [CrossRef]
55. El-Shimi, M.S.; Awad, H.A.; Abdelwahed, M.A.; Mohamed, M.H.; Khafagy, S.M.; Saleh, G. Enteral L-arginine and glutamine supplementation for prevention of NEC in preterm neonates. *Int. J. Pediatr.* **2015**, *2015*, 856091. [CrossRef]
56. Brown, J.; Moe-Byrne, T.; McGuire, W. Glutamine supplementation for young infants with severe gastrointestinal disease. *Cochrane Database Syst. Rev.* **2007**, CD005947. [CrossRef]

57. Moe-Byrne, T.; Brown, J.V.E.; McGuire, W. Glutamine supplementation to prevent morbidity and mortality in preterm infants. *Cochrane Database Syst. Rev.* **2016**, *4*, CD001457.
58. Zhou, L.; Yoshimura, Y.; Huang, Y.; Suzuki, R.; Yokoyama, M.; Okabe, M.; Shimamura, M. Two independent pathways of maternal cell transmission to offspring: Through placenta during pregnancy and by breast-feeding after birth. *Immunology* **2000**, *101*, 570–580. [CrossRef]
59. Lewis, E.D.; Richard, C.; Larsen, B.M.; Field, C.J. The importance of human milk for immunity in preterm infants. *Clin. Perinatol.* **2017**, *44*, 23–47. [CrossRef]
60. Trend, S.; de Jong, E.; Lloyd, M.L.; Kok, C.H.; Richmond, P.; Doherty, D.A.; Simmer, K.; Kakulas, F.; Strunk, T.; Currie, A. Leukocyte populations in human preterm and term breast milk identified by multicolour flow cytometry. *PLoS ONE* **2015**, *10*, e0135580. [CrossRef]
61. Cabinian, A.; Sinsimer, D.; Tang, M.; Zumba, O.; Mehta, H.; Toma, A.; Sant'Angelo, D.; Laouar, Y.; Laouar, A. Transfer of maternal immune cells by breastfeeding: Maternal cytotoxic T lymphocytes present in breast milk localize in the peyer's patches of the nursed infant. *PLoS ONE* **2016**, *11*, e0156762. [CrossRef] [PubMed]
62. Riskin, A.; Almog, M.; Peri, R.; Halasz, K.; Srugo, I.; Kessel, A. Changes in immunomodulatory constituents of human milk in response to active infection in the nursing infant. *Pediatr. Res.* **2012**, *71*, 220–225. [CrossRef] [PubMed]
63. Ustundag, B.; Yilmaz, E.; Dogan, Y.; Akarsu, S.; Canatan, H.; Halifeoglu, I.; Cikim, G.; Aygun, A.D. Levels of cytokines (IL-1beta, IL-2, IL-6, IL-8, TNF-alpha) and trace elements (Zn, Cu) in breast milk from mothers of preterm and term infants. *Mediators Inflamm.* **2005**, *2005*, 331–336. [CrossRef] [PubMed]
64. Minekawa, R.; Takeda, T.; Sakata, M.; Hayashi, M.; Isobe, A.; Yamamoto, T.; Tasaka, K.; Murata, Y. Human breast milk suppresses the transcriptional regulation of IL-1beta-induced NF-kappaB signaling in human intestinal cells. *Am. J. Physiol. Cell Physiol.* **2004**, *287*, C1404–C1411. [CrossRef]
65. Bryan, D.-L.; Forsyth, K.D.; Gibson, R.A.; Hawkes, J.S. Interleukin-2 in human milk: A potential modulator of lymphocyte development in the breastfed infant. *Cytokine* **2006**, *33*, 289–293. [CrossRef]
66. Hassan, J.; Reen, D.J. Reduced primary antigen-specific T-cell precursor frequencies in neonates is associated with deficient interleukin-2 production. *Immunology* **1996**, *87*, 604–608. [CrossRef]
67. Saito, S.; Maruyama, M.; Kato, Y.; Moriyama, I.; Ichijo, M. Detection of IL-6 in human milk and its involvement in IgA production. *J. Reprod. Immunol.* **1991**, *20*, 267–276. [CrossRef]
68. Rudloff, H.E.; Schmalstieg, F.C.; Palkowetz, K.H.; Paszkiewicz, E.J.; Goldman, A.S. Interleukin-6 in human milk. *J. Reprod. Immunol.* **1993**, *23*, 13–20. [CrossRef]
69. Maheshwari, A.; Lu, W.; Lacson, A.; Barleycorn, A.A.; Nolan, S.; Christensen, R.D.; Calhoun, D.A. Effects of interleukin-8 on the developing human intestine. *Cytokine* **2002**, *20*, 256–267. [CrossRef]
70. Polat, A.; Tunc, T.; Erdem, G.; Yerebasmaz, N.; Tas, A.; Beken, S.; Basbozkurt, G.; Saldir, M.; Zenciroglu, A.; Yaman, H. Interleukin-8 and its receptors in human milk from mothers of full-term and premature infants. *Breastfeed. Med.* **2016**, *11*, 247–251. [CrossRef]
71. Fiorentino, D.F.; Bond, M.W.; Mosmann, T.R. Two types of mouse T helper cell. IV. Th2 clones secrete a factor that inhibits cytokine production by Th1 clones. *J. Exp. Med.* **1989**, *170*, 2081–2095. [CrossRef] [PubMed]
72. Garofalo, R.; Chheda, S.; Mei, F.; Palkowetz, K.H.; Rudloff, H.E.; Schmalstieg, F.C.; Rassin, D.K.; Goldman, A.S. Interleukin-10 in human milk. *Pediatr. Res.* **1995**, *37*, 444–449. [CrossRef] [PubMed]
73. Fiorentino, D.F.; Zlotnik, A.; Mosmann, T.R.; Howard, M.; O'Garra, A. IL-10 inhibits cytokine production by activated macrophages. *J. Immunol.* **1991**, *147*, 3815–3822. [PubMed]
74. Jinquan, T.; Larsen, C.G.; Gesser, B.; Matsushima, K.; Thestrup-Pedersen, K. Human IL-10 is a chemoattractant for $CD8^+$ T lymphocytes and an inhibitor of IL-8-induced $CD4^+$ T lymphocyte migration. *J. Immunol.* **1993**, *151*, 4545–4551. [PubMed]
75. Fluckiger, A.C.; Garrone, P.; Durand, I.; Galizzi, J.P.; Banchereau, J. Interleukin 10 (IL-10) upregulates functional high affinity IL-2 receptors on normal and leukemic B lymphocytes. *J. Exp. Med.* **1993**, *178*, 1473–1481. [CrossRef]
76. Ballard, O.; Morrow, A.L. Human milk composition: Nutrients and bioactive factors. *Pediatr. Clin. N. Am.* **2013**, *60*, 49–74. [CrossRef]
77. Beaurepaire, C.; Smyth, D.; McKay, D.M. Interferon-gamma regulation of intestinal epithelial permeability. *J. Interferon Cytokine Res.* **2009**, *29*, 133–144. [CrossRef]

78. Hui, L.; Dai, Y.; Guo, Z.; Zhang, J.; Zheng, F.; Bian, X.; Wu, Z.; Jiang, Q.; Guo, M.; Ma, K.; et al. Immunoregulation effects of different γδT cells and toll-like receptor signaling pathways in neonatal necrotizing enterocolitis. *Medicine (Baltimore)*. **2017**, *96*, e6077. [CrossRef]
79. Yu, J.C.; Khodadadi, H.; Malik, A.; Davidson, B.; da Salles, É.S.L.; Bhatia, J.; Hale, V.L.; Baban, B. Innate immunity of neonates and infants. *Front. Immunol.* **2018**, *9*, 1759. [CrossRef]
80. Buescher, E.S.; Malinowska, I. Soluble receptors and cytokine antagonists in human milk. *Pediatr. Res.* **1996**, *40*, 839–844. [CrossRef]
81. Castellote, C.; Casillas, R.; Ramírez-Santana, C.; Pérez-Cano, F.J.; Castell, M.; Moretones, M.G.; López-Sabater, M.C.; Franch, A. Premature delivery influences the immunological composition of colostrum and transitional and mature human milk. *J. Nutr.* **2011**, *141*, 1181–1187. [CrossRef] [PubMed]
82. Chokshi, N.K.; Guner, Y.S.; Hunter, C.J.; Upperman, J.S.; Grishin, A.; Ford, H.R. The role of nitric oxide in intestinal epithelial injury and restitution in neonatal necrotizing enterocolitis. *Semin. Perinatol.* **2008**, *32*, 92–99. [CrossRef] [PubMed]
83. Nankervis, C.A.; Giannone, P.J.; Reber, K.M. The neonatal intestinal vasculature: Contributing factors to necrotizing enterocolitis. *Semin. Perinatol.* **2008**, *32*, 83–91. [CrossRef] [PubMed]
84. Akçay, F.; Aksoy, H.; Memişoğullari, R. Effect of breast-feeding on concentration of nitric oxide in breast milk. *Ann. Clin. Biochem.* **2002**, *39*, 68–69. [CrossRef] [PubMed]
85. Ford, H.; Watkins, S.; Reblock, K.; Rowe, M. The role of inflammatory cytokines and nitric oxide in the pathogenesis of necrotizing enterocolitis. *J. Pediatr. Surg.* **1997**, *32*, 275–282. [CrossRef]
86. Yazji, I.; Sodhi, C.P.; Lee, E.K.; Good, M.; Egan, C.E.; Afrazi, A.; Neal, M.D.; Jia, H.; Lin, J.; Ma, C.; et al. Endothelial TLR4 activation impairs intestinal microcirculatory perfusion in necrotizing enterocolitis via eNOS-NO-nitrite signaling. *Proc. Natl. Acad. Sci. USA* **2013**, *110*, 9451–9456. [CrossRef]
87. Bravi, F.; Wiens, F.; Decarli, A.; Dal Pont, A.; Agostoni, C.; Ferraroni, M. Impact of maternal nutrition on breast-milk composition: A systematic review. *Am. J. Clin. Nutr.* **2016**, *104*, 646–662. [CrossRef]
88. Gay, M.C.L.; Koleva, P.T.; Slupsky, C.M.; du Toit, E.; Eggesbo, M.; Johnson, C.C.; Wegienka, G.; Shimojo, N.; Campbell, D.E.; Prescott, S.L.; et al. Worldwide variation in human milk metabolome: Indicators of breast physiology and maternal lifestyle? *Nutrients* **2018**, *10*, 1151. [CrossRef]

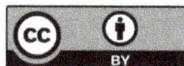

© 2019 by the authors. Licensee MDPI, Basel, Switzerland. This article is an open access article distributed under the terms and conditions of the Creative Commons Attribution (CC BY) license (http://creativecommons.org/licenses/by/4.0/).

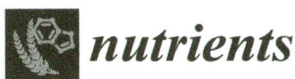 

*Review*

# Bioactive Factors in Human Breast Milk Attenuate Intestinal Inflammation during Early Life

Julie D. Thai [1,*] and Katherine E. Gregory [2]

1. Division of Newborn Medicine, Boston Children's Hospital, Boston, MA 02115, USA
2. Department of Pediatric Newborn Medicine, Department of Nursing, Brigham and Women's Hospital, Boston, MA 02115, USA; kgregory1@bwh.harvard.edu
* Correspondence: julie.d.thai@gmail.com; Tel.: +1-617-919-2341

Received: 31 January 2020; Accepted: 16 February 2020; Published: 23 February 2020

**Abstract:** Human breast milk is well known as the ideal source of nutrition during early life, ensuring optimal growth during infancy and early childhood. Breast milk is also the source of many unique and dynamic bioactive components that play a key role in the development of the immune system. These bioactive components include essential microbes, human milk oligosaccharides (HMOs), immunoglobulins, lactoferrin and dietary polyunsaturated fatty acids. These factors all interact with intestinal commensal bacteria and/or immune cells, playing a critical role in establishment of the intestinal microbiome and ultimately influencing intestinal inflammation and gut health during early life. Exposure to breast milk has been associated with a decreased incidence and severity of necrotizing enterocolitis (NEC), a devastating disease characterized by overwhelming intestinal inflammation and high morbidity among preterm infants. For this reason, breast milk is considered a protective factor against NEC and aberrant intestinal inflammation common in preterm infants. In this review, we will describe the key microbial, immunological, and metabolic components of breast milk that have been shown to play a role in the mechanisms of intestinal inflammation and/or NEC prevention.

**Keywords:** human milk; breast milk; intestinal inflammation; bioactive; necrotizing enterocolitis

## 1. Introduction

Human breast milk is well known as the optimal source of nutrition during early life, as a result of a nutritional content that evolves with the needs of the growing infant [1,2]. Equally important to its nutritional attributes, human breast milk contains several bioactive factors that promote immune health, protecting against infectious and inflammatory disease processes throughout childhood [2–11]. In this review, we will focus on specific microbial, immunological and metabolic factors and the role they play in attenuating inflammation during early life.

Inflammation is the result of a complex cascade of chemical signals released by immune cells. [12] It is a necessary and protective process of the innate immune system, required for physiological responses, such as initiating tissue repair and eliminating pathogenic insults [13]. However, evidence suggests that uncontrolled inflammation plays a prominent role in many common and chronic diseases, such as arthritis, inflammatory bowel disease, cardiovascular disease, Alzheimer's, Parkinson's disease, cancer, and metabolic syndrome [14]. Furthermore, inflammation early in life may lead to adverse neurodevelopmental outcomes, underscoring the importance of mitigating inflammation during the newborn period [15].

The intestine, which plays a critical role in the overall inflammatory response, is the largest immune organ in the body and, due to its large surface area, has the greatest exposure to the outside environment [16]. The newborn intestine is equipped with all the basic functional structures, but in order to fully mature, it undergoes rapid mucosal differentiation and development with exposure to enteral nutrition, namely human breast milk [16,17]. The newborn intestinal immune system is also notably immature, relying on maternal passive antibodies, particularly secretory immunoglobulin A (sIgA), for protection in the first weeks of life. In the first months of infancy, the intestinal immune system develops the ability to distinguish between foreign pathogens and safe nutrient proteins or commensal organisms [16–18].

The preterm infant's intestine is more immature in structure and immune function when compared to full-term born infants, and is characterized by the elicitation of an exaggerated inflammatory response towards potential insults [19]. For example, the preterm intestine exhibits high expression of Toll-like receptor 4 (TLR4), an immune receptor expressed on leukocyte membranes that recognize molecular patterns in potential pathogens and, in turn, upregulate and suppress genes that orchestrate an inflammatory response [20,21]. This exaggerated inflammatory response has been implicated in the pathogenesis of necrotizing enterocolitis (NEC), a disease characterized by overwhelming intestinal inflammation and a major contributor to neonatal morbidity and mortality [19,22]. Breast milk has been shown to be protective against NEC in a dose-dependent manner, though the mechanism is unclear [4,23,24]. This protection is likely a result of the many bioactive components found in human breast milk that have been shown to regulate the immune system and attenuate inflammation, specifically within preterm infant intestinal biology [25–29] (Table 1). NEC is an extreme example of intestinal inflammation, underpinning the importance of bioactive factors in human milk.

## 2. Methods

*Literature Search*

The literature review was conducted using the PubMed and Google Scholar databases, as well as hand searches for primary studies investigating bioactive factors in human milk and their effects on intestinal inflammation. The literature search was conducted using key words, including combinations of human milk, intestinal inflammation, microbiome, *Bifdobacteria*, *Lactobacillus*, human milk oligosaccharides, immunoglobulins, secretory IgA, IgG, cytokines, growth factors, epidermal growth factor, heparin binding growth factor, vascular endothelial growth factor, lactoferrin, lactadherin, lysozyme, metabolic factors, fatty acids, antioxidants, and anti-proteases.

## 3. Microbiome and Microbial Factors

*3.1. Microbiome and Probiotics*

Humans have evolved to develop a symbiotic relationship with the commensal bacteria comprising the intestinal microbiome. Despite the close and potentially health-compromising proximity between the many bacterial communities and the host's intestinal surface, the host's intestinal immune system has developed to contain and work together with the intestinal microbiota in order to maintain intestinal health homeostasis [30]. Mounting evidence suggests that exposure to commensal bacteria in early life is crucial to appropriate development of the immune system [13]. Disruption of this symbiotic relationship has been shown to lead to intestinal inflammation and disease [30].

The main functions of gut microbiota include facilitating the breakdown of food substances to liberate nutrients for the host to absorb, promoting host cell differentiation, protecting the host from pathogenic colonization and modulating the immune system [31]. Disruption of gut microbiota homeostasis causes shifts in microbiota balance or dysbiosis. Intestinal dysbiosis has been shown to be associated with long-term health consequences, such as obesity, diabetes and inflammatory bowel disease, as well as NEC in preterm infants [19,31]. Furthermore, germ free animals are unable to exhibit clinical signs of NEC as animals with conventional gut microbial colonization do, indicating the importance of microbial composition in the development of NEC [32]. The intestinal microbial composition of infants who develop NEC consists of unusual intestinal microbial species and overall decreased diversity of microbiota [19,33]. Therefore, the acquisition of appropriate intestinal microbiota is essential to intestinal health and prevention from inflammation and disease.

Human breast milk has been shown to have its own unique microbiome and contains one of the main sources of bacteria to the intestine of a primarily breastfed infant [34]. Breast milk is estimated to provide 25% of a breastfed infant's intestinal microbiota by 1 month of age as a result of exposing the infant to approximately $1 \times 10^5$ to $1 \times 10^7$ bacteria and over 700 species of bacteria daily [8,32,35]. Thus, the human milk microbiota influences the acquisition and establishment of the intestinal microbiome during infancy and is thought to be a major factor involved in innate immunity during early life [36].

The most commonly reported genera in human milk include *Staphylococcus*, *Streptococcus*, *Lactobacillus*, *Enterococcus*, *Bifidobacterium*, *Propionibacterium*, as well as the family *Enterobacteriaceae* [36–38]. However, the types and amounts of bacteria in human milk are likely impacted by many factors including genetics, maternal health and diet, stage of lactation and geographic location [39]. In a study performed by Cabrera-Rubio et al., mothers with higher body mass indexes (BMI) had higher levels of *Lactobacillus* in colostrum and lower numbers of *Bifidobacterium* in their breast milk at 6 months postpartum. Moreover, mothers who delivered via cesarean section had decreased amounts of *Leuconostocaceae*, a family of bacteria within the order of *Lactobacillus*, in their breast milk, compared to mothers who delivered vaginally [40].

*Bifidobacteria* have been shown to modulate inflammation and increase colonic luminal short chain fatty acid production (SCFA) in both mice and humans [41,42]. Interestingly, a lack of *Bifidobacterium* has been shown to be associated with NEC [43]. The role of *Bifidobacterium* in attenuating intestinal inflammation has been highlighted in multiple probiotic studies. In a study done by Underwood et al. in 2014, mice fed with formula and *Bifidobacterium longum* subspecies *Infantis* had decreased incidence of NEC, as well as decreased expression of pro-inflammatory mediators, interleukin (IL)-6, chemokine-1 (CXCL-1), tumor necrosis factor alpha (TNF-α), and IL-23, as well as inducible nitric oxide synthase, an important microbial pattern sensor that triggers an inflammatory response [44].

*Lactobacillus rhamnosus* SHA113, isolated from breast milk, was shown to inhibit multidrug resistant *Escherichia coli* (multi-drug resistant (MDR) *E. coli*) intestinal infection in vitro and in vivo, through blocking pro-inflammatory pathways and restoring homeostasis in the intestinal microbiota. Specifically, serum pro-inflammatory cytokines, TNF-α and IL-6, were reduced and anti-inflammatory cytokine IL-10 was increased in mice receiving *Lactobacillus rhamnosus* SHA113 following MDR *E. coli* infection when compared to those who received no treatment. Furthermore, *Lactobacillus rhamnosus* reversed the increased abundance of Proteobacteria observed in the MDR *E. coli* infected mice [45].

A study by Guo et al. showed that a combination of *Lactobacillus acidophilus* and *Bifidobacterium longum* species exposed to immature human enterocytes and immature human intestinal xenografts showed a decrease in pro-inflammatory mediators IL-8 and IL-6, as well as alteration of genes in the nuclear factor kappa beta (NF-κB) signaling pathway, a critical pathway in the maintenance of immune homeostasis and a strong pro-inflammatory signaling cascade [46,47]. Specifically, there was a decrease in positive inductors of the pathway, including Toll-like receptor 2 (TLR2) and TLR4 mRNA, and an increase in negative regulators—single immunoglobulin IL-1 related receptor (SIGIRR) and Toll-interacting protein (TOLLIP)—characteristic of a matured innate immune response [48]. Bacteria within breast milk can influence the intestinal microbiome, which has important roles in regulating inflammation.

**Table 1.** Bioactive Components in Breast Milk and Roles in Attenuating Intestinal Inflammation.

| Bioactive Components in Breast Milk | Role in Intestinal Inflammation Regulation or Prevention | Effect | References |
|---|---|---|---|
| **Microbial or microbial modulating factors** | | | |
| Lactobacillus spp, | -Inhibit NF-κB pathway<br>-decrease pro-inflammatory cytokines, TNF-α, IL-6<br>-reverse intestinal dysbiosis in bacterial intestinal infection | -decrease inflammatory response<br>-Restore intestinal microbiome homeostasis | [41–44] |
| Bifidobacterium spp | -increase SCFA production<br>-Decrease pro-inflammatory CK release (IL-6, CXCL-1, TNF-α, IL-23) and iNOS | -promote anti-inflammatory commensal bacteria proliferation<br>-decrease inflammatory response | [45–48] |
| Human Milk Oligosaccharides | -regulate commensal bacteria<br>-act as decoy receptors for pathogens<br>-modulate immune signaling pathways, TLR3, TLR5, PAMP | -promote healthy intestinal microbiota with anti-inflammatory properties<br>-prevent and decrease inflammatory response | [32,49–53] |
| **Immunological factors** | | | |
| Secretory IgA | -bind to pathogens and commensal bacteria | -prevention of typical inflammatory response, or immune exclusion<br>-influence intestinal microbiome | [29,54] |
| IgG | -opsonization, agglutination of bacteria | -prevention of typical acute inflammatory response | [52,55–57] |
| IL-10 | -inhibit Th1, NK cell, macrophages | -provide immunoregulation and prevent inflammation | [18,58–61] |
| TGF-β | -inhibit differentiation of naïve T cells into Th1, Th2 cells<br>-Stabilize FOXP3 expression | -decrease pro-inflammatory cytokine expression and inflammation<br>-inhibit immune response and decrease inflammation | [18,60,62–64] |
| ILRA-1<br>TNFR I and II<br>soluble TLR2 | -compete with IL-1 receptor for IL-1<br>-directly bind, inhibit TNF-α<br>-decoy receptor to inhibit IL-8, TNF | -prevent pro-inflammatory cytokine expression and inflammation | [52,60,65–67] |
| EGF<br>HB-EGF<br>VEGF | -upregulate IL-10 expression<br>-bind to bacteria<br>-stimulate angiogenesis- | -decrease pro-inflammatory cytokine expression<br>-prevent intestinal edema | [68–74] |
| Lactoferrin | -direct cytotoxicity on pathogens by forming lactoferricin<br>-inhibit IL-1, IL-6, TNF-α, IL-8<br>-promote growth of probiotics | -eliminate trigger for acute inflammatory response<br>-decrease pro-inflammatory cytokine expression and inflammation<br>-regulate intestinal microbiome | [18,75–77] |
| Lactadherin | -enhance phagocytosis of apoptotic cells<br>-blocks NF-κB pathway via TLR4 inhibition<br>-promote healing during intestinal inflammation | -eliminate trigger for acute inflammatory response<br>-prevent pro-inflammatory signaling and decreasing inflammatory response<br>-limit degree of intestinal inflammation | [78,79] |
| Lysozyme | -degrades GP bacteria outer wall<br>-kill GN bacteria with lactoferrin | -eliminate trigger for acute inflammatory response | [18,80] |
| **Metabolic factors** | | | |
| Adiponectin | -suppress mature macrophage function | -decrease inflammatory response | [52,81] |
| Leptin | -stimulates T cells<br>-influence polarization of macrophages to anti-inflammatory phenotype | -regulate immune response and prevent inflammation | [81–84] |
| Omega 3 PUFA | -decrease NF-κB, bind to PPAR-γ<br>-increase proliferation of Lactobacillus and Bifidobacterium<br>-change membrane PL concentration<br>-inhibit leukocyte migration | -downregulate pro-inflammatory genes<br>-promote anti-inflammatory commensal bacteria proliferation<br>-decrease degree of inflammatory response | [13,85–90] |
| Antioxidants | -scavenge free radicals | -prevent injury and inflammation | [60] |
| Anti-proteases | -metabolize proteases produced by inflammatory cells | -prevent excessive inflammatory response | [60] |

Abbreviations: Nuclear factor kappa B (NF-κB); tumor necrosis factor alpha (TNF-α); interleukin (IL); short chain fatty acid (SCFA); cytokine (CK); chemokine-1 (CXCL-1); inducible nitric oxide synthase (iNOS); Toll-like receptor (TLR); pathogen-associated molecular pattern (PAMP); Immunoglobulin (Ig); T-helper (Th) cell; natural killer cell (NK); transformation growth factor beta (TGF-β); forkhead box P3 (FOXP3); interleukin receptor antagonist 1 (ILRA-1); tumor necrosis factor receptor (TNFR); epidermal growth factor (EGF); heparin-binding epidermal growth factor (HB-EGF)-like growth factor; vascular endothelial growth factor (VEGF); gram positive (GP); gram negative (GN); polyunsaturated fatty acid (PUFA); peroxisome proliferator-activated receptor gamma (PPAR-γ); phospholipid (PL).

## 3.2. Human Milk Oligosaccharides and Glycans

Human milk oligosaccharides (HMOs) are within the group of glycans, which are potent antimicrobial factors in human milk. HMOs comprise an abundant and diverse component of breast milk, being not only the third largest solid component of milk, but also constituting more than 200 different structural types. Each HMO is also structurally distinct, consisting of a mixture of glucose, galactose, N-acetylglucosamine, fucose and/or sialic acid [49]. They range from three to 32 monosaccharides in size and are undigestible by the host [50–52]. HMOs and glycans vary by maternal genotype and change over the course of lactation [32]. Interestingly, the maternal milk of preterm infants has higher HMO concentrations than term milk [49].

HMOs have a prebiotic role, arriving to the distal intestine undigested and able to support the growth of mutualistic bacteria, specifically certain *Bifidobacteria* taxa and *Bacteroides* species. HMOs are the sole carbon source of these certain *Bifidobacterial* taxa. These microbes ferment the prebiotic glycan into small organic acids for sustenance [32]. Given the long and diverse structure of HMOs, microbial communities can act in concordance to metabolize HMOs. [31]. HMOs and glycans also act to inhibit infection by acidifying the gut lumen [32]. HMOs produce bacteriocins and organic acids which have been proved useful for preventing the growth of pathogens [49]. They also supply fucose and sialic acid [91]. HMOs and glucosaminoglycans function as pathogen-binding inhibitors that function as "decoy" receptors for pathogens that have an affinity for binding oligosaccharide receptors expressed on the infant's intestinal surface [2,50–53]. This mechanism modulates expression of immune signaling genes, which have been shown to repress inflammation at the mucosal surface [75]. The antiadhesive activity and prebiotic activity secondarily reduce inflammation within the intestine [32].

Colostrum HMOs have been shown to modulate immune signaling pathways, including TLR3, TLR5, and IL-1β-dependent pathogen-associated molecular pathways (PAMP), and subsequently decrease acute phase inflammatory cytokine secretion. For example, 3'-galactosyllactose, directly inhibits polyinosine–polycytidylic acid, which, in turn, decreases levels of the potent proinflammatory cytokine, IL-8. Another glycan, diasialyllacto-N-tetraose (DSLNT) has been shown to suppress NEC-like inflammation in neonatal rats [32]. Supplementation with HMOs has also been shown to attenuate intestinal inflammation. In a study on preterm pigs, a formula diet consisting of HMOs was shown to decrease lipopolysaccharide-induced cytokine secretion relative to controls. Pigs who received HMO also showed higher levels of anti-inflammatory cytokines (IL-10, IL-12, TGF-β). Whether it is in promoting anti-inflammatory bacteria or directly preventing a pathogen-induced immune response, HMOs play a significant role in attenuating inflammation within the gut.

## 4. Immunological Factors: Immunoglobulins and Immunological Proteins

### 4.1. Immunoglobulins

Human milk provides the only source of sIgA for the first 4 weeks of life due to the lack of functioning plasma cells in the infant. sIgA is formed by cleavage of IgA in the mammary gland, allowing its release into breast milk and subsequent consumption by the infant [92]. sIgA comprises up to 80%–90% of the immunoglobulins present in breast milk and is at its highest concentrations in colostrum and in the breast milk of mothers who deliver early [65,93,94]. In contrast, other major immunoglobulin isotypes (IgM), whose roles include promoting inflammation, are present in modest or very low concentrations. Immunoglobulin E, IgE, is absent in human milk [95].

sIgA comprises the first line of antigen-specific immune defense and its actions are fundamentally local. They bind to commensal or pathogenic microorganisms, toxins, viruses and other antigenic materials, like lipopolysaccharide (LPS), preventing adherence and penetration into epithelium without triggering inflammatory reactions that could be harmful during early life. This phenomenon is known as immune exclusion. Because sIgA coinhabit the outer intestinal mucosal layer with commensal bacteria, its ability to effectively recognize and eliminate pathogens while, at the same time, maintaining a mutually beneficial relationship with commensal bacteria, is crucial. Interestingly, 74% of bacteria in the gut lumen are coated with sIgA [54]. Given this role, it is not surprising that sIgA influences the composition of the intestinal microbiome and, furthermore, promotes intestinal homeostasis by preventing inappropriate inflammatory responses to pathogenic microbes and nutritional antigens.

In a recent study by Gopalakrishna et al., maternal milk-fed infants had higher percentages of IgA that were bound to bacteria compared to formula-fed infants. In addition, higher percentages of IgA bound to bacteria in the intestine of preterm infants was associated with lower rates of NEC. Furthermore, it was observed that lower levels of IgA-bound bacteria were inversely associated with abundance of enterobacteria among infants who developed NEC. Thus, IgA binding to bacteria presumably plays a protective role against NEC, likely by limiting inflammation induced by *Enterobacteriaceae*. Mice who were fed maternal milk that lacked IgA were indistinguishable from formula-fed controls, implying that maternal milk is only protective against NEC when containing IgA. While the protective mechanism by which IgA binds bacteria is unknown, it is hypothesized that IgA may limit the ability of the bacteria to gain access to the intestinal epithelium. IgA also has a role in modifying the expression of bacterial surface proteins and motility of bacteria [29].

Though comprising a small proportion of immunoglobulins in breastmilk, immunoglobulin G (IgG) plays an anti-inflammatory role by direct binding, opsonization and agglutination of pathogens [52,55]. IgG is mainly transferred via the placenta from mother to fetus, but IgG is also produced in the mammary gland and detected in a majority of colostrum samples of mothers, adding to the much-needed immunological protection to the vulnerable infant [56,57].

### 4.2. Cytokines and Growth Factors

Many cytokines, including transformation growth factor beta (TGF-$\beta$), interleukin 1B (IL-1B), IL-6, I-10, IL-12, TNF-$\alpha$, interferon gamma (IFN-$\gamma$), and granulocyte-macrophage colony-stimulating factor (GM-CSF) are present in human milk [18,96]. These cytokines are small proteins or peptides that act as intercellular messengers and elicit a particular response after binding to a receptor on a target cell. Responses include mediation and regulation of immunity, hematopoiesis and inflammation. IL-10, TGF-$\beta$, IL-1 receptor antagonist (IL-1RA), Tumor necrosis factor receptor I and II (TNFR I and II) all have been shown to have anti-inflammatory roles [18].

IL-10 is an important anti-inflammatory and immunoregulatory cytokine present in high concentrations in both the aqueous phase and in the lipid layer of human milk [18]. It specifically inhibits T-helper 1 (Th1) effector cell activity, natural killer cells and macrophages, resulting in immune homeostasis [58]. In a study of mice who were genetically unable to produce IL-10, an unexpected immune response was mounted to a normal intestinal microbiota in the gut. These mice ultimately developed an enterocolitis that was similar to ulcerative colitis and celiac disease in humans, emphasizing IL-10's importance in suppressing inflammation [59,60]. Similar results were observed in IL-10-deficient mice who underwent a NEC-inducing regimen of formula feeding, hypoxia and hypothermia [61].

The TGF-$\beta$ family comprise the most abundant cytokines of human milk. The highest levels are present in colostrum and decline substantially by 4-6 weeks of life [97]. They include 3 isoforms, with TGF-$\beta$2 being the most predominant. TGF-$\beta$ has many immunomodulatory properties, including stimulating intestinal maturation and defense by switching immunoglobulin classes from IgM to IgA in B lymphocytes, immunoglobulin production in the mammary gland and gastrointestinal tract of the newborn, assistance with intestinal mucosal repair, and induction of oral tolerance [18]. It is known to regulate inflammation by decreasing pro-inflammatory cytokine expression. In a study of pediatric patients with Crohn's disease, a feeding trial consisting of supplemental TGF-$\beta$ resulted in decreased mucosal IL-1 mRNA and clinical remission in 79% of patients [60,62]. TGF-$\beta$ inhibits naïve T cells from differentiation into Th1 and Th2 subtypes, which promote cell mediated immune responses by secreting pro-inflammatory cytokines and promote IgE and eosinophilic responses, respectively. TGF-$\beta$ also helps stabilize forkhead box P3 (FOXP3) expression and maintains the differentiation of T-regulatory cells which inhibit immune responses and temper inflammation [63]. In preterm infants, lower TGF-β levels preceded NEC development, underlining the significance of TGF-β in immune and inflammation regulation [64]. In addition to essential immunoregulatory roles in the newborn, studies have suggested the association between human milk TGF-β and allergic diseases in infancy and childhood, including asthma, eczema, food allergy, and allergic rhinitis. However, a recent systemic review by Khaleva suggested that studies were too heterogenous to deduce a clear association and that larger prospective studies are needed [97].

Other cytokines serve as direct antagonists to pro-inflammatory signaling. IL-1 receptor antagonist (IL-1RA) is also present in human milk and limits inflammation by competing with the pro-inflammatory cytokine, IL-1, for receptor binding. In a study of rats with colitis, those fed human milk instead of formula had similar inflammatory responses compared to those who were fed formula [60]. TNFRI and II, though present in small quantities in human milk, directly bind and inhibit TNF-α, a proinflammatory cytokine produced by a wide range of immune cells [52,65]. Soluble TLR2 is present at high concentrations in breast milk and acts as a negative regulatory mechanism for cytokines and chemokines. By acting as a decoy receptor, sTLR2 has been shown to inhibit IL-8 and TNF production by monocytes stimulated with bacterial lipopeptide, which is an agonist of TLR2 [66,67].

Epidermal growth factor (EGF) is a peptide that is abundant in breast milk and is important for preserving intestinal barrier function, improving nutrient transport and increasing intestinal enzyme activity [68]. Studies have shown that rats with experimental NEC who were treated with EGF had decreased intestinal inflammation and particularly decreased levels of proinflammatory cytokine, IL-18, at the site of intestinal injury, as well as IL-18 mRNA levels. IL-18 dysregulation has been associated with inflammatory diseases of the small intestine. EGF has also been shown to have indirect anti-inflammatory effects by upregulation of IL-10 [68,69]. Heparin-binding epidermal growth factor-like growth factor (HB-EGF), a member of the EGF family of growth factors, also protects against intestinal injury in the developing intestine by binding to pathogenic bacteria [70,71]. In rats who underwent ischemic/reperfusion injury had less pro-inflammatory cytokine expression, particularly TNF-α and IL-6, in vivo [71,72].

Similarly, vascular endothelial growth factor is a glycoprotein present in breast milk, at higher levels in the colostrum and breast milk of mothers with preterm infants than those with term infants [73]. Its primary role is mediating formation of new blood vessels, a process called angiogenesis, but it has been suggested that VEGF may also have anti-inflammatory effects. In a study performed by Karatepe et al., rats induced with NEC and given subcutaneous VEGF had less villous atrophy and less intestinal edema, as well as lower TNF-α and IL-6 levels when compared to NEC-induced rats who were not treated with VEGF [74].

Pro-inflammatory cytokines, including TNF-α, IL-6, IL-8 and IFN-γ a, are also present in mother's milk, but at lower levels than the immunoregulatory cytokines mentioned. These pro-inflammatory cytokines also decrease overtime. Certain pro-inflammatory cytokines, IL-1B, IL-6, TNF-α, are decreased in the breastmilk of preterm infants when compared to that of breastmilk of term infants [98]. This suggests that human milk cytokine composition helps regulate intestinal inflammation in newborns and may be tailored to the particular immune system needs in the infant.

*4.3. Lactoferrin, Lactadherin, and Lysozyme*

Lactoferrin is a single-chain metal binding glycoprotein that is abundant in breast milk with highest concentrations in colostrum that decline throughout lactation [76]. It is partially degraded in the intestine and has bacteriostatic function in the intestinal mucosa of the newborn. It specifically binds to iron, preventing growth of various pathogens who are reliant on iron for further proliferation [75]. Lactoferrin has also been shown to inhibit microbial adhesion to host cells and has direct cytotoxic effects against bacteria, viruses and fungi, specifically by forming lactoferricin, a potent cationic peptide with bactericidal activity formed during digestion of lactoferrin [77]. In regard to inflammation, lactoferrin helps limit excessive immune responses by blocking many pro-inflammatory cytokines, including IL-1β, IL-6, TNF-α and IL-8, as well as suppressing free-radical activity [18,77].

Furthermore, lactoferrin has been shown to promote the growth of probiotic bacteria, regulating intestinal homeostasis. Lactoferrin supplementation in newborns has been promising, with multiple studies showing decreased NEC and late onset sepsis rates in newborns [99]. However, in a recent large randomized control trial of 2203 infants, lactoferrin supplementation did not decrease NEC or infection rates [77]. This suggests that the etiology of NEC is multifactorial and that human milk components in their collective teamwork, rather than the individual roles, protect against NEC.

Lactadherin, also known as milk fat globule-epidermal growth factor 8, is a glycoprotein found in human milk that prevents inflammation by enhancing phagocytosis of apoptotic cells. It specifically stimulates a signaling cascade that blocks NF-κB via the TLR4 blockade, resulting in decreased inflammation [78,79]. It is also noted to promote healing during intestinal inflammation. It was shown that lactadherin administration restored enterocyte migration in septic mice, suggesting the potential benefit of lactadherin in the treatment of intestinal injuries [78].

Lysozyme is an enzyme that has primarily antibacterial effects. It degrades the outer wall of gram-positive bacteria by hydrolyzing beta 1,4 bonds from the residues of N-acetylmuramic acid and N-acetylglucosamine. It also has been reported to have some antiviral activity [80]. In conjunction with lactoferrin, lysozyme can also kill gram negative bacteria in vitro. Lactoferrin binds to lipopolysaccharide in the outer bacterial membrane, removing it and allowing lysozyme to access and degrade the internal proteoglycan matrix of the membrane [18]. These proteins, through their direct effects on pathogens, help to prevent excessive inflammation at the intestinal surface.

## 5. Metabolic Factors

### 5.1. Adipokines

Adipokines are a group of mediators primarily released by adipocytes that regulate metabolic functions within adipose tissue, liver, brain and muscle, but are also present in breast milk. Furthermore, adipokines have been recently shown to attenuate intestinal inflammation by immunoregulatory mechanisms. For example, adiponectin is an adipokine available in large quantities in human milk and crosses the intestinal barrier. It has been shown to actively regulate insulin sensitivity, as well as suppressing mature macrophage function, thereby decreasing the inflammatory response. It is available in large quantities in human milk and crosses the intestinal barrier [52,81]. Interestingly, adiponectin-deficient mice exhibited more severe colitis, decreased intestinal epithelial proliferation, increased apoptosis and cellular stress when induced with dextran sulfate sodium (DSS). This colitis was reversed in vitro when adiponectin was present [100]. However, in vivo models have suggested conflicting results and require further study.

Leptin, another adipokine, is also present in breast milk and has been implicated in infant metabolism and weight regulation. It also has immunoregulatory functions, including T cell stimulation. Interestingly, leptin is upregulated in the mesenteric fat of Crohn's disease patients and influences the polarization of tissue macrophages towards an anti-inflammatory phenotype [81–83]. Leptin-deficient mice were also protected from DSS-induced colitis and leptin administration reversed disease susceptibility [84]. In addition to metabolic functions, adipokines have an immunomodulatory role that protects against intestinal inflammation.

### 5.2. Antioxidants and Anti-Proteases

Antioxidants scavenge free radicals, or reactive oxygen species, that are produced during the normal metabolic activity of cells. Free radicals damage cells by lipid peroxidation and alteration of protein or nucleic acid structures. Antioxidants in breast milk include α-tocepherol, β-carotene, cysteine, ascorbic acid, catalase and glutathione peroxidase [60].

Inflammatory cells produce proteases, which allow them to enter the injured tissue area. Human milk contains anti-proteases, including alpha-1-antitrypsin, alpha-1-antichymotrypsin, and elastase inhibitor, which limit the ability for pathogens to enter the body, thereby limiting inflammation locally [60].

*5.3. Dietary Fatty Acids*

Fatty acid concentrations in breast milk vary considerably over the course of lactation and are likely affected by maternal diet intake. Certain structures of fatty acids have been known to alter the host inflammatory response, particularly those following infection [13]. There are three main types of fatty acids: saturated, monounsaturated and polyunsaturated, which differ according to the number of double bonds in the acyl chain structure. Omega-6 and omega-3 polyunsaturated fatty acids (PUFAs) are the two essential fatty acids in animal cells and comprise 12% to 26% and 0.8% to 3.6% of fatty acids in mature human milk, respectively [85]. Breast milk contains a high proportion of omega-3 PUFAs, which have been shown to decrease production of inflammatory cytokines. Specifically, omega-3 PUFAs decrease the activity of NF-κB, a transcription factor that induces a range of pro-inflammatory genes, including COX-2, intercellular adhesion molecule-1, vascular cell adhesion molecule-1, E-selectin, TNF-α, IL-1B, inducible nitric oxide synthase, and acute phase protein. Omega-3 PUFA binding to the nuclear receptor, peroxisome proliferator-activated receptor, PPAR-γ, has been shown to be involved in regulating immune and inflammatory responses by inhibiting the induction of inflammatory genes by LPS, IL-1B and IFN-γ [86,87]. Omega-3 PUFAs increase anti-inflammatory microbes, such as *Lactobacillus* and *Bifidobacterium* species [13,88]. They change membrane phospholipid composition by increasing arachidonic acid, an omega-6 PUFA, subsequently decreasing the systemic inflammatory response syndrome. Omega-3 PUFAS also inhibit migration of leukocytes to site of infection by lowering expression of intracellular adhesion molecule 1 on monocytes and decreasing chemotaxis in neutrophils and monocytes [13,89,90]. In addition, specialized pro-resolving mediators (SPMs), derived from omega-3 PUFAs, specifically resolve inflammation by stopping polymorphonuclear cell migration and protect against chronic inflammatory conditions, including colitis, neuroinflammation and arthritis [101].

Diets rich in omega-6 PUFAS have been shown to be associated with *Enterobacteriaceae* blooms, which have in turn been associated with intestinal inflammatory responses, oxidative stress and intestinal barrier dysfunction. Arachidonic acid, the most well-known omega-6 PUFA, is the origin for inflammatory mediators, such as prostaglandins, leukotrienes and thromboxanes. Similarly, diets of saturated fat have been shown to increase activation of Toll-like receptors which have been linked to increased inflammatory response and intestinal injury [13]. Supplementation of a combination of omega-3 and omega-6 PUFAs decreased the incidence of NEC and intestinal inflammation via decreased platelet activating factor (PAF)-induced TLR4 activation in mice [102,103].

## 6. Conclusions

Although intestinal inflammation has a vital role in the neonatal immune response, excessive inflammation may lead to decreased gastrointestinal function and injury. The most prime example is NEC, which continues to be the most devastating gastrointestinal illness and a major cause of morbidity and mortality in the newborn population. Human milk is the ideal form of nutrition and its use has been associated with decreased incidences of NEC. As outlined in this review, human milk provides a variety of protective factors that each have a role in attenuating inflammation in the intestine (Figure 1). Specific commensal bacteria, such as *Bifidobacterium* and *Lactobacillus*, directly decrease inflammatory responses in the intestine by inhibiting activation of the pro-inflammatory NF-κB signaling pathway. HMOs promote the proliferation of inflammation, regulating commensal bacteria, and act as decoy receptors for otherwise threatening pathogens. Immunoregulatory cytokines prevent the activation of pro-inflammatory signaling pathways. Antimicrobial factors, such as lactoferrin, lactadherin and lysozyme, eliminate pathogens directly. Metabolic factors, like omega-3 PUFAs, have a multifunctional role, decreasing pro-inflammatory cytokine production and signaling, while promoting the proliferation of anti-inflammatory commensals.

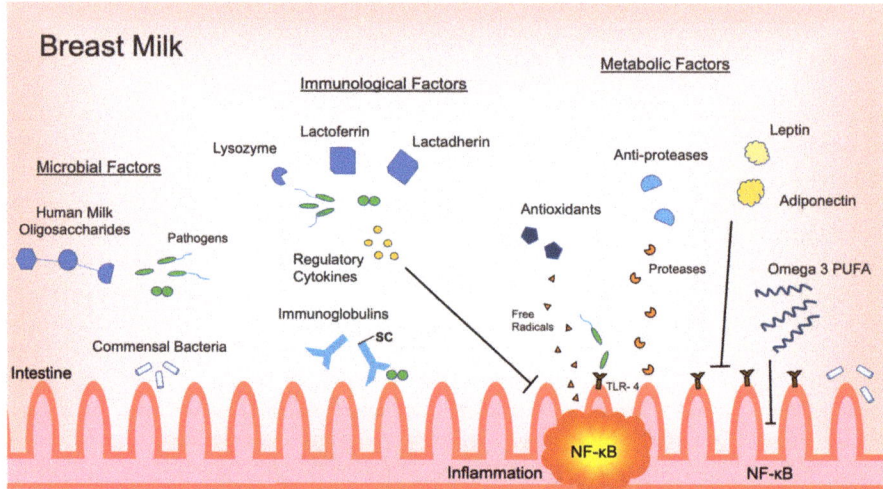

**Figure 1.** Summary of microbiologic, immunological and metabolic factors in breast milk with effects on regulating intestinal inflammation. Abbreviations: secretory component (SC); Toll-like receptor 4 (TLR4); nuclear factor kappa B (NF-κB); polyunsaturated fatty acid (PUFA).

Though each factor has a specific role in decreasing intestinal inflammation, the interaction among the intestinal microbiota, human milk oligosaccharides, immunological factors and metabolic components together foster optimal intestinal biology and a healthy functioning gastrointestinal tract, free of overt inflammation and infection. For breast milk-fed infants, additional inflammatory regulation is not only protective in the preterm period, but also likely has implications in decreasing risk of acquiring long-term chronic inflammatory illnesses. Though the connection between human milk's attenuation of intestinal inflammation and the development of these chronic illnesses in adulthood is not yet clear, emerging evidence suggests that providing human milk is crucial to optimizing both short-term and long-term health outcomes for newborns.

**Author Contributions:** J.D.T. and K.E.G. conceived the subject of the manuscript. J.D.T. contributed to the literature review and writing of the original draft. J.D.T. and K.E.G. reviewed and edited the final manuscript. All authors have read and agreed to the published version of the manuscript.

**Funding:** This research received no external funding.

**Acknowledgments:** K.E.G. is supported by R21NR017256 from the National Institutes of Health.

**Conflicts of Interest:** The authors have no conflicts of interest in the writing of this manuscript.

## References

1. Eldelman, A.I.; Schandler, R.J. Breastfeeding and the use of human milk. *Pediatrics* **2012**, *129*, e827–e841. [CrossRef]
2. Underwood, M.A. Human milk for the premature infant. *Pediatr. Clin. North Am.* **2013**, *60*, 189–207. [CrossRef] [PubMed]
3. Schanler, R.J.; Shulman, R.J.; Lau, C. Feeding strategies for premature infants: beneficial outcomes of feeding fortified human milk versus preterm formula. *Pediatrics* **1999**, *103*, 1150–1157. [CrossRef] [PubMed]
4. Cortez, J.; Makker, K.; Kraemer, D.F.; Neu, J.; Sharma, R.; Hudak, M.L. Maternal milk feedings reduce sepsis, necrotizing enterocolitis and improve outcomes of premature infants. *J. Perinatol.* **2018**, *38*, 71–74. [CrossRef] [PubMed]
5. Sisk, P.M.; A Lovelady, C.; Dillard, R.G.; Gruber, K.; O'Shea, T.M. Early human milk feeding is associated with a lower risk of necrotizing enterocolitis in very low birth weight infants. *J. Perinatol.* **2007**, *27*, 428–433. [CrossRef]

6. Meinzen-Derr, J.; Poindexter, B.; Wrage, L.; Morrow, A.L.; Stoll, B.; Donovan, E.F. Role of human milk in extremely low birth weight infants' risk of necrotizing enterocolitis or death. *J. Perinatol.* **2009**, *29*, 57–62. [CrossRef]
7. Hermansson, H.; Kumar, H.; Collado, M.C.; Salminen, S.; Isolauri, E.; Rautava, S. Breast Milk Microbiota Is Shaped by Mode of Delivery and Intrapartum Antibiotic Exposure. *Front. Nutr.* **2019**, *6*, 4. [CrossRef]
8. Pannaraj, P.S.; Li, F.; Cerini, C.; Bender, J.M.; Yang, S.; Rollie, A.; Adisetiyo, H.; Zabih, S.; Lincez, P.J.; Bittinger, K.; et al. Association Between Breast Milk Bacterial Communities and Establishment and Development of the Infant Gut Microbiome. *JAMA Pediatr.* **2017**, *171*, 647–654. [CrossRef]
9. Arrieta, M.-C.; Stiemsma, L.T.; Dimitriu, P.A.; Thorson, L.; Russell, S.; Yurist-Doutsch, S.; Kuzeljevic, B.; Gold, M.J.; Britton, H.; Lefebvre, D.L.; et al. Early infancy microbial and metabolic alterations affect risk of childhood asthma. *Sci. Transl. Med.* **2015**, *7*, 307ra152. [CrossRef]
10. Turnbaugh, P.J.; Hamady, M.; Yatsunenko, T.; Cantarel, B.L.; Duncan, A.; Ley, R.E.; Sogin, M.L.; Jones, W.J.; Roe, B.A.; Affourtit, J.P.; et al. A core gut microbiome in obese and lean twins. *Nature.* **2009**, *457*, 480–484. [CrossRef]
11. Fujimura, K.E.; Sitarik, A.R.; Havstad, S.; Lin, D.L.; LeVan, S.; Fadrosh, D.; Panzer, A.R.; LaMere, B.; Rackaityte, E.; Lukacs, N.W.; et al. Neonatal gut microbiota associates with childhood multisensitized atopy and T cell differentiation. *Nat. Med.* **2016**, *22*, 1187–1191. [CrossRef] [PubMed]
12. Lordan, R.; Zabetakis, I. Invited review: The anti-inflammatory properties of dairy lipids. *J. Dairy Sci.* **2017**, *100*, 4197–4212. [CrossRef] [PubMed]
13. Quin, C.; Gibson, D. Dietary Fatty Acids and Host–Microbial Crosstalk in Neonatal Enteric Infection. *Nutr.* **2019**, *11*, 2064. [CrossRef] [PubMed]
14. Serhan, C.N.; Levy, B.D. Resolvins in inflammation: Emergence of the pro-resolving superfamily of mediators. *J. Clin. Investig.* **2018**, *128*, 2657–2669. [CrossRef] [PubMed]
15. Kuban, K.C.; O'Shea, T.M.; Allred, E.N.; Fichorova, R.N.; Heeren, T.; Paneth, N.; Hirtz, D.; Dammann, O.; Leviton, A.; ELGAN Study Investigators. The breadth and type of systemic inflammation and the risk of adverse neurological outcomes in extremely low gestation newborns. *Pediatr. Neurol.* **2015**, *52*, 42–48. [CrossRef]
16. McElroy, S.J.; Frey, M.R.; Torres, B.A.; Maheshwari, A. Innate and Mucosal Immunity in the Developing Gastrointestinal Tract. In *Avery's Disease of the Newborn*, 10th ed.; Elsevier: Philadelphia, PA, USA, 2017; pp. 1054–1067.
17. McElroy, S.J.; Weitkamp, J.-H. Innate Immunity in the Small Intestine of the Preterm Infant. *NeoReviews* **2011**, *12*, e517–e526. [CrossRef]
18. Palmeira, P.; Carneiro-Sampaio, M. Immunology of breast milk. *Revista da Associação Médica Brasileira* **2016**, *62*, 584–593. [CrossRef]
19. Neu, J.; Walker, W.A. Necrotizing Enterocolitis. *N. Engl. J. Med.* **2011**, *364*, 255–264. [CrossRef]
20. Hackam, D.J.; Good, M.; Sodhi, C.P.; Sodhi, C.P. Mechanisms of gut barrier failure in the pathogenesis of necrotizing enterocolitis: Toll-like receptors throw the switch. *Semin. Pediatr. Surg.* **2013**, *22*, 76–82. [CrossRef]
21. Maheshwari, A.; Kelly, D.R.; Nicola, T.; Ambalavanan, N.; Jain, S.K.; Murphy–Ullrich, J.; Athar, M.; Shimamura, M.; Bhandari, V.; Aprahamian, C.; et al. TGF-β2 Suppresses Macrophage Cytokine Production and Mucosal Inflammatory Responses in the Developing Intestine. *Gastroenterology* **2011**, *140*, 242–253. [CrossRef]
22. Patel, R.M.; Kandefer, S.; Walsh, M.C.; Bell, E.F.; Carlo, W.A.; Laptook, A.R.; Sanchez, P.J.; Shankaran, S.; Van Meurs, K.P.; Ball, M.B.; et al. Causes and timing of death in extremely premature infants from 2000 through 2011. *New Engl. J. Med.* **2015**, *372*, 331–340. [CrossRef] [PubMed]
23. Lucas, A.; Cole, T. Breast milk and neonatal necrotising enterocolitis. *Lancet* **1990**, *336*, 1519–1523. [CrossRef]
24. Furman, L.; Taylor, G.; Minich, N.; Hack, M. The effect of maternal milk on neonatal morbidity of very low-birth-weight infants. *Arch. Pediatr. Adolesc. Med.* **2003**, *157*, 66–71. [CrossRef] [PubMed]
25. Pammi, M.; Cope, J.; Tarr, P.I.; Warner, B.B.; Morrow, A.L.; Mai, V.; Gregory, K.E.; Kroll, J.S.; McMurtry, V.; Ferris, M.J.; et al. Intestinal dysbiosis in preterm infants preceding necrotizing enterocolitis: a systematic review and meta-analysis. *Microbiome* **2017**, *5*, 31. [CrossRef]
26. Underwood, M.A. Probiotics and the prevention of necrotizing enterocolitis. *J. Pediatr. Surg.* **2019**, *54*, 405–412. [CrossRef]

27. Dunne-Castagna, V.P.; Taft, D.H. Mother's Touch: Milk IgA and Protection from Necrotizing Enterocolitis. *Cell Host Microbe* **2019**, *26*, 147–148. [CrossRef]
28. Bode, L. Human Milk Oligosaccharides in the Prevention of Necrotizing Enterocolitis: A Journey From in vitro and in vivo Models to Mother-Infant Cohort Studies. *Front. Pediatr.* **2018**, *6*, 385. [CrossRef]
29. Gopalakrishna, K.P.; Macadangdang, B.R.; Rogers, M.B.; Tometich, J.T.; Firek, B.A.; Baker, R.; Ji, J.; Burr, A.H.P.; Ma, C.; Good, M.; et al. Maternal IgA protects against the development of necrotizing enterocolitis in preterm infants. *Nat. Med.* **2019**, *25*, 1110–1115. [CrossRef]
30. Hooper, L.V.; Littman, D.R.; MacPherson, A.J. Interactions Between the Microbiota and the Immune System. *Sci.* **2012**, *336*, 1268–1273. [CrossRef]
31. Milani, C.; Duranti, S.; Bottacini, F.; Casey, E.; Turroni, F.; Mahony, J.; Belzer, C.; Palacio, S.D.; Montes, S.A.; Mancabelli, L.; et al. The First Microbial Colonizers of the Human Gut: Composition, Activities, and Health Implications of the Infant Gut Microbiota. *Microbiol. Mol. Boil. Rev.* **2017**, *81*, e00036-17. [CrossRef]
32. Newburg, D.; He, Y. Neonatal Gut Microbiota and Human Milk Glycans Cooperate to Attenuate Infection and Inflammation. *Clin. Obstet. Gynecol.* **2015**, *58*, 814–826. [CrossRef] [PubMed]
33. Mshvildadze, M.; Neu, J.; Shuster, J.; Theriaque, U.; Li, N.; Mai, V. Intestinal Microbial Ecology in Premature Infants Assessed with Non–Culture-Based Techniques. *J. Pediatr.* **2010**, *156*, 20–25. [CrossRef] [PubMed]
34. Hunt, K.M.; Foster, J.A.; Forney, L.J.; Schütte, U.M.E.; Beck, D.L.; Abdo, Z.; Fox, L.K.; Williams, J.E.; McGuire, M.; McGuire, M.A. Characterization of the Diversity and Temporal Stability of Bacterial Communities in Human Milk. *PLoS ONE* **2011**, *6*, e21313. [CrossRef] [PubMed]
35. Fernández, L.; Langa, S.; Martin, V.; Maldonado, A.; Jiménez, E.; Martín, R.; Rodríguez, J. The human milk microbiota: Origin and potential roles in health and disease. *Pharmacol. Res.* **2013**, *69*, 1–10. [CrossRef] [PubMed]
36. Fitzstevens, J.L.; Smith, K.C.; Hagadorn, J.I.; Caimano, M.J.; Matson, A.P.; Brownell, E.A. Systematic review of the human milk microbiota. *Nutr. Clin. Pract.* **2017**, *32*, 354–364. [CrossRef]
37. Schwab, C.; Voney, E.; Garcia, A.R.; Vischer, M.; Lacroix, C. Characterization of the Cultivable Microbiota in Fresh and Stored Mature Human Breast Milk. *Front. Microbiol.* **2019**, *10*, 2666. [CrossRef]
38. Urbaniak, C.; Angelini, M.; Gloor, G.B.; Reid, G. Human milk microbiota profiles in relation to birthing method, gestation and infant gender. *Microbiome* **2016**, *4*, 1. [CrossRef]
39. Gallego, C.G.; Garcia-Mantrana, I.; Salminen, S.; Collado, M.C. The human milk microbiome and factors influencing its composition and activity. *Semin. Fetal Neonatal Med.* **2016**, *21*, 400–405. [CrossRef]
40. Cabrera-Rubio, R.; Collado, M.C.; Laitinen, K.; Salminen, S.; Isolauri, E.; Mira, A.; Miras, A.; Jackson, R.N.; Goldstone, A.P.; Olbers, T.; et al. The human milk microbiome changes over lactation and is shaped by maternal weight and mode of delivery. *Am. J. Clin. Nutr.* **2012**, *96*, 544–551. [CrossRef]
41. Smith, P.M.; Howitt, M.R.; Panikov, N.; Michaud, M.; Gallini, C.A.; Bohlooly-Y, M.; Glickman, J.N.; Garrett, W.S. The Microbial Metabolites, Short-Chain Fatty Acids, Regulate Colonic Treg Cell Homeostasis. *Sci.* **2013**, *341*, 569–573. [CrossRef]
42. Fukuda, S.; Toh, H.; Hase, K.; Oshima, K.; Nakanishi, Y.; Yoshimura, K.; Tobe, T.; Clarke, J.; Topping, D.L.; Suzuki, T.; et al. Bifidobacteria can protect from enteropathogenic infection through production of acetate. *Nat.* **2011**, *469*, 543–547. [CrossRef] [PubMed]
43. Embleton, N.; Berrington, J.E.; Dorling, J.; Ewer, A.K.; Juszczak, E.; Kirby, J.A.; Lamb, C.A.; Lanyon, C.; McGuire, W.; Probert, C.S.; et al. Mechanisms Affecting the gut of preterm infants in enteral feeding trials. *Front. Nutr.* **2017**, *4*, 14. [CrossRef] [PubMed]
44. Underwood, M.A.; Arriola, J.; Gerber, C.W.; Kaveti, A.; Kalanetra, K.M.; Kananurak, A.; Bevins, C.L.; Mills, D.A.; Dvořák, B. Bifidobacterium longum subsp. infantis in experimental necrotizing enterocolitis: alterations in inflammation, innate immune response, and the microbiota. *Pediatr. Res.* **2014**, *76*, 326–333. [CrossRef] [PubMed]
45. Li, N.; Pang, B.; Liu, G.; Zhao, X.; Xu, X.; Jiang, C.; Yang, B.; Liu, Y.; Li, N. Lactobacillus rhamnosus from human breast milk shows therapeutic function against foodborne infection by multi-drug resistant Escherichia coli in mice. *Food Funct.* **2020**, *11*, 435–447. [CrossRef]
46. Guo, S.; Guo, Y.; Ergun, A.; Lü, L.; Walker, W.A.; Ganguli, K. Secreted Metabolites of Bifidobacterium infantis and Lactobacillus acidophilus Protect Immature Human Enterocytes from IL-1β-Induced Inflammation: A Transcription Profiling Analysis. *PLoS ONE* **2015**, *10*, e0124549. [CrossRef]
47. Pasparakis, M. Role of NF-κB in epithelial biology. *Immunol. Rev.* **2012**, *246*, 346–358. [CrossRef]

48. Ganguli, K.; Meng, D.; Rautava, S.; Lu, L.; Walker, W.A.; Nanthakumar, N. Probiotics prevent necrotizing enterocolitis by modulating enterocyte genes that regulate innate immune-mediated inflammation. *Am. J. Physiol. Gastrointest. Liver Physiol.* **2013**, *304*, G132–G141. [CrossRef]
49. Plaza-Díaz, J.; Fontana, L.; Gil, A. Human Milk Oligosaccharides and Immune System Development. *Nutr.* **2018**, *10*, 1038. [CrossRef]
50. Newburg, D.S.; Ruiz-Palacios, G.M.; Morrow, A.L. HUMAN MILK GLYCANS PROTECT INFANTS AGAINST ENTERIC PATHOGENS. *Annu. Rev. Nutr.* **2005**, *25*, 37–58. [CrossRef]
51. Morrow, A.L.; Ruiz-Palacios, G.M.; Jiang, X.; Newburg, D.S. Human-Milk Glycans That Inhibit Pathogen Binding Protect Breast-feeding Infants against Infectious Diarrhea. *J. Nutr.* **2005**, *135*, 1304–1307. [CrossRef]
52. Ballard, O.; Morrow, A.L. Human milk composition: nutrients and bioactive factors. *Pediatr. Clin. North Am.* **2013**, *60*, 49–74. [CrossRef] [PubMed]
53. Gabrielli, O.; Zampini, L.; Galeazzi, T.; Padella, L.; Santoro, L.; Peila, C.; Giuliani, F.; Bertino, E.; Fabris, C.; Coppa, G.V. Preterm milk oligosaccharides during the first month of lactation. *Pediatrics* **2011**, *128*, e1520–e1531. [CrossRef] [PubMed]
54. Rogier, E.; Frantz, A.L.; Bruno, M.E.C.; Kaetzel, C. Secretory IgA is concentrated in the outer layer of colonic mucus along with gut bacteria. *Pathogens* **2014**, *3*, 390–403. [CrossRef] [PubMed]
55. Cianga, P.; Medesan, C.; Richardson, J.A.; Ghetie, V.; Ward, E.S. Identification and function of neonatal Fc receptor in mammary gland of lactating mice. *Eur. J. Immunol.* **1999**, *29*, 2515–2523. [CrossRef]
56. Gross, S.J.; Buckley, R.H.; Wakil, S.S.; McAllister, D.C.; David, R.J.; Faix, R.G. Elevated IgA concentration in milk produced by mothers delivered of preterm infants. *J. Pediatr.* **1981**, *99*, 389–393. [CrossRef]
57. Mathur, N.B.; Dwarkadas, A.M.; Sharma, V.K.; Saha, K.; Jain, N. Anti-Infective Factors in Preterm Human Colostrum. *Acta Paediatr.* **1990**, *79*, 1039–1044. [CrossRef]
58. Garofalo, R.; Chheda, S.; Mei, F.; Palkowetz, K.H.; E Rudloff, H.; Schmalstieg, F.C.; Rassin, D.K.; Goldman, A.S. Interleukin-10 in Human Milk. *Pediatr. Res.* **1995**, *37*, 444–449. [CrossRef]
59. Sydora, B.C.; Tavernini, M.M.; Wessler, A.; Jewell, L.D.; Fedorak, R. Lack of interleukin-10 leads to intestinal inflammation, independent of the time at which luminal microbial colonization occurs. *Inflamm. Bowel Dis.* **2003**, *9*, 87–97. [CrossRef]
60. Lepage, P.; Van De Perre, P. The Immune System of Breast Milk: Antimicrobial and Anti-inflammatory Properties. *Adv. Exp. Med. Biol.* **2012**, *743*, 121–137.
61. Emami, C.N.; Chokshi, N.; Wang, J.; Hunter, C.J.; Guner, Y.; Goth, K.; Wang, L.; Grishin, A.; Ford, H.R. Role of interleukin-10 in the pathogenesis of necrotizing enterocolitis. *Am. J. Surg.* **2012**, *203*, 428–435. [CrossRef]
62. Fell, J.M.; Paintin, M.; Arnaud-Battandier, F.; Beattie, R.M.; Hollis, A.; Kitching, P.; Donnet-Hughes, A.; MacDonald, T.T.; Walker-Smith, J.A. Mucosal healing and a fall in mucosal pro-inflammatory cytokine mRNA induced by a specific oral polymeric diet in paediatric Crohn's disease. *Ailm. Pharmacol. Ther.* **2000**, *14*, 281–289. [CrossRef] [PubMed]
63. Dawod, B.; Marshall, J. Cytokines and soluble receptors in breast milk as enhancers of oral tolerance development. *Front. Immunol.* **2019**, *10*, 16. [CrossRef] [PubMed]
64. Maheshwari, A.; for the Eunice Kennedy Shriver National Institute of Child Health and Human Development Neonatal Research Network; Schelonka, R.L.; Dimmitt, R.A.; Carlo, W.A.; Munoz-Hernandez, B.; Das, A.; McDonald, S.A.; Thorsen, P.; Skogstrand, K.; et al. Cytokines associated with necrotizing enterocolitis in extremely-low-birth-weight infants. *Pediatr. Res.* **2014**, *76*, 100–108. [CrossRef] [PubMed]
65. Castellote, C.; Casillas, R.; Ramírez-Santana, C.; Pérez-Cano, F.J.; Castell, M.; Moretones, M.G.; López-Sabater, M.C.; Franch, À. Premature Delivery Influences the Immunological Composition of Colostrum and Transitional and Mature Human Milk. *J. Nutr.* **2011**, *141*, 1181–1187. [CrossRef]
66. Liew, F.Y.; Xu, D.; Brint, E.; O'Neill, L.A. Negative regulation of Toll-like receptor-mediated immune responses. *Nat. Rev. Immunol.* **2005**, *5*, 446–458. [CrossRef]
67. Henrick, B.M.; Nag, K.; Yao, X.-D.; Drannik, A.G.; Aldrovandi, G.M.; Rosenthal, K.L. Milk Matters: Soluble Toll-Like Receptor 2 (sTLR2) in Breast Milk Significantly Inhibits HIV-1 Infection and Inflammation. *PLoS ONE* **2012**, *7*, e40138. [CrossRef]
68. Coursodon, C.F.; Dvořák, B. Epidermal growth factor and necrotizing enterocolitis. *Curr. Opin. Pediatr.* **2012**, *24*, 160–164. [CrossRef]

69. Halpern, M.D.; Holubec, H.; Dominguez, J.A.; Williams, C.S.; Meza, Y.G.; McWilliam, D.L.; Payne, C.M.; McCuskey, R.S.; Besselsen, D.G.; Dvorak, B. Up-regulation of IL-18 and IL-12 in the ileum of neonatal rats with necrotizing enterocolitis. *Pediatr. Res.* **2002**, *51*, 733–739. [CrossRef]
70. Dvorak, B. Milk Epidermal Growth Factor and Gut Protection. *J. Pediatr.* **2010**, *156*, S31–S35. [CrossRef]
71. Chatterton, D.E.; Nguyen, D.N.; Bering, S.B.; Sangild, P.T. Anti-inflammatory mechanisms of bioactive milk proteins in the intestine of newborns. *Int. J. Biochem. Cell. Biol.* **2013**, *45*, 1730–1747. [CrossRef]
72. Rocourt, R.V.; Mehta, V.B.; Besner, G.E. Heparin-Binding EGF-like Growth Factor Decreases Inflammatory Cytokine Expression After Intestinal Ischemia/Reperfusion Injury. *J. Surg. Res.* **2007**, *139*, 269–273. [CrossRef] [PubMed]
73. Ozgurtas, T.; Aydin, I.; Turan, O.; Koç, E.; Hirfanoglu, I.M.; Acikel, C.H.; Akyol, M.; Erbil, M.K. Vascular endothelial growth factor, basic fibroblast growth factor, insulin-like growth factor-I and platelet-derived growth factor levels in human milk of mothers with term and preterm neonates. *Cytokine* **2010**, *50*, 192–194. [CrossRef]
74. Karatepe, H.Ö.; Kilincaslan, H.; Berber, M.; Ozen, A.; Saricoban, H.E.; Ustek, D.; Kemik, A.S.; Adas, M.; Bakar, F. The effect of vascular endothelial growth factor overexpression in experimental necrotizing enterocolitis. *Pediatr. Surg. Int.* **2014**, *30*, 327–332. [CrossRef] [PubMed]
75. Buescher, E.S. Anti-inflammatory characteristics of human milk: how, where, why. *Single Mol. Single Cell Seq.* **2001**, *501*, 207–222.
76. Albenzio, M.; Santillo, A.; Stolfi, I.; Manzoni, P.; Iliceto, A.; Rinaldi, M.; Magaldi, R. Lactoferrin Levels in Human Milk after Preterm and Term Delivery. *Am. J. Perinatol.* **2016**, *33*, 1085–1089. [CrossRef] [PubMed]
77. Griffiths, J.; Jenkins, P.; Vargova, M.; Bowler, U.; Juszczak, E.; King, A.; Linsell, L.; Murray, D.; Partlett, C.; Patel, M.; et al. Enteral lactoferrin supplementation for very preterm infants: a randomised placebo-controlled trial. *Lancet* **2019**, *393*, 423–433. [CrossRef]
78. Bu, H.-F.; Zuo, X.-L.; Wang, X.; Ensslin, M.A.; Koti, V.; Hsueh, W.; Raymond, A.S.; Shur, B.D.; Tan, X.-D. Milk fat globule–EGF factor 8/lactadherin plays a crucial role in maintenance and repair of murine intestinal epithelium. *J. Clin. Investig.* **2007**, *117*, 3673–3683. [CrossRef]
79. He, Y.; Lawlor, N.; Newburg, D. Human Milk Components Modulate Toll-Like Receptor-Mediated Inflammation. *Adv. Nutr.* **2016**, *7*, 102–111. [CrossRef]
80. Lee-Huang, S.; Huang, P.L.; Sun, Y.; Huang, P.L.; Kung, H.F.; Blithe, D.L.; Chen, H.C. Lysozyme and RNases as anti-HIV components in beta-core preparations of human chorionic gonadotropin. *Proc. Natl. Acad. Sci. USA* **1999**, *96*, 2678–2681. [CrossRef]
81. Weidinger, C.; Ziegler, J.F.; Letizia, M.; Schmidt, F.; Siegmund, B. Adipokines and their role in intestinal inflammation. *Front. Immunol.* **2018**, *9*, 1974. [CrossRef]
82. Zulian, A.; Cancello, R.; Micheletto, G.; Gentilini, D.; Gilardini, L.; Danelli, P.; Invitti, C. Visceral adipocytes: old actors in obesity and new protagonists in Crohn's disease? *Gut* **2012**, *61*, 86–94. [CrossRef] [PubMed]
83. Kredel, L.I.; Batra, A.; Stroh, T.; Kühl, A.A.; Zeitz, M.; Erben, U.; Siegmund, B. Adipokines from local fat cells shape the macrophage compartment of the creeping fat in Crohn's disease. *Gut.* **2013**, *62*, 852–862. [CrossRef] [PubMed]
84. Siegmund, B.; Lehr, H.A.; Fantuzzi, G. Leptin: A pivotal mediator of intestinal inflammation in mice. *Gastroenterol.* **2002**, *122*, 2011–2025. [CrossRef] [PubMed]
85. Delplanque, B.; Gibson, R.; Koletzko, B.; Lapillonne, A.; Strandvik, B. Lipid Quality in Infant Nutrition: Current Knowledge and Future Opportunities. *J. Pediatr. Gastroenterol. Nutr.* **2015**, *61*, 8–17. [CrossRef] [PubMed]
86. Valledor, A.F.; Ricote, M. Nuclear receptor signaling in macrophages. *Biochem. Pharmacol.* **2004**, *67*, 201–212. [CrossRef] [PubMed]
87. Gottrand, F. Long-Chain Polyunsaturated Fatty Acids Influence the Immune System of Infants. *J. Nutr.* **2008**, *138*, 1807S–1812S. [CrossRef]
88. Ghosh, S.; DeCoffe, D.; Brown, K.; Rajendiran, E.; Estaki, M.; Dai, C.; Yip, A.; Gibson, D. Fish Oil Attenuates Omega-6 Polyunsaturated Fatty Acid-Induced Dysbiosis and Infectious Colitis but Impairs LPS Dephosphorylation Activity Causing Sepsis. *PLoS ONE* **2013**, *8*, e55468. [CrossRef]
89. Hughes, D.; Pinder, A.C.; Piper, Z.; Johnson, I.; Lund, E.K. Fish oil supplementation inhibits the expression of major histocompatibility complex class II molecules and adhesion molecules on human monocytes. *Am. J. Clin. Nutr.* **1996**, *63*, 267–272. [CrossRef]

90. Schmidt, E.; Pedersen, J.; Ekelund, S.; Grunnet, N.; Jersild, C.; Dyerberg, J. Cod liver oil inhibits neutrophil and monocyte chemotaxis in healthy males. *Atherosclerosis* **1989**, *77*, 53–57. [CrossRef]
91. Bode, L. Human milk oligosaccharides: Every baby needs a sugar mama. *Glycobiology* **2012**, *22*, 1147–1162. [CrossRef]
92. Rogier, E.W.; Frantz, A.L.; Bruno, M.E.C.; Wedlund, L.; Cohen, N.A.; Stromberg, A.J.; Kaetzel, C.S. Secretory antibodies in breast milk promote long-term intestinal homeostasis by regulating the gut microbiota and host gene expression. *Proc. Natl. Acad. Sci. USA* **2014**, *111*, 3074–3079. [CrossRef] [PubMed]
93. Araújo, E.D.; Gonçalves, A.K.; Cornetta, M.D.C.; Cunha, H.; Cardoso, M.L.; Morais, S.S.; Giraldo, P.C. Evaluation of the secretory immunoglobulin A levels in the colostrum and milk of mothers of term and pre-term newborns. *Braz. J. Infect. Dis.* **2005**, *9*, 357–362. [CrossRef] [PubMed]
94. Ballabio, C.; Bertino, E.; Coscia, A.; Fabris, C.; Fuggetta, D.; Molfino, S.; Testa, T.; Sgarrella, M.; Sabatino, G.; Restani, P. Immunoglobulin-A Profile in Breast Milk from Mothers Delivering Full Term and Preterm Infants. *Int. J. Immunopathol. Pharmacol.* **2007**, *20*, 119–128. [CrossRef] [PubMed]
95. Goldman, A.S.; Goldblum, R.M.; Hanson, L.Å. Anti-Inflammatory Systems in Human Milk. *Adv. Exp. Med. Biol.* **1990**, *262*, 69–76. [PubMed]
96. Lewis, E.D.; Richard, C.; Larsen, B.; Field, C. The Importance of Human Milk for Immunity in Preterm Infants. *Clin. Perinatol.* **2017**, *44*, 23–47. [CrossRef] [PubMed]
97. Khaleva, E.; Gridneva, Z.; Geddes, D.T.; Oddy, W.H.; Colicino, S.; Blyuss, O.; Boyle, R.J.; Warner, J.O.; Munblit, D. Transforming growth factor beta in human milk and allergic outcomes in children: A systematic review. *Clin. Exp. Allergy* **2019**, *49*, 1201–1213. [CrossRef]
98. Ustundag, B. Levels of cytokines (IL-1beta, IL-2, IL-6, IL-8, TNF-alpha) and trace elements (Zn, Cu) in breast milk from mothers of preterm and term infants. *Mediat. Inflamm.* **2005**, *2005*, 331–336. [CrossRef]
99. Pammi, M.; Suresh, G. Enteral lactoferrin supplementation for prevention of sepsis and necrotizing enterocolitis in preterm infants. *Cochrane Database Syst. Rev.* **2017**, *2017*, CD007137. [CrossRef]
100. Obeid, S.; Wankell, M.; Charrez, B.; Sternberg, J.; Kreuter, R.; Esmaili, S.; Ramezani-Moghadam, M.; Devine, C.; Read, S.; Bhathal, P.; et al. Adiponectin confers protection from acute colitis and restricts a B cell immune response. *J. Boil. Chem.* **2017**, *292*, 6569–6582. [CrossRef]
101. Serhan, C.N.; Clish, C.B.; Brannon, J.; Colgan, S.P.; Chiang, N.; Gronert, K. Novel Functional Sets of Lipid-Derived Mediators with Antiinflammatory Actions Generated from Omega-3 Fatty Acids via Cyclooxygenase 2–Nonsteroidal Antiinflammatory Drugs and Transcellular Processing. *J. Exp. Med.* **2000**, *192*, 1197–1204. [CrossRef]
102. Caplan, M.S.; Russell, T.; Xiao, Y.; Amer, M.; Kaup, S.; Jilling, T. Effect of Polyunsaturated Fatty Acid (PUFA) Supplementation on Intestinal Inflammation and Necrotizing Enterocolitis (NEC) in a Neonatal Rat Model. *Pediatr. Res.* **2001**, *49*, 647–652. [CrossRef] [PubMed]
103. Lu, J.; Jilling, T.; Li, D.; Caplan, M.S. Polyunsaturated fatty acid supplementation alters proinflammatory gene expression and reduces the incidence of necrotizing enterocolitis in a neonatal rat model. *Pediatr. Res.* **2007**, *61*, 427–432. [CrossRef] [PubMed]

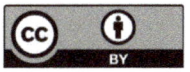

© 2020 by the authors. Licensee MDPI, Basel, Switzerland. This article is an open access article distributed under the terms and conditions of the Creative Commons Attribution (CC BY) license (http://creativecommons.org/licenses/by/4.0/).

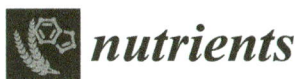 

*Review*

# Breast Milk Lipids and Fatty Acids in Regulating Neonatal Intestinal Development and Protecting against Intestinal Injury

**David Ramiro-Cortijo** [1,†], **Pratibha Singh** [1,†], **Yan Liu** [1], **Esli Medina-Morales** [1], **William Yakah** [2], **Steven D. Freedman** [1,3] **and Camilia R. Martin** [2,3,*]

1. Division of Gastroenterology, Beth Israel Deaconess Medical Center, Harvard Medical School, 330 Brookline Avenue, Boston, MA 02215, USA; dramiro@bidmc.harvard.edu (D.R.-C.); psingh6@bidmc.harvard.edu (P.S.); yliu19@seas.harvard.edu (Y.L.); jemedina@bidmc.harvard.edu (E.M.-M.); sfreedma@bidmc.harvard.edu (S.D.F.)
2. Department of Neonatology, Beth Israel Deaconess Medical Center, Harvard Medical School, 330 Brookline Avenue, Boston, MA 02215, USA; wyakah@bidmc.harvard.edu
3. Division of Translational Research, Beth Israel Deaconess Medical Center, Harvard Medical School, 330 Brookline Avenue, Boston, MA 02215, USA
* Correspondence: cmartin1@bidmc.harvard.edu
† These authors have equal contribution.

Received: 31 January 2020; Accepted: 16 February 2020; Published: 19 February 2020

**Abstract:** Human breast milk is the optimal source of nutrition for infant growth and development. Breast milk fats and their downstream derivatives of fatty acids and fatty acid-derived terminal mediators not only provide an energy source but also are important regulators of development, immune function, and metabolism. The composition of the lipids and fatty acids determines the nutritional and physicochemical properties of human milk fat. Essential fatty acids, including long-chain polyunsaturated fatty acids (LCPUFAs) and specialized pro-resolving mediators, are critical for growth, organogenesis, and regulation of inflammation. Combined data including in vitro, in vivo, and human cohort studies support the beneficial effects of human breast milk in intestinal development and in reducing the risk of intestinal injury. Human milk has been shown to reduce the occurrence of necrotizing enterocolitis (NEC), a common gastrointestinal disease in preterm infants. Preterm infants fed human breast milk are less likely to develop NEC compared to preterm infants receiving infant formula. Intestinal development and its physiological functions are highly adaptive to changes in nutritional status influencing the susceptibility towards intestinal injury in response to pathological challenges. In this review, we focus on lipids and fatty acids present in breast milk and their impact on neonatal gut development and the risk of disease.

**Keywords:** breast milk; milk fat globule; long chain polyunsaturated fatty acids; premature infants; necrotizing enterocolitis

## 1. Introduction

Human milk is a complex matrix of bioactive proteins, lipids, enzymes, hormones, and vitamins that collectively optimize infant development [1]. Understanding the lipid nutritional composition of breast milk provides guidance for defining adequate nutrient intake in critically ill infants, given that human breast milk fat provides almost 50% of energy intake for neonates up to 6 months of age [2]. Multiple lipid classes and compounds also found in human milk have been associated with neonatal health outcomes [3], such as adequate growth, neurocognitive development and function, regulation of inflammation and infection risk, and reduced risk of later metabolic and cardiovascular disease in adulthood. Exposure to these compounds during infancy varies, however, as it is now well understood that human milk composition is highly variable between individuals with some key determinant factors being maternal health and dietary patterns [4]. In this review, we will discuss (1) lipid and fatty acid content in breast milk, and (2) how these compounds contribute to gut development and gut health.

## 2. Lipids and Fatty Acid Composition in Human Breast Milk

### 2.1. Concentrations of Breast Milk Lipids and Fatty Acids

Breast milk fat content increases with time or "maturation". In mothers of full-term infants, colostrum fat content is 2.2 g/100 mL, increasing to 3.0 g/100 mL in transitional milk, and 3.4 g/100 mL in mature milk [5]. In contrast, mothers with preterm neonates have higher breast milk fat concentrations [6] with values of 2.6, 3.6, and 3.9 g/100 mL in colostrum, transitional, and mature milk, respectively [7]. Saturated fatty acid content in breast milk lipids represents 53.2% in colostrum, 62.1% in transitional milk, and 58.0% in mature milk [8,9]. Table 1 shows the relative contribution of principal saturated and monounsaturated fatty acids in breast milk. Palmitic acid (C16:0), a major saturated fatty acid, provides approximately 25% of all milk fatty acids [9]. The proportion of monounsaturated fatty acids is more stable than saturated fatty acids and make up about 45%–50% of breast milk during lactation [9]. Thirty-six percent of the monounsaturated fatty acids in breast milk is oleic acid (C18:1n-9) and provides an important function in reducing the melting point of triglycerides, thus providing the liquidity required for the formation, transport, and metabolism of the milk fat globule [10,11]. Long chain polyunsaturated fatty acids (LCPUFAs) represent about 15% of the total lipids in breast milk and have been extensively studied for their developmental, cardioprotective, anti-cancer, anti-inflammatory, and antioxidant biological functions [12,13].

**Table 1.** Fatty acid profile of breast milk across lactation stages.

|  | Term Infants | | | Preterm Infants | | |
| --- | --- | --- | --- | --- | --- | --- |
|  | Colostrum | Transitional | Mature | Colostrum | Transitional | Mature |
| *Saturated Fatty Acids* | | | | | | |
| Caprylic acid (C8:0) | 0.07–0.19 | 0.2–0.31 | 0.2–0.3 | 0.03–0.03 | 0.09–0.11 | 0.16–0.16 |
| Capric acid (C10:0) | 0.5–1.04 | 1.2–1.6 | 1.5–1.8 | 0.09–0.09 | 1.0–1.7 | 1.2–2.1 |
| Lauric acid (C12:0) | 2.8–3.5 | 5.4–6.6 | 5.7–6.5 | 3.2–4.6 | 5.7–7.5 | 5.7–8.1 |
| Myristic acid (C14:0) | 5.4–6.0 | 6.6–7.5 | 6.5–7.1 | 5.8–7.2 | 8.0–9.2 | 7.4–9.0 |
| Palmitic acid (C16:0) | 24.3–25.5 | 21.9–23.3 | 21.7–22.7 | 22.5–24.1 | 21.5–23.5 | 20.9–22.3 |
| Stearic acid (C18:0) | 6.2–6.6 | 6.1–6.7 | 6.3–6.6 | 5.8–6.5 | 6.0–6.9 | 6.2–7.1 |
| Arachidic acid (C20:0) | 0.19–0.25 | 0.20–0.32 | 0.20–0.26 | 0.16–0.18 | 0.15–0.15 | 0.20–0.30 |
| *Monounsaturated Fatty Acids* | | | | | | |
| Myristoleic acid (C14:1n-5) | 0.13–0.23 | 0.19–0.25 | 0.18–0.22 | 0.11–0.13 | 0.22–0.22 | 0.21–0.21 |
| Palmitoleic acid (C16:1n-7) | 1.9–2.2 | 2.0–2.4 | 2.2–2.4 | 1.7–1.8 | 2.1–2.5 | 2.0–2.5 |
| Oleic acid (C18:1n-9) | 34.7–35.9 | 31.2–33.2 | 32.2–33.6 | 30.6–33.7 | 30.5–34.3 | 31.7–36.7 |
| Vaccenic acid (C18:1n-7) | 2.6–2.8 | 1.9–2.0 | 1.7–2.1 | 2.3–2.4 | 2.5–2.6 | 2.1–2.2 |
| Erucic acid (C22:1n-9) | 0.20–0.24 | 0.14–0.28 | 0.10–0.12 | 0.16–0.16 | 0.10–0.14 | 0.08–0.05 |
| *n-3 Polyunsaturated fatty acids (n-3 LCPUFAs)* | | | | | | |
| α-Linolenic acid (C18:3n-3) | 0.74–0.90 | 0.84–1.06 | 0.91–1.03 | 0.69–1.09 | 0.70–1.02 | 0.85–1.13 |
| Eicosapentaenoic acid (C20:5n-3) | 0.08–0.12 | 0.11–0.17 | 0.08–0.10 | 0.06–0.10 | 0.10–0.16 | 0.08–0.16 |
| Clupanodonic acid (C22:5n-3) | 0.27–0.33 | 0.19–0.25 | 0.14–0.16 | 0.30–0.34 | 0.24–0.36 | 0.16–0.24 |
| Docosahexaenoic acid (C22:6n-3) | 0.47–0.55 | 0.40–0.52 | 0.28–0.34 | 0.43–0.71 | 0.47–0.67 | 0.31–0.49 |
| *n-6 Polyunsaturated fatty acids (n-6 LCPUFAs)* | | | | | | |
| Linoleic acid (C18:2n-6) | 13.5–15.3 | 13.4–14.8 | 14.3–15.7 | 13.7–16.3 | 11.4–13.6 | 12.3–14.4 |
| γ-Linolenic acid (C18:3n-6) | 0.07–0.11 | 0.10–0.18 | 0.14–0.20 | 0.07–0.07 | 0.09–0.13 | 0.11–0.21 |
| Eicosadienoic acid (C20:2n-6) | 0.82–0.96 | 0.53–0.63 | 0.35–0.41 | 0.89–0.95 | 0.28–0.30 | 0.24–0.24 |
| Dihomo-γ-Linolenic acid (C20:3n-6) | 0.56–0.64 | 0.46–0.52 | 0.39–0.43 | 0.69–0.81 | 0.47–0.55 | 0.40–0.50 |
| Arachidonic acid (C20:4n-6) | 0.73–0.81 | 0.61–0.69 | 0.45–0.51 | 0.68–0.90 | 0.54–0.68 | 0.48–0.58 |
| Docosatetraenoic acid (C22:4n-6) | 0.29–0.39 | 0.19–0.25 | 0.09–0.11 | 0.44–0.49 | 0.22–0.22 | 0.13–0.17 |
| Adrenic acid (C22:5n-6) | 0.13–0.21 | 0.09–0.13 | 0.06–0.10 | 0.15–0.17 | 0.05–0.05 | 0.05–0.09 |

Data shows the relative proportion in total lipids (%) between mothers who had term and preterm infants. Colostrum = 0–5 days of postnatal life (DPL); Transitional = 6–15 DPL; Mature = 16–60 DPL. Data abstracted from [6].

## 2.2. Breast Milk Fat Globules

Lipids in breast milk are present in the form of milk fat globules homogenously distributed within the aqueous phase of milk. The average size of milk fat globules, depending on the stage of lactation, varies between 0.1 and 15 μm. Breast milk fat globules are larger during the 24 h postpartum and the size reduces to similar sizes in transitional and mature milk [14,15]. Fat globules possess a core-shell structure, as illustrated in Figure 1. The membranes of a fat globule are composed of a unique tri-layer structure. The formation of a fat globule follows a coordinated sequence of synthesis and secretion. Briefly, the triglyceride core is first synthesized at the endoplasmic reticulum, and the first closely packed single layer is formed during secretion into the cytoplasm. The second, outer phospholipid bilayer is formed during secretion from the epithelial cell of the lactocyte [16,17]. These layers, also known as milk fat globule membranes (MFGM), are 8–10 nm thick and contains 70% protein, 25% phospholipid, and 5% cerebrosides/cholesterol. The phospholipid composition is distinctive between the layers, the major phospholipid components are phosphatidylethanolamine (30%) in the single layer, and phosphatidylcholine (35%) and sphingomyelin (25%) in the double layer. The MFGM also contains important proteins such as mucin-1, butyrophilin, xanthine oxidoreductase, glycoprotein bovine lactadherin 6/7, selectively placed in the double layer, which are important in infant health and have been discussed comprehensively in another review [18–20].

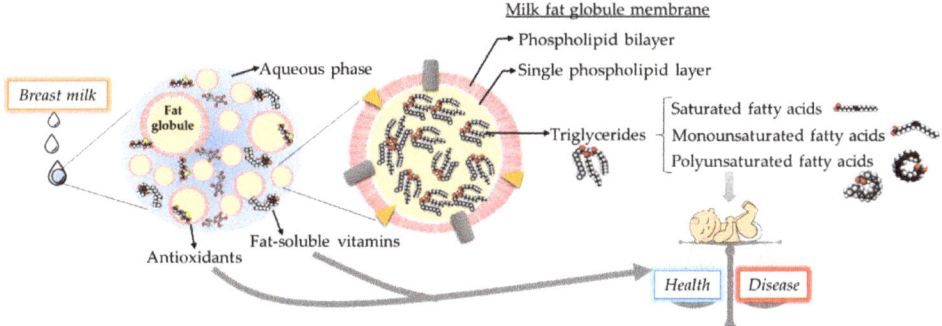

**Figure 1.** Breast milk fat components and relationship with neonatal health-disease balance. Scheme of fat globule illustrating of the core-shell structure.

Bovine milk based infant formulas have attempted to closely mimic the lipid composition of naturally originated breast milk. However, large differences still exist in physiochemical properties between the fat globule in breast milk and the fat globule found in formula. Fat globules in conventional infant formulas are smaller (0.1–1.0 μm) in milk protein (caseins and whey proteins), dominated membranes induced by the manufacturing process of centrifugation, homogenization, and heat treatment [21–23]. Adding bovine milk phospholipids to an amount of 1.5% of total fat with modified processing procedures have shown to yield infant formulas with larger fat globules [23,24]. In addition, in human milk sphingomyelin is the dominant phospholipid versus phosphatidylcholine and phosphatidylethanolamine in formula [18,23]. While researchers are still making efforts to understand the functionalities of MFGM, there are already commercialized products supplementing MFGMs from bovine milk cream. The effectiveness of supplementation of MFGM in formula has been demonstrated in several independent cellular and animal studies, and clinical trials [25–28]. In mouse and rat studies, bovine MFGMs showed cognitive and neuronal development improvement and this observation was further illustrated in multiple clinical trials, suggesting bovine MFGMs have positive effects on cognitive development and protection against bacterial infection.

The downstream physiochemical properties of milk fat globules are dependent on the efficiency of fat digestion in infants. The interfacial structure, which is represented by the distribution of complex lipids in the MFGM, and the available fat area, defined as the globule size, are of primary importance for adequate lipolysis and digestion in the neonate [21,29]. In preterm infants, human milk fat globules were digested faster than preterm formulas in a digestive time range of 10 to 50 min [30]. It has been postulated that the difference in the digestion rate is caused by the variation of fat globule size and membrane composition in human milk versus preterm formulas [22]. Research in the MFGM field continues to garner interest as data indicate that breast milk fat globules could provide the right vehicle for bioactive factors, such as vitamin E and digestive enzymes, to be effectively delivered optimizing bioavailability. The MFGM fraction may have important biological roles for the development of physiological neonatal systems and immune function [9].

*2.3. Complex Lipids in Breast Milk*

Although about 98%–99% of lipids found in breast milk are in the form of triglycerides, other complex lipid types such as glycerophospholipids (e.g., phosphatidylethanolamine, phosphatidylcholine) and sphingolipids account for 0.2%–1.0%, or 100–400 mg/l of breast milk lipids [31]. These lipids are mostly located in MFGMs and extracellular vesicles such as exosomes in breast milk. Sphingolipids share a similar sphingosine backbone, but the type of headgroup attached determines the type of sphingolipid (sphingomyelin, glucosyl and lactosylceramides, or gangliosides). Quantification of complex lipids in human milk shows that sphingomyelin is the most abundant, making up about 36% of complex lipids, followed by glycerophospholipids, phosphatidylethanolamine (29%), and phosphatidylcholine (25%) [23,32,33]. Exosomes are also enriched with sphingolipids, particularly ceramide and sphingomyelin, and glycerophospholipids such as phosphatidylserine [34]. Like fatty acid levels, the composition of sphingolipids in breast milk can also be modified by diet. Lopez et al. demonstrated an increase in phospholipid and sphingolipid content in MFGM from cows fed with diets rich in LCPUFAs [35].

## 3. Breast Milk Lipids Enhance Neonatal Intestinal Development and Protect against Injury

The impact of lipids and fatty acids on gut development is not as well studied as in other organ systems. To date, the contribution of lipids and essential fatty acids on early postnatal gut development and subsequent host responses after an inciting event remain unknown. Understanding the changes in intestinal development in response to early priming with varying lipids and fatty acids during a pre-injurious state will be helpful to investigate the underlying mechanisms by which fatty acids may modulate the risk of intestinal injury and inflammation.

*3.1. Saturated and Monounsaturated Fatty Acids*

*Role in intestinal development and injury.* Dietary saturated and monounsaturated fatty acids have been shown to influence the microbiota diversity of human breast milk and neonatal gut [36]. Breast milk fatty acid composition changes rapidly in response to fat intake in the maternal diet. Higher levels of monounsaturated fatty acids in breast milk resulted in a decrease of *Staphylococcus*, *Pseudomonas*, *Lactobacillus*, and *Bifidobacterium*, while the level of saturated fatty acids in breast milk was negatively correlated with *Streptococcus*. The fatty acid composition of human milk along with specific microbial constitution likely affect the developmental programming of immune ontogeny in infants. *Bifidobacterium* and *Lactobacillus* spp. are crucial for immunological functions and mucosal barrier homeostasis, including tolerance, mucus production, tight junction expression, and T-helper cell balance [37].

In human breast milk triglycerides, the sn-2 position is commonly occupied by palmitic acid. In contrast, in palm-oil based human infant formula, palmitic acid is mainly present at the sn-1 or sn-3 position. The difference in sn- position leads to impaired absorption of calcium and fat, which negatively influence early bone accretion [38]. When human infant formula contains palmitic acid at the sn-2 position, improved absorption of fat and calcium with absorption rates similar to those seen in breastmilk-fed infants is observed [39]. Consequently, a low palmitic acid formula has been developed to reduce the amount of sn-1, 3 palmitic acids thus enabling higher absorption of calcium and fat in neonates [40,41].

Palmitic acid at the sn-2 position of the triacylglycerol backbone imparts benefits for neonatal intestinal and immunological health outcomes [42]. Lu et al. examined the effect of diet with sn-2 palmitic acids using Muc2 deficient mice, an animal model for spontaneous enterocolitis. Compared to sn-1,3 palmitic acids of triglycerides, sn-2 palmitic acids resulted in decreased intestinal injury and inflammation by upregulation of PPAR-γ, antioxidant enzymes (superoxide dismutase, glutathione peroxidase), and induction of an immunosuppressive T-regulatory cell response [43]. These data support the role of the saturated fatty acid, palmitic acid, specifically in sn-2 configuration, as being important for intestinal mucosal homeostasis, gut microbiome, and immune response [44]. However, the lack of evidence in clinical trials to establish a cause and effect relationship between the palmitic acid at sn-2 position and neonatal health outcomes, led the European Society for Paediatric Gastroenterology, Hepatology, and Nutrition to recommend that the inclusion of high sn-2 palmitic acid cannot be considered essential in human infant formula [45,46].

Among monounsaturated fatty acids, oleic acid has been shown to possess an immunomodulatory function. However, the role of oleic acid in immune responses is still controversial. An olive oil-based diet in adult mice showed improved immune responses against bacterial infection with enhanced phagocytic activity by macrophages [47,48]. In vitro, human lymphocytes treated with oleic acid resulted in increased neutral lipid accumulation thought to protect against lipid toxicity [49]. However, these studies also demonstrated oleic acid-induced cell death and necrosis mediated by caspase-3 activation. The role of oleic acid remains largely unexplored in infants [49].

### 3.2. Polyunsaturated Fatty Acids

*Role in intestinal development.* It is well-documented that in the early postnatal period of preterm infants, whole blood docosahexaenoic acid (DHA, C22:6n-3) and arachidonic acid (ARA, C20:4n-6) deficits and linoleic acid (LA, C18:2n-6) excesses occur within the first postnatal week [50]. Although these altered fatty acid profiles have been linked to the increased risk of developing bronchopulmonary dysplasia, retinopathy of prematurity, and late onset sepsis, the impact of these altered fatty acid profiles on intestinal development has just recently been described [50–52].

Singh et al. took advantage of the fat-1 transgenic mouse model to examine the differences in postnatal gut development in mouse pups in control, wild-type dam fed mice versus dam fed fat-1 transgenic mice [52]. Relative to the wild-type group, fat-1 mice had a greater n-3 shift in their intestinal fatty acid levels with an increase in DHA and eicosapentaenoic acid (EPA, C20:5n-3), and a decrease in ARA in the pre-weaning period. Of clinical importance is the parallel of the wild-type fatty acid levels with systemic levels observed in the postnatal period of preterm infants and the parallel of fat-1 fatty acid levels to systemic levels observed in preterm infants supplemented with enteral or parenteral fish oil [53]. This study confirmed that fatty acid exposure and intestinal levels do impact postnatal intestinal development and that a balance between both n-3 and n-6 may be critical in this early developmental period. In the pre-weaning period, while an n-3 dominant pattern increased gene expression of cell differentiation markers (EphB2, Fzd5) and fatty acid metabolism (fatty acid binding protein 2 and 6), this n-3 dominant pattern also decreased villus height over time and reduced expression of markers that inform innate host defenses, such as a reduced number of acidic mucin filled goblet cells, reduced expression of tight-junction genes (claudin 3 and 7), and reduced gene expression of muc2, trefoil factor 3, toll like receptor 9, and cathelicidin antimicrobial peptide [52]. These data suggest that that LCPUFA changes reflective of those seen in neonatal intensive care units likely influence the trajectory of postnatal intestinal development.

In a preterm piglet model evaluating the effect of an enteral complex lipid emulsion containing LCPUFAs on early postnatal fatty acid levels, it was demonstrated that an ARA:DHA ratio >1.0 compared to a ratio <1.0 uniquely prevented the postnatal deficit of ARA while also demonstrating increased ileal villus height and muscular thickness compared to the control soybean-oil and ARA:DHA

<1.0 groups [54]. In contrast, parenteral nutrition did not show an effect on intestinal morphology and function in preterm piglet models, suggesting postnatal intestinal adaptation is driven more by enterally administered fatty acids versus parenteral delivery [55]. Wang et al. showed that both triglyceride (fish oil, DHA, and EPA) and phospholipid-derived n-3 LCPUFAs (DHA and EPA) enriched diets led to improved small intestine villus to crypt depth ratio in 4-week old mice. The villus to crypt depth ratio was significantly increased in the LCPUFA supplemented group compared to the control group, and this increase was more pronounced in the phospholipid-derived n-3 LCPUFAs compared to the triglyceride-derived n-3 group. Moreover, higher enrichment of gut- microbiota was observed in response to phospholipid-derived n-3 LCPUFAs [56].

*Role in intestinal injury.* Potential benefits of LCPUFAs have been reported in inflammatory bowel disease, a disease with similar pathology as necrotizing enterocolitis (NEC) [57,58]. However, human studies investigating the role of n-3 fatty acids in the prevention, treatment, and maintenance of remission inflammatory bowel disease have shown mixed results [59–65].

In vitro studies have consistently demonstrated anti-inflammatory actions of LCPUFAs. ARA and DHA treatment to intestinal epithelial cells blocked platelet-activating factor-induced toll like receptor 4 (TLR4) and platelet-activating factor receptor expression in intestinal epithelial cells [66]. Similarly, LCPUFA treated human fetal and adult intestinal epithelial cells demonstrated that DHA and ARA treatment led to a decreased IL-1β-induced pro-inflammatory response [67]. The protective effect of LCPUFAs in intestinal inflammatory disease could be partly explained by their effect on gut barrier function [68]. Although in vitro studies have shown mixed results about the impact of LCPUFAs on intestinal permeability [52,69,70], LCPUFA treatment to human intestinal epithelial cells resulted in improved intestinal barrier by decreasing the impairment in intestinal permeability induced by cytokines [71,72].

In vivo studies support the role of LCPUFAs in reducing inflammation and modulating the risk for NEC. Studies evaluating the effect of n-3 fatty acids and their derivatives in adult mice and a rat model of colitis showed beneficial effects by reducing the expression of inflammatory mediators [73–78]. Furthermore, Gobbetti et al. showed the protective effect of n-6, but not n-3 LCPUFA containing diet on ischemia/perfusion induced intestinal injury in an adult murine model. Three-week-old mice supplemented with n-6 enriched diet for 9 weeks showed reduced intestinal damage and inflammation and this effect was mediated by increased level of lipoxin A4, suggesting the anti-inflammatory role of lipoxin A4 in ischemia/perfusion induced intestinal injury [79]. These results suggest that ARA is not only a precursor of pro-inflammatory lipid mediators but also plays a critical role in generating anti-inflammatory lipid mediators [80]. Altogether, the balance of n-3 and n-6 LCPUFAs plays a critical role in regulating intestinal pathophysiology and inflammation.

Several animal studies using experimental models of NEC have shown that LCPUFA supplementation results in reduced NEC incidence and its severity by regulating multiple pathways associated with intestinal inflammation/injury and necrosis, including TLR4, platelet-activating factor, and nuclear factor-κB [81–83]. Preterm rats born to dams who were fed a DHA or EPA enriched diet and subjected to an NEC induction protocol showed significant decreased NEC-like colitis incidence [84]. In a different study, LCPUFA supplementation significantly reduced the incidence of NEC in a neonatal rat model compared with controls by downregulating phospholipase A(2)-II and platelet-activating factor receptor at 24 and 48 h, respectively [81]. Compared to a control formula, three different LCPUFA supplementation strategies (ARA and DHA, egg phospholipid, DHA) showed reduced NEC incidence in a neonatal rat model of NEC by downregulating TLR4 expression [66]. Similarly, young mice supplemented with 10% fish oil for 4 weeks showed protective effects against hypoxia-induced NEC with a reduction in platelet-activating factor as well as leukotriene B4 [85].

Several clinical trials have evaluated the impact of LCPUFAs in term and preterm infants. However, the data about the role of LCPUFAs in NEC is limited. Furthermore, in many of these studies, the assessment of the risk of NEC with nutritional intervention was a secondary outcome analysis. Differences in LCPUFA formulation, dosing, and study populations results in inconclusive data about the use of LCPUFA in the prevention of NEC. Despite promising results of LCPUFAs in experimental NEC in animal models, results in preterm human infants are mixed and limited.

A summary of LCPUFA supplemented feedings and NEC risk in preterm infants is shown in Table 2. The systemic review by Smithers et al. did not find any benefit of n-3 LCPUFA supplemented formula in the risk of NEC. In this work, the studies were not limited to preterm infants who are at the highest risk of developing NEC [86]. Fewtrell et al. included infants who received human milk, which could be a confounding factor in this study [87]. In the Carlson et al. study, no infant received human milk and the preterm infants were randomly assigned into two groups receiving either experimental formula containing egg phospholipids (0.13% DHA and 0.41% ARA) or control group. The egg phospholipid-containing formula resulted in a significant decrease in NEC incidence compared to the control formula [88]. Currently, this is the only single-center human study demonstrated to decrease NEC incidence in response to LCPUFA supplementation. It is important to note that none of the trials looked at NEC incidence as a primary outcome. In addition, what is unclear is whether a potential benefit would be seen in a population of largely human milk fed infants, which is the current standard.

Table 2. Human studies of long-chain polyunsaturated fatty acid (LCPUFA) supplementation in preterm infants and necrotizing enterocolitis (NEC) risk.

| Reference | Study Design | Population | n | Powerful and Prevalence of NEC | Principal Finding in NEC |
|---|---|---|---|---|---|
| Smithers et al. (2008) [86] | Systematic review | <37 GA | 1333 | RR = [0.62–2.04] | No benefit of n-3 LCPUFA supplemented formula |
| Zhang et al. (2014) [89] | Systemic review | <32 GA | 900 | RR = [0.23–1.10] | No benfit of n-3 LCPUFA supplementation |
| *Double-blinded randomized clinical trials* | | | | | |
| Carlson et al. (1998) [88] | Formula supplemented with 0.41% ARA + 0.13% DHA | <32 GA BW between 725–1375 g | 119 | Control = 17.6% Experimental = 2.9% | Significantly decreased |
| Fewtrell et al. (2002) [90] | Formula supplemented with 0.31% ARA + 0.17% DHA | <37 GA BW <1750 g | 197 | Control = 11% Experimental = 19% | No significant difference |
| Innis et al. (2002) [91] | BM supplemented with DHA BM supplemented with ARA + DHA | BW between 846–1560 g | 194 | Control = 1.6% Experimental = 1.5% | No significant difference |
| Fewtrell et al. (2004) [87] | Formula supplemented with 0.31% ARA + 0.17% DHA | <35 GA BW ≤2000 g | 238 | Control = 2% Experimental = 4% | No significant difference |
| Clandinin et al. (2005) [92] | Formula supplemented with DHA + ARA | <35 GA | 361 | Control = 3% Experimental = 5% | No significant difference |
| Henriksen et al. (2008) [93] | BM supplemented with 6.7% ARA + 6.9% DHA | BW <1500 g | 141 | Control = 3% Experimental = 1.5% | No significant difference |
| Makrides et al. (2009) [94] | High DHA (1%) Low DHA (0.3%) | <33 GA | 657 | Adj. OR = [0.87–5.22] | No significant difference |
| Collins et al. (2016) [95] | Formula supplemented with different doses of DHA | <30 GA | 53 | Control = 9% Experimental = 9% | No significant difference |
| Collins et al. (2017) [96] | BM supplemented with 60 mg/kg/day DHA | <29 WGA | 1273 | Adj. OR = [0.79–1.69] | No significant difference |

In the double-blinded randomized clinical trials, the control group was no supplementation feeding. Breast milk (BM); birth weight (BW); weeks of gestational age (GA); the relative risk (RR) or adjusted odd ratio (OR) shown as 95% confidence interval.

### 3.3. Milk Fat Globule Membranes

*Role in intestinal development.* MFGM proteins have been identified [18] that exert multiple biological functions critical for intestinal development and health. Mucin 1 interacts with molecule-3-grabbing non-integrin, expressed by dendritic cells, in the infant gastrointestinal tract and subsequently inhibits binding of certain intestinal pathogenic bacteria to dendritic cells [97]. Moreover, mucin 1 demonstrates anti-viral properties against rotavirus infection [98]. Xanthine oxidoreductase, a predominant protein of MFGM, possesses antimicrobial activity and has been shown to inhibit the growth of *Escherichia coli* and *Salmonella enteritides* by generating superoxide and peroxide, thus providing protection to the neonatal gut [99]. Lactadherin, also known as milk fat globule–EGF factor 8, aids in the clearance of dead cells by macrophages through phagocytosis [100]. Exogenous administration of lactadherin decreased the inflammatory response and injury by enhancing phagocytosis of apoptotic cells in experimental sepsis and ischemia/perfusion injury models [101–103]. Furthermore, lactadherin deficient mice showed more severe injury in response to dextran sulfate sodium, which induces colitis, and the administration of human lactadherin attenuated the dextran sulfate sodium injury [104]. Results from in vitro and in vivo studies showed that lactadherin deficiency results in delayed epithelial cell renewal and turnover [105]. Together, these results suggest the importance of lactadherin in intestinal homeostasis and imply that the provision of lactadherin in human or bovine milk could be beneficial against intestinal injury/inflammation. Butyrophilin, another quantitatively major protein in human MFGM, has been considered as a potentially important regulator for immune function. In addition to its effect on the secretion of milk fat globules [106], butyrophilin induces apoptosis and promotes T cell response [107]. Finally, in rat pups, the addition of MFGM to formula resulted in an enteric microbiome and intestinal development pattern (measured by villus height, crypt depth, crypt cell proliferation, paneth and goblet cell counts, and tight junction proteins) more similar to breastfed rats compared to rats fed with formula without MFGM [108]. Collectively, these results suggest the important role of MFGM and MFGM proteins in shaping the gastrointestinal tract immune system and maintaining immune homeostasis.

*Role in intestinal injury.* MFGM supplemented formula in rat pups protects against *C. difficile* toxin [108] and LPS-induced intestinal inflammation [109]. In the latter study, MFGM supplementation protected against histological changes in the intestine, reduced inflammatory cytokines, and increased tight junction proteins. In an asphyxia, cold stress model of NEC in neonatal rat pups, MFGM supplementation reduced NEC incidence and severity with a concurrent reduction in TLR4 expression [110]. Clinical trials of MFGM supplementation have not been conducted in preterm infants. In 6–12-month-old infants supplemented daily with MFGM, the number of bloody diarrheal episodes was reduced significantly by almost 50% [111]. Rapidly evolving and emerging evidence from animal model studies and clinical trials indicates the potential of beneficial effects of the combination of bioactive compounds or any specific component of MFGM to optimize postnatal intestinal development in the preterm infant and to protect against disease.

*3.4. Complex Lipids*

*Role in intestinal development and injury.* Breast milk provides complex lipids through the delivery of MFGMs and exosomes. Published data support the role of extracellular vesicles on intestinal development and protection from intestinal injury such as NEC [112–114]. When evaluated in totality versus in individual components, human milk-derived exosomes attenuate oxidative stress-induced cell death in intestinal epithelial cells [115] and enhance proliferation and migration of intestinal epithelial cells in preterm infants compared to those with full term birth [116].

Breast milk sphingolipids, such as sphingomyelin and gangliosides, are important modulators of neonatal intestinal development, the establishment of the gut microbiome, and inflammation [117]. Sphingomyelin is digested by nucleotide phosphodiesterase pyrophosphatase 7 (NPP7), a brush border enzyme of the intestinal epithelium, and generates ceramide, sphingosine, and sphingosine-1-phosphate [118,119]. In contrast to sphingomyelin and ceramide, sphingosine is rapidly absorbed and largely converted to palmitic acid in the mucosa [120]. NPP7 is specifically expressed in intestinal mucosa and is highly expressed in the middle part of the jejunum and the lower colon.

NPP7 possesses phospholipase C activity against platelet activating factor, a pro-inflammatory lipid mediator produced by gut epithelial cells [121]. Higher levels of platelet activating factor have been shown in inflammatory bowel disease, ischemic colitis and NEC [118]. Intrarectal administration of recombinant NPP7 significantly reduced the intestinal injury and inflammation against colitis in an adult rat model [122]. It is possible that NPP7 expression is dependent on gestational age or the changes in enzymatic activity that occur later after birth, which may predispose the preterm infant to intestinal injury. However, similar expression of NPP7 was observed in the meconium of term and preterm infants [123]. The anti-inflammatory benefits of sphingomyelin might be mediated through the induced changes in the microbiome. In an adult murine model, a diet containing 0.25% (wt/wt) milk sphingomyelin had lower fecal Gram-negative bacteria and higher fecal *Bifidobacterium* compared to mice fed with a high fat diet, and these changes were accompanied by reduced serum lipopolysaccharide levels in the sphingomyelin group [124].

Gangliosides have been reported to reduce pro-inflammatory signaling in the intestine [125] and protect the bowel in an infant model of necrotizing enterocolitis [126]. Weaning rats fed with ganglioside-enriched diets demonstrated increased ganglioside levels in the intestinal brush border and reduced levels of the pro-inflammatory mediator platelet activating factor [127]. In a follow-up study, rats fed with dietary gangliosides compared to controls exhibited reduced expression of pro-inflammatory mediators such prostaglandin E2, LTB4, IL-1β, TNF-α in the intestinal mucosa following lipopolysaccharide-induced inflammation [128]. Similar to sphingomyelin, some of this mediation may be due to induced microbiome changes in the gut. In preterm infants, fecal *Escherichia coli* counts were lower and *Bifidobacterial* counts were higher in infants fed with a ganglioside-supplemented diet compared to infants fed a control milk formula [129].

Together, these studies support the role of sphingolipids, particularly sphingomyelin and gangliosides, as important mediators of intestinal development and protection against intestinal injury.

## 4. Scientific Gaps and Future Directions

Dietary lipids and fatty acids are of critical importance in several developmental processes such as immune responses, organogenesis, and central nervous system development. Although after a term pregnancy adipose stores and human milk continue to supply the infant with critical lipids and fatty acids, preterm infants do not have these sustainable sources with a lack of adipose tissue and minimal enteral feeding volumes. To prevent postnatal deficits of these critical nutrients, the preterm infant will likely require additional dietary supplementation. The specific content of such supplementation and the chemical composition to ensure adequate absorption remains to be defined. Based on the available data, infant formula should provide both ARA and DHA, and in an ARA:DHA ratio >1. Providing solely DHA or DHA exceeding ARA may induce undesirable health outcomes in infants, leading to adverse effects on growth and immune development [130,131].

The precise mechanisms by which lipids and fatty acids mediate their effects on the developing intestine still need to be fully characterized. It is possible that dietary intervention may have different effects across different exposure times and different clinical contexts (during acute illness versus convalescence). As a result, studies that examine timing, composition, and dosing, including desirable target levels, are needed.

The role of human milk-derived vesicles, including the human milk fat globule and exosomes, may reveal an opportunity to present multiple critical molecules simultaneously and ensuring delivery and bioavailability to the intended site.

The biggest challenge in translational research is reconciling the disparate results obtained from animal models versus human clinical trials. Establishing animal models that better reflect the preterm neonatal experience, as well as refinement of humanoid model systems, will be essential in bridging the gap from bench to bedside.

## 5. Conclusions

The lipid and fatty acid content in human milk inform investigators and clinicians of the important nutrient pathways that facilitate growth, development, and resistance to disease. The preterm infant is uniquely vulnerable to nutrient deprivation, and parenteral and enteral feedings alone may not be sufficient to close the nutrient gaps that develop early after delivery. The science of breast milk will likely open new avenues of therapeutic options to minimize the health consequences of such nutrient gaps. An improvement in the experimental model systems will iteratively close the gap in translation from bench to bedside.

**Author Contributions:** Conceptualization and validation, S.D.F. and C.R.M.; investigation, resources and writing—original draft preparation, D.R.-C., P.S., Y.L., E.M.-M. and W.Y.; writing—review and editing, D.R.-C., S.D.F. and C.R.M.; supervision, C.R.M.; funding acquisition, C.R.M. All authors have read and agreed to the published version of the manuscript.

**Funding:** This research was funded by Charles H and Judy Hood Family Infant Health Research Program and National Institute of Diabetes and Digestive and Kidney Diseases (NIH R01 DK104346).

**Conflicts of Interest:** Martin and Freedman have grant support from Alcresta Therapeutics, Inc., and serve on the scientific advisory board of Prolacta Biosciences. Martin has grant support from Feihe International and Mead Johnson Nutrition; and serves on the scientific advisory boards of Fresenius Kabi and LUCA Biologics. The funders had no role in the writing of the manuscript, or in the decision to publish the results.

## References

1. Gila-Diaz, A.; Arribas, S.M.; Algara, A.; Martin-Cabrejas, M.A.; Lopez de Pablo, A.L.; Saenz de Pipaon, M.; Ramiro-Cortijo, D. A review of bioactive factors in human breastmilk: A focus on prematurity. *Nutrients* **2019**, *11*, 1307. [CrossRef] [PubMed]
2. Grote, V.; Verduci, E.; Scaglioni, S.; Vecchi, F.; Contarini, G.; Giovannini, M.; Koletzko, B.; Agostoni, C.; European Childhood Obesity, P. Breast milk composition and infant nutrient intakes during the first 12 months of life. *Eur. J. Clin. Nutr.* **2016**, *70*, 250–256. [CrossRef] [PubMed]
3. Munblit, D.; Verhasselt, V.; Warner, J.O. Editorial: Human milk composition and health outcomes in children. *Front. Pediatr.* **2019**, *7*, 319. [CrossRef]
4. Miliku, K.; Duan, Q.L.; Moraes, T.J.; Becker, A.B.; Mandhane, P.J.; Turvey, S.E.; Lefebvre, D.L.; Sears, M.R.; Subbarao, P.; Field, C.J.; et al. Human milk fatty acid composition is associated with dietary, genetic, sociodemographic, and environmental factors in the CHILD Cohort Study. *Am. J. Clin. Nutr.* **2019**, *110*, 1370–1383. [CrossRef] [PubMed]
5. Gidrewicz, D.A.; Fenton, T.R. A systematic review and meta-analysis of the nutrient content of preterm and term breast milk. *BMC Pediatr.* **2014**, *14*, 216. [CrossRef]
6. Floris, L.M.; Stahl, B.; Abrahamse-Berkeveld, M.; Teller, I.C. Human milk fatty acid profile across lactational stages after term and preterm delivery: A pooled data analysis. *Prostaglandins Leukot. Essent. Fat. Acids* **2019**, 102023. [CrossRef] [PubMed]
7. Boyce, C.; Watson, M.; Lazidis, G.; Reeve, S.; Dods, K.; Simmer, K.; McLeod, G. Preterm human milk composition: A systematic literature review. *Br. J. Nutr.* **2016**, *116*, 1033–1045. [CrossRef]
8. Lopez-Lopez, A.; Lopez-Sabater, M.C.; Campoy-Folgoso, C.; Rivero-Urgell, M.; Castellote-Bargallo, A.I. Fatty acid and sn-2 fatty acid composition in human milk from Granada (Spain) and in infant formulas. *Eur. J. Clin. Nutr.* **2002**, *56*, 1242–1254. [CrossRef]
9. Koletzko, B. Human Milk Lipids. *Ann. Nutr. Metab.* **2016**, *69* (Suppl. 2), 28–40. [CrossRef]
10. Jensen, R.G. Lipids in human milk. *Lipids* **1999**, *34*, 1243–1271. [CrossRef]
11. Martin, C.R.; Ling, P.R.; Blackburn, G.L. Review of infant feeding: Key features of breast milk and infant formula. *Nutrients* **2016**, *8*, 279. [CrossRef]
12. Mozaffarian, D.; Ascherio, A.; Hu, F.B.; Stampfer, M.J.; Willett, W.C.; Siscovick, D.S.; Rimm, E.B. Interplay between different polyunsaturated fatty acids and risk of coronary heart disease in men. *Circulation* **2005**, *111*, 157–164. [CrossRef] [PubMed]
13. Aglago, E.K.; Huybrechts, I.; Murphy, N.; Casagrande, C.; Nicolas, G.; Pischon, T.; Fedirko, V.; Severi, G.; Boutron-Ruault, M.C.; Fournier, A.; et al. Consumption of fish and long-chain n-3 polyunsaturated fatty acids is associated with reduced risk of colorectal cancer in a large European cohort. *Clin. Gastroenterol. Hepatol.* **2019**, *18*, 654–666. [CrossRef] [PubMed]
14. Michalski, M.C.; Briard, V.; Michel, F.; Tasson, F.; Poulain, P. Size distribution of fat globules in human colostrum, breast milk, and infant formula. *J. Dairy Sci.* **2005**, *88*, 1927–1940. [CrossRef]
15. Zou, X.Q.; Guo, Z.; Huang, J.H.; Jin, Q.Z.; Cheong, L.Z.; Wang, X.G.; Xu, X.B. Human milk fat globules from different stages of lactation: A lipid composition analysis and microstructure characterization. *J. Agric. Food Chem.* **2012**, *60*, 7158–7167. [CrossRef]

16. Bionaz, M.; Loor, J.J. Gene networks driving bovine milk fat synthesis during the lactation cycle. *BMC Genom.* **2008**, *9*, 366. [CrossRef]
17. Truchet, S.; Honvo-Houeto, E. Physiology of milk secretion. *Best Pract. Res. Clin. Endocrinol. Metab.* **2017**, *31*, 367–384. [CrossRef]
18. Mather, I.H. A review and proposed nomenclature for major proteins of the milk-fat globule membrane. *J. Dairy Sci.* **2000**, *83*, 203–247. [CrossRef]
19. Dewettinck, K.R.; Thienpont, N.; Thien Le, T.; Messens, K.; Van Camp, J. Nutritional and technological aspects of milk fat globule membrane material. *Int. Dairy J.* **2008**, *18*, 436–457. [CrossRef]
20. Chatterton, D.E.; Nguyen, D.N.; Bering, S.B.; Sangild, P.T. Anti-inflammatory mechanisms of bioactive milk proteins in the intestine of newborns. *Int. J. Biochem. Cell. Biol.* **2013**, *45*, 1730–1747. [CrossRef]
21. Bourlieu, C.D.; Deglaire, A.; De Oliveira, S.C.; Ménard, O.; Le Gouar, Y.; Carrière, F.; Dupont, D. Towards infant formula biomimetic of human milk structure and digestive behavior. *Proceedings* **2017**, *24*, 17. [CrossRef]
22. Bourlieu, C.; Menard, O.; De La Chevasnerie, A.; Sams, L.; Rousseau, F.; Madec, M.N.; Robert, B.; Deglaire, A.; Pezennec, S.; Bouhallab, S.; et al. The structure of infant formulas impacts their lipolysis, proteolysis and disintegration during in vitro gastric digestion. *Food Chem.* **2015**, *182*, 224–235. [CrossRef] [PubMed]
23. Wei, W.; Yang, J.; Yang, D.; Wang, X.; Yang, Z.; Jin, Q.; Wang, M.; Lai, J.; Wang, X. Phospholipid composition and fat globule structure i: Comparison of human milk fat from different gestational ages, lactation stages, and infant formulas. *J. Agric. Food Chem.* **2019**, *67*, 13922–13928. [CrossRef]
24. Gallier, S.; Vocking, K.; Post, J.A.; Van De Heijning, B.; Acton, D.; Van Der Beek, E.M.; Van Baalen, T. A novel infant milk formula concept: Mimicking the human milk fat globule structure. *Colloids Surf. B Biointerfaces* **2015**, *136*, 329–339. [CrossRef] [PubMed]
25. Moukarzel, S.; Dyer, R.A.; Garcia, C.; Wiedeman, A.M.; Boyce, G.; Weinberg, J.; Keller, B.O.; Elango, R.; Innis, S.M. Milk fat globule membrane supplementation in formula-fed rat pups improves reflex development and may alter brain lipid composition. *Sci. Rep.* **2018**, *8*, 15277. [CrossRef] [PubMed]
26. Ji, X.; Xu, W.; Cui, J.; Ma, Y.; Zhou, S. Goat and buffalo milk fat globule membranes exhibit better effects at inducing apoptosis and reduction the viability of HT-29 cells. *Sci. Rep.* **2019**, *9*, 2577. [CrossRef]
27. Hernell, O.; Domellof, M.; Grip, T.; Lonnerdal, B.; Timby, N. Physiological effects of feeding infants and young children formula supplemented with milk fat globule membranes. *Nestle Nutr. Inst. Workshop Ser.* **2019**, *90*, 35–42. [CrossRef]
28. Li, F.; Wu, S.S.; Berseth, C.L.; Harris, C.L.; Richards, J.D.; Wampler, J.L.; Zhuang, W.; Cleghorn, G.; Rudolph, C.D.; Liu, B.; et al. Improved Neurodevelopmental outcomes associated with bovine milk fat globule membrane and lactoferrin in infant formula: A randomized, controlled trial. *J. Pediatr.* **2019**, *215*, 24–31. [CrossRef]
29. Oosting, A.; van Vlies, N.; Kegler, D.; Schipper, L.; Abrahamse-Berkeveld, M.; Ringler, S.; Verkade, H.J.; van der Beek, E.M. Effect of dietary lipid structure in early postnatal life on mouse adipose tissue development and function in adulthood. *Br. J. Nutr.* **2014**, *111*, 215–226. [CrossRef]
30. Armand, M.; Hamosh, M.; Mehta, N.R.; Angelus, P.A.; Philpott, J.R.; Henderson, T.R.; Dwyer, N.K.; Lairon, D.; Hamosh, P. Effect of human milk or formula on gastric function and fat digestion in the premature infant. *Pediatr. Res.* **1996**, *40*, 429–437. [CrossRef]
31. Delplanque, B.; Gibson, R.; Koletzko, B.; Lapillonne, A.; Strandvik, B. Lipid quality in infant nutrition: Current knowledge and future opportunities. *J. Pediatr. Gastroenterol. Nutr.* **2015**, *61*, 8–17. [CrossRef]
32. Giuffrida, F.; Cruz-Hernandez, C.; Fluck, B.; Tavazzi, I.; Thakkar, S.K.; Destaillats, F.; Braun, M. Quantification of phospholipids classes in human milk. *Lipids* **2013**, *48*, 1051–1058. [CrossRef] [PubMed]
33. Tavazzi, I.; Fontannaz, P.; Lee, L.Y.; Giuffrida, F. Quantification of glycerophospholipids and sphingomyelin in human milk and infant formula by high performance liquid chromatography coupled with mass spectrometer detector. *J. Chromatogr. B Anal. Technol. Biomed. Life Sci.* **2018**, *1072*, 235–243. [CrossRef] [PubMed]
34. Dinkins, M.B.; Wang, G.; Bieberich, E. Sphingolipid-enriched extracellular vesicles and alzheimer's disease: A decade of research. *J. Alzheimers Dis.* **2017**, *60*, 757–768. [CrossRef] [PubMed]
35. Lopez, C.; Briard-Bion, V.; Menard, O.; Rousseau, F.; Pradel, P.; Besle, J.M. Phospholipid, sphingolipid, and fatty acid compositions of the milk fat globule membrane are modified by diet. *J. Agric. Food Chem.* **2008**, *56*, 5226–5236. [CrossRef]

36. Moossavi, S.; Atakora, F.; Miliku, K.; Sepehri, S.; Robertson, B.; Duan, Q.L.; Becker, A.B.; Mandhane, P.J.; Turvey, S.E.; Moraes, T.J.; et al. Integrated analysis of human milk microbiota with oligosaccharides and fatty acids in the CHILD cohort. *Front. Nutr.* **2019**, *6*, 58. [CrossRef]
37. Walker, W.A.; Iyengar, R.S. Breast milk, microbiota, and intestinal immune homeostasis. *Pediatr. Res.* **2015**, *77*, 220–228. [CrossRef]
38. Leite, M.E.; Lasekan, J.; Baggs, G.; Ribeiro, T.; Menezes-Filho, J.; Pontes, M.; Druzian, J.; Barreto, D.L.; de Souza, C.O.; Mattos, A.; et al. Calcium and fat metabolic balance, and gastrointestinal tolerance in term infants fed milk-based formulas with and without palm olein and palm kernel oils: A randomized blinded crossover study. *BMC Pediatr.* **2013**, *13*, 215. [CrossRef]
39. Carnielli, V.P.; Luijendijk, I.H.; van Beek, R.H.; Boerma, G.J.; Degenhart, H.J.; Sauer, P.J. Effect of dietary triacylglycerol fatty acid positional distribution on plasma lipid classes and their fatty acid composition in preterm infants. *Am. J. Clin. Nutr.* **1995**, *62*, 776–781. [CrossRef]
40. Petit, V.; Sandoz, L.; Garcia-Rodenas, C.L. Importance of the regiospecific distribution of long-chain saturated fatty acids on gut comfort, fat and calcium absorption in infants. *Prostaglandins Leukot. Essent. Fat. Acids* **2017**, *121*, 40–51. [CrossRef]
41. Beghin, L.; Marchandise, X.; Lien, E.; Bricout, M.; Bernet, J.P.; Lienhardt, J.F.; Jeannerot, F.; Menet, V.; Requillart, J.C.; Marx, J.; et al. Growth, stool consistency and bone mineral content in healthy term infants fed sn-2-palmitate-enriched starter infant formula: A randomized, double-blind, multicentre clinical trial. *Clin. Nutr.* **2019**, *38*, 1023–1030. [CrossRef] [PubMed]
42. Miles, E.A.; Calder, P.C. The influence of the position of palmitate in infant formula triacylglycerols on health outcomes. *Nutr. Res.* **2017**, *44*, 1–8. [CrossRef] [PubMed]
43. Lu, P.; Bar-Yoseph, F.; Levi, L.; Lifshitz, Y.; Witte-Bouma, J.; de Bruijn, A.C.; Korteland-van Male, A.M.; van Goudoever, J.B.; Renes, I.B. High beta-palmitate fat controls the intestinal inflammatory response and limits intestinal damage in mucin Muc2 deficient mice. *PLoS ONE* **2013**, *8*, e65878. [CrossRef] [PubMed]
44. Jiang, T.; Liu, B.; Li, J.; Dong, X.; Lin, M.; Zhang, M.; Zhao, J.; Dai, Y.; Chen, L. Association between sn-2 fatty acid profiles of breast milk and development of the infant intestinal microbiome. *Food Funct.* **2018**, *9*, 1028–1037. [CrossRef]
45. Bronsky, J.; Campoy, C.; Embleton, N.; Fewtrell, M.; Mis, N.F.; Gerasimidis, K.; Hojsak, I.; Hulst, J.; Indrio, F.; Lapillonne, A.; et al. Palm oil and beta-palmitate in infant formula: A position paper by the european society for paediatric gastroenterology, hepatology, and nutrition (ESPGHAN) committee on nutrition. *J. Pediatr. Gastroenterol. Nutr.* **2019**, *68*, 742–760. [CrossRef]
46. Zou, L.; Pande, G.; Akoh, C.C. Infant formula fat analogs and human milk fat: New focus on infant developmental needs. *Annu. Rev. Food Sci. Technol.* **2016**, *7*, 139–165. [CrossRef]
47. Sales-Campos, H.; Souza, P.R.; Peghini, B.C.; da Silva, J.S.; Cardoso, C.R. An overview of the modulatory effects of oleic acid in health and disease. *Mini Rev. Med. Chem.* **2013**, *13*, 201–210.
48. Cruz-Chamorro, L.; Puertollano, E.; de Cienfuegos, G.A.; Puertollano, M.A.; de Pablo, M.A. Acquired resistance to Listeria monocytogenes during a secondary infection in a murine model fed dietary lipids. *Nutrition* **2011**, *27*, 1053–1060. [CrossRef]
49. Cury-Boaventura, M.F.; Gorjao, R.; de Lima, T.M.; Newsholme, P.; Curi, R. Comparative toxicity of oleic and linoleic acid on human lymphocytes. *Life Sci.* **2006**, *78*, 1448–1456. [CrossRef]
50. Martin, C.R.; Dasilva, D.A.; Cluette-Brown, J.E.; Dimonda, C.; Hamill, A.; Bhutta, A.Q.; Coronel, E.; Wilschanski, M.; Stephens, A.J.; Driscoll, D.F.; et al. Decreased postnatal docosahexaenoic and arachidonic acid blood levels in premature infants are associated with neonatal morbidities. *J. Pediatr.* **2011**, *159*, 743–749.e2. [CrossRef]
51. Lofqvist, C.A.; Najm, S.; Hellgren, G.; Engstrom, E.; Savman, K.; Nilsson, A.K.; Andersson, M.X.; Hard, A.L.; Smith, L.E.H.; Hellstrom, A. Association of retinopathy of prematurity with low levels of arachidonic acid: A secondary analysis of a randomized clinical trial. *JAMA Ophthalmol.* **2018**, *136*, 271–277. [CrossRef]
52. Singh, P.; Ochoa-Allemant, P.; Brown, J.; Perides, G.; Freedman, S.D.; Martin, C.R. Effect of polyunsaturated fatty acids on postnatal ileum development using the fat-1 transgenic mouse model. *Pediatr. Res.* **2019**, *85*, 556–565. [CrossRef] [PubMed]

53. Najm, S.; Lofqvist, C.; Hellgren, G.; Engstrom, E.; Lundgren, P.; Hard, A.L.; Lapillonne, A.; Savman, K.; Nilsson, A.K.; Andersson, M.X.; et al. Effects of a lipid emulsion containing fish oil on polyunsaturated fatty acid profiles, growth and morbidities in extremely premature infants: A randomized controlled trial. *Clin. Nutr. ESPEN* **2017**, *20*, 17–23. [CrossRef] [PubMed]
54. Akinsulire, O.; Perides, G.; Anez-Bustillos, L.; Cluette-Brown, J.; Nedder, A.; Pollack, E.; Singh, P.; Liu, Y.; Sanchez-Fernandez, L.L.; Obregon, E.; et al. Early enteral administration of a complex lipid emulsion supplement prevents postnatal deficits in docosahexaenoic and arachidonic acids and increases tissue accretion of lipophilic nutrients in preterm piglets. *JPEN J. Parenter. Enteral. Nutr.* **2020**, *44*, 69–79. [CrossRef]
55. Vegge, A.; Thymann, T.; Lauritzen, L.; Bering, S.B.; Wiinberg, B.; Sangild, P.T. Parenteral lipids and partial enteral nutrition affect hepatic lipid composition but have limited short term effects on formula-induced necrotizing enterocolitis in preterm piglets. *Clin. Nutr.* **2015**, *34*, 219–228. [CrossRef]
56. Wang, X.; Liu, F.; Wang, Y.M.; Xue, C.H.; Tang, Q.J. The modulation effect of triglyceride type and phospholipids type ω-3 LCPUFA on mice gut microbiota. *J. Biosci. Med.* **2017**, *5*, 11. [CrossRef]
57. Calder, P.C. Marine omega-3 fatty acids and inflammatory processes: Effects, mechanisms and clinical relevance. *Biochim. Biophys. Acta* **2015**, *1851*, 469–484. [CrossRef]
58. Marion-Letellier, R.; Savoye, G.; Beck, P.L.; Panaccione, R.; Ghosh, S. Polyunsaturated fatty acids in inflammatory bowel diseases: A reappraisal of effects and therapeutic approaches. *Inflamm. Bowel Dis.* **2013**, *19*, 650–661. [CrossRef]
59. John, S.; Luben, R.; Shrestha, S.S.; Welch, A.; Khaw, K.T.; Hart, A.R. Dietary n-3 polyunsaturated fatty acids and the aetiology of ulcerative colitis: A UK prospective cohort study. *Eur. J. Gastroenterol. Hepatol.* **2010**, *22*, 602–606. [CrossRef]
60. Barbosa, D.S.; Cecchini, R.; El Kadri, M.Z.; Rodriguez, M.A.; Burini, R.C.; Dichi, I. Decreased oxidative stress in patients with ulcerative colitis supplemented with fish oil omega-3 fatty acids. *Nutrition* **2003**, *19*, 837–842. [CrossRef]
61. Chan, S.S.; Luben, R.; Olsen, A.; Tjonneland, A.; Kaaks, R.; Lindgren, S.; Grip, O.; Bergmann, M.M.; Boeing, H.; Hallmans, G.; et al. Association between high dietary intake of the n-3 polyunsaturated fatty acid docosahexaenoic acid and reduced risk of Crohn's disease. *Aliment. Pharmacol. Ther.* **2014**, *39*, 834–842. [CrossRef] [PubMed]
62. Chan, S.S.; Hart, A.R. Commentary: The association between high dietary intake of docosahexaenoic acid and reduced risk of Crohn's disease–authors' reply. *Aliment. Pharmacol. Ther.* **2014**, *39*, 1332. [CrossRef] [PubMed]
63. Dichi, I.; Frenhane, P.; Dichi, J.B.; Correa, C.R.; Angeleli, A.Y.; Bicudo, M.H.; Rodrigues, M.A.; Victoria, C.R.; Burini, R.C. Comparison of omega-3 fatty acids and sulfasalazine in ulcerative colitis. *Nutrition* **2000**, *16*, 87–90. [CrossRef]
64. Lev-Tzion, R.; Griffiths, A.M.; Leder, O.; Turner, D. Omega 3 fatty acids (fish oil) for maintenance of remission in Crohn's disease. *Cochrane Database Syst. Rev.* **2014**. [CrossRef]
65. Feagan, B.G.; Sandborn, W.J.; Mittmann, U.; Bar-Meir, S.; D'Haens, G.; Bradette, M.; Cohen, A.; Dallaire, C.; Ponich, T.P.; McDonald, J.W.; et al. Omega-3 free fatty acids for the maintenance of remission in Crohn disease: The EPIC randomized controlled trials. *JAMA* **2008**, *299*, 1690–1697. [CrossRef]
66. Lu, J.; Jilling, T.; Li, D.; Caplan, M.S. Polyunsaturated fatty acid supplementation alters proinflammatory gene expression and reduces the incidence of necrotizing enterocolitis in a neonatal rat model. *Pediatr. Res.* **2007**, *61*, 427–432. [CrossRef]
67. Wijendran, V.; Brenna, J.T.; Wang, D.H.; Zhu, W.; Meng, D.; Ganguli, K.; Kothapalli, K.S.; Requena, P.; Innis, S.; Walker, W.A. Long-chain polyunsaturated fatty acids attenuate the IL-1beta-induced proinflammatory response in human fetal intestinal epithelial cells. *Pediatr. Res.* **2015**, *78*, 626–633. [CrossRef]
68. Whiting, C.V.; Bland, P.W.; Tarlton, J.F. Dietary n-3 polyunsaturated fatty acids reduce disease and colonic proinflammatory cytokines in a mouse model of colitis. *Inflamm. Bowel Dis.* **2005**, *11*, 340–349. [CrossRef]
69. Usami, M.; Muraki, K.; Iwamoto, M.; Ohata, A.; Matsushita, E.; Miki, A. Effect of eicosapentaenoic acid (EPA) on tight junction permeability in intestinal monolayer cells. *Clin. Nutr.* **2001**, *20*, 351–359. [CrossRef]
70. Ferrer, R.; Moreno, J.J. Role of eicosanoids on intestinal epithelial homeostasis. *Biochem. Pharmacol.* **2010**, *80*, 431–438. [CrossRef]
71. Li, Q.; Zhang, Q.; Wang, M.; Zhao, S.; Xu, G.; Li, J. n-3 polyunsaturated fatty acids prevent disruption of epithelial barrier function induced by proinflammatory cytokines. *Mol. Immunol.* **2008**, *45*, 1356–1365. [CrossRef]

72. Willemsen, L.E.; Koetsier, M.A.; Balvers, M.; Beermann, C.; Stahl, B.; van Tol, E.A. Polyunsaturated fatty acids support epithelial barrier integrity and reduce IL-4 mediated permeability in vitro. *Eur. J. Nutr.* **2008**, *47*, 183–191. [CrossRef] [PubMed]
73. Charpentier, C.; Chan, R.; Salameh, E.; Mbodji, K.; Ueno, A.; Coeffier, M.; Guerin, C.; Ghosh, S.; Savoye, G.; Marion-Letellier, R. Dietary n-3 PUFA may attenuate experimental colitis. *Mediat. Inflamm.* **2018**, *2018*, 8430614. [CrossRef] [PubMed]
74. Bento, A.F.; Claudino, R.F.; Dutra, R.C.; Marcon, R.; Calixto, J.B. Omega-3 fatty acid-derived mediators 17(R)-hydroxy docosahexaenoic acid, aspirin-triggered resolvin D1 and resolvin D2 prevent experimental colitis in mice. *J. Immunol.* **2011**, *187*, 1957–1969. [CrossRef] [PubMed]
75. Marcon, R.; Bento, A.F.; Dutra, R.C.; Bicca, M.A.; Leite, D.F.; Calixto, J.B. Maresin 1, a proresolving lipid mediator derived from omega-3 polyunsaturated fatty acids, exerts protective actions in murine models of colitis. *J. Immunol.* **2013**, *191*, 4288–4298. [CrossRef] [PubMed]
76. Cho, J.Y.; Chi, S.G.; Chun, H.S. Oral administration of docosahexaenoic acid attenuates colitis induced by dextran sulfate sodium in mice. *Mol. Nutr. Food Res.* **2011**, *55*, 239–246. [CrossRef]
77. Camuesco, D.; Comalada, M.; Concha, A.; Nieto, A.; Sierra, S.; Xaus, J.; Zarzuelo, A.; Galvez, J. Intestinal anti-inflammatory activity of combined quercitrin and dietary olive oil supplemented with fish oil, rich in EPA and DHA (n-3) polyunsaturated fatty acids, in rats with DSS-induced colitis. *Clin. Nutr.* **2006**, *25*, 466–476. [CrossRef] [PubMed]
78. Camuesco, D.; Galvez, J.; Nieto, A.; Comalada, M.; Rodriguez-Cabezas, M.E.; Concha, A.; Xaus, J.; Zarzuelo, A. Dietary olive oil supplemented with fish oil, rich in EPA and DHA (n-3) polyunsaturated fatty acids, attenuates colonic inflammation in rats with DSS-induced colitis. *J. Nutr.* **2005**, *135*, 687–694. [CrossRef]
79. Gobbetti, T.; Ducheix, S.; le Faouder, P.; Perez, T.; Riols, F.; Boue, J.; Bertrand-Michel, J.; Dubourdeau, M.; Guillou, H.; Perretti, M.; et al. Protective effects of n-6 fatty acids-enriched diet on intestinal ischaemia/reperfusion injury involve lipoxin A4 and its receptor. *Br. J. Pharmacol.* **2015**, *172*, 910–923. [CrossRef] [PubMed]
80. Dufton, N.; Perretti, M. Therapeutic anti-inflammatory potential of formyl-peptide receptor agonists. *Pharmacol. Ther.* **2010**, *127*, 175–188. [CrossRef]
81. Caplan, M.S.; Russell, T.; Xiao, Y.; Amer, M.; Kaup, S.; Jilling, T. Effect of polyunsaturated fatty acid (PUFA) supplementation on intestinal inflammation and necrotizing enterocolitis (NEC) in a neonatal rat model. *Pediatr. Res.* **2001**, *49*, 647–652. [CrossRef] [PubMed]
82. De Plaen, I.G.; Liu, S.X.; Tian, R.; Neequaye, I.; May, M.J.; Han, X.B.; Hsueh, W.; Jilling, T.; Lu, J.; Caplan, M.S. Inhibition of nuclear factor-kappaB ameliorates bowel injury and prolongs survival in a neonatal rat model of necrotizing enterocolitis. *Pediatr. Res.* **2007**, *61*, 716–721. [CrossRef]
83. Caplan, M.S.; Jilling, T. The role of polyunsaturated fatty acid supplementation in intestinal inflammation and neonatal necrotizing enterocolitis. *Lipids* **2001**, *36*, 1053–1057. [CrossRef] [PubMed]
84. Ohtsuka, Y.; Okada, K.; Yamakawa, Y.; Ikuse, T.; Baba, Y.; Inage, E.; Fujii, T.; Izumi, H.; Oshida, K.; Nagata, S.; et al. omega-3 fatty acids attenuate mucosal inflammation in premature rat pups. *J. Pediatr. Surg.* **2011**, *46*, 489–495. [CrossRef] [PubMed]
85. Akisu, M.; Baka, M.; Coker, I.; Kultursay, N.; Huseyinov, A. Effect of dietary n-3 fatty acids on hypoxia-induced necrotizing enterocolitis in young mice. n-3 fatty acids alter platelet-activating factor and leukotriene B4 production in the intestine. *Biol. Neonate* **1998**, *74*, 31–38. [CrossRef]
86. Smithers, L.G.; Gibson, R.A.; McPhee, A.; Makrides, M. Effect of long-chain polyunsaturated fatty acid supplementation of preterm infants on disease risk and neurodevelopment: A systematic review of randomized controlled trials. *Am. J. Clin. Nutr.* **2008**, *87*, 912–920. [CrossRef]
87. Fewtrell, M.S.; Abbott, R.A.; Kennedy, K.; Singhal, A.; Morley, R.; Caine, E.; Jamieson, C.; Cockburn, F.; Lucas, A. Randomized, double-blind trial of long-chain polyunsaturated fatty acid supplementation with fish oil and borage oil in preterm infants. *J. Pediatr.* **2004**, *144*, 471–479. [CrossRef]
88. Carlson, S.E.; Montalto, M.B.; Ponder, D.L.; Werkman, S.H.; Korones, S.B. Lower incidence of necrotizing enterocolitis in infants fed a preterm formula with egg phospholipids. *Pediatr. Res.* **1998**, *44*, 491–498. [CrossRef]
89. Zhang, P.; Lavoie, P.M.; Lacaze-Masmonteil, T.; Rhainds, M.; Marc, I. Omega-3 long-chain polyunsaturated fatty acids for extremely preterm infants: A systematic review. *Pediatrics* **2014**, *134*, 120–134. [CrossRef]
90. Fewtrell, M.S.; Morley, R.; Abbott, R.A.; Singhal, A.; Isaacs, E.B.; Stephenson, T.; MacFadyen, U.; Lucas, A. Double-blind, randomized trial of long-chain polyunsaturated fatty acid supplementation in formula fed to preterm infants. *Pediatrics* **2002**, *110*, 73–82. [CrossRef]

91. Innis, S.M.; Adamkin, D.H.; Hall, R.T.; Kalhan, S.C.; Lair, C.; Lim, M.; Stevens, D.C.; Twist, P.F.; Diersen-Schade, D.A.; Harris, C.L.; et al. Docosahexaenoic acid and arachidonic acid enhance growth with no adverse effects in preterm infants fed formula. *J. Pediatr.* **2002**, *140*, 547–554. [CrossRef] [PubMed]
92. Clandinin, M.T.; Van Aerde, J.E.; Merkel, K.L.; Harris, C.L.; Springer, M.A.; Hansen, J.W.; Diersen-Schade, D.A. Growth and development of preterm infants fed infant formulas containing docosahexaenoic acid and arachidonic acid. *J. Pediatr.* **2005**, *146*, 461–468. [CrossRef] [PubMed]
93. Henriksen, C.; Haugholt, K.; Lindgren, M.; Aurvag, A.K.; Ronnestad, A.; Gronn, M.; Solberg, R.; Moen, A.; Nakstad, B.; Berge, R.K.; et al. Improved cognitive development among preterm infants attributable to early supplementation of human milk with docosahexaenoic acid and arachidonic acid. *Pediatrics* **2008**, *121*, 1137–1145. [CrossRef] [PubMed]
94. Makrides, M.; Gibson, R.A.; McPhee, A.J.; Collins, C.T.; Davis, P.G.; Doyle, L.W.; Simmer, K.; Colditz, P.B.; Morris, S.; Smithers, L.G.; et al. Neurodevelopmental outcomes of preterm infants fed high-dose docosahexaenoic acid: A randomized controlled trial. *JAMA* **2009**, *301*, 175–182. [CrossRef]
95. Collins, C.T.; Gibson, R.A.; Makrides, M.; McPhee, A.J.; Sullivan, T.R.; Davis, P.G.; Thio, M.; Simmer, K.; Rajadurai, V.S.; Team, N.R.I. The N3RO trial: A randomised controlled trial of docosahexaenoic acid to reduce bronchopulmonary dysplasia in preterm infants < 29 weeks' gestation. *BMC Pediatr.* **2016**, *16*, 72. [CrossRef]
96. Collins, C.T.; Makrides, M.; McPhee, A.J.; Sullivan, T.R.; Davis, P.G.; Thio, M.; Simmer, K.; Rajadurai, V.S.; Travadi, J.; Berry, M.J.; et al. Docosahexaenoic acid and bronchopulmonary dysplasia in preterm infants. *N. Engl. J. Med.* **2017**, *376*, 1245–1255. [CrossRef]
97. Koning, N.; Kessen, S.F.; Van Der Voorn, J.P.; Appelmelk, B.J.; Jeurink, P.V.; Knippels, L.M.; Garssen, J.; Van Kooyk, Y. Human milk blocks DC-SIGN-pathogen interaction via MUC1. *Front. Immunol.* **2015**, *6*, 112. [CrossRef]
98. Yolken, R.H.; Peterson, J.A.; Vonderfecht, S.L.; Fouts, E.T.; Midthun, K.; Newburg, D.S. Human milk mucin inhibits rotavirus replication and prevents experimental gastroenteritis. *J. Clin. Investig.* **1992**, *90*, 1984–1991. [CrossRef]
99. Stevens, C.R.; Millar, T.M.; Clinch, J.G.; Kanczler, J.M.; Bodamyali, T.; Blake, D.R. Antibacterial properties of xanthine oxidase in human milk. *Lancet* **2000**, *356*, 829–830. [CrossRef]
100. Hanayama, R.; Tanaka, M.; Miwa, K.; Shinohara, A.; Iwamatsu, A.; Nagata, S. Identification of a factor that links apoptotic cells to phagocytes. *Nature* **2002**, *417*, 182–187. [CrossRef]
101. Miksa, M.; Wu, R.; Dong, W.; Das, P.; Yang, D.; Wang, P. Dendritic cell-derived exosomes containing milk fat globule epidermal growth factor-factor VIII attenuate proinflammatory responses in sepsis. *Shock* **2006**, *25*, 586–593. [CrossRef] [PubMed]
102. Cui, T.; Miksa, M.; Wu, R.; Komura, H.; Zhou, M.; Dong, W.; Wang, Z.; Higuchi, S.; Chaung, W.; Blau, S.A.; et al. Milk fat globule epidermal growth factor 8 attenuates acute lung injury in mice after intestinal ischemia and reperfusion. *Am. J. Respir. Crit. Care Med.* **2010**, *181*, 238–246. [CrossRef] [PubMed]
103. Matsuda, A.; Jacob, A.; Wu, R.; Zhou, M.; Nicastro, J.M.; Coppa, G.F.; Wang, P. Milk fat globule-EGF factor VIII in sepsis and ischemia-reperfusion injury. *Mol. Med.* **2011**, *17*, 126–133. [CrossRef]
104. Chogle, A.; Bu, H.F.; Wang, X.; Brown, J.B.; Chou, P.M.; Tan, X.D. Milk fat globule-EGF factor 8 is a critical protein for healing of dextran sodium sulfate-induced acute colitis in mice. *Mol. Med.* **2011**, *17*, 502–507. [CrossRef]
105. Bu, H.F.; Zuo, X.L.; Wang, X.; Ensslin, M.A.; Koti, V.; Hsueh, W.; Raymond, A.S.; Shur, B.D.; Tan, X.D. Milk fat globule-EGF factor 8/lactadherin plays a crucial role in maintenance and repair of murine intestinal epithelium. *J. Clin. Investig.* **2007**, *117*, 3673–3683. [CrossRef]
106. Ogg, S.L.; Weldon, A.K.; Dobbie, L.; Smith, A.J.; Mather, I.H. Expression of butyrophilin (Btn1a1) in lactating mammary gland is essential for the regulated secretion of milk-lipid droplets. *Proc. Natl. Acad. Sci. USA* **2004**, *101*, 10084–10089. [CrossRef]
107. Rhodes, D.A.; Reith, W.; Trowsdale, J. Regulation of Immunity by Butyrophilins. *Annu. Rev. Immunol.* **2016**, *34*, 151–172. [CrossRef]
108. Bhinder, G.; Allaire, J.M.; Garcia, C.; Lau, J.T.; Chan, J.M.; Ryz, N.R.; Bosman, E.S.; Graef, F.A.; Crowley, S.M.; Celiberto, L.S.; et al. Milk Fat globule membrane supplementation in formula modulates the neonatal gut microbiome and normalizes intestinal development. *Sci. Rep.* **2017**, *7*, 45274. [CrossRef]
109. Huang, S.; Wu, Z.; Liu, C.; Han, D.; Feng, C.; Wang, S.; Wang, J. Milk fat globule membrane supplementation promotes neonatal growth and alleviates inflammation in low-birth-weight mice treated with lipopolysaccharide. *Biomed. Res. Int.* **2019**, *2019*, 4876078. [CrossRef]

110. Zhang, D.; Wen, J.; Zhou, J.; Cai, W.; Qian, L. Milk fat globule membrane ameliorates necrotizing enterocolitis in neonatal rats and suppresses lipopolysaccharide-induced inflammatory response in IEC-6 enterocytes. *JPEN J. Parenter. Enteral. Nutr.* **2019**, *43*, 863–873. [CrossRef]
111. Zavaleta, N.; Kvistgaard, A.S.; Graverholt, G.; Respicio, G.; Guija, H.; Valencia, N.; Lonnerdal, B. Efficacy of an MFGM-enriched complementary food in diarrhea, anemia, and micronutrient status in infants. *J. Pediatr. Gastroenterol. Nutr.* **2011**, *53*, 561–568. [CrossRef] [PubMed]
112. Miyake, H.; Lee, C.; Chusilp, S.; Bhalla, M.; Li, B.; Pitino, M.; Seo, S.; O'Connor, D.L.; Pierro, A. Human breast milk exosomes attenuate intestinal damage. *Pediatr. Surg. Int.* **2020**, *36*, 155–163. [CrossRef] [PubMed]
113. Gao, R.; Zhang, R.; Qian, T.; Peng, X.; He, W.; Zheng, S.; Cao, Y.; Pierro, A.; Shen, C. A comparison of exosomes derived from different periods breast milk on protecting against intestinal organoid injury. *Pediatr. Surg. Int.* **2019**, *35*, 1363–1368. [CrossRef] [PubMed]
114. Matei, A.C.; Antounians, L.; Zani, A. Extracellular Vesicles as a potential therapy for neonatal conditions: State of the art and challenges in clinical translation. *Pharmaceutics* **2019**, *11*, 404. [CrossRef] [PubMed]
115. Martin, C.; Patel, M.; Williams, S.; Arora, H.; Brawner, K.; Sims, B. Human breast milk-derived exosomes attenuate cell death in intestinal epithelial cells. *Innate Immun.* **2018**, *24*, 278–284. [CrossRef] [PubMed]
116. Wang, X.; Yan, X.; Zhang, L.; Cai, J.; Zhou, Y.; Liu, H.; Hu, Y.; Chen, W.; Xu, S.; Liu, P.; et al. Identification and peptidomic profiling of exosomes in preterm human milk: Insights into necrotizing enterocolitis prevention. *Mol. Nutr. Food Res.* **2019**, *16*, 1801247. [CrossRef]
117. Norris, G.H.; Milard, M.; Michalski, M.C.; Blesso, C.N. Protective properties of milk sphingomyelin against dysfunctional lipid metabolism, gut dysbiosis, and inflammation. *J. Nutr. Biochem.* **2019**, *73*, 108224. [CrossRef]
118. Nilsson, A. Role of sphingolipids in infant gut health and immunity. *J. Pediatr.* **2016**, *173*, S53–S59. [CrossRef]
119. Zhang, Y.; Cheng, Y.; Hansen, G.H.; Niels-Christiansen, L.L.; Koentgen, F.; Ohlsson, L.; Nilsson, A.; Duan, R.D. Crucial role of alkaline sphingomyelinase in sphingomyelin digestion: A study on enzyme knockout mice. *J. Lipid Res.* **2011**, *52*, 771–781. [CrossRef]
120. Nilsson, A. The presence of spingomyelin- and ceramide-cleaving enzymes in the small intestinal tract. *Biochim. Biophys. Acta* **1969**, *176*, 339–347. [CrossRef]
121. Wu, J.; Nilsson, A.; Jonsson, B.A.; Stenstad, H.; Agace, W.; Cheng, Y.; Duan, R.D. Intestinal alkaline sphingomyelinase hydrolyses and inactivates platelet-activating factor by a phospholipase C activity. *Biochem. J.* **2006**, *394*, 299–308. [CrossRef]
122. Andersson, D.; Kotarsky, K.; Wu, J.; Agace, W.; Duan, R.D. Expression of alkaline sphingomyelinase in yeast cells and anti-inflammatory effects of the expressed enzyme in a rat colitis model. *Dig. Dis. Sci.* **2009**, *54*, 1440–1448. [CrossRef]
123. Duan, R.D.; Cheng, Y.; Jonsson, B.A.; Ohlsson, L.; Herbst, A.; Hellstrom-Westas, L.; Nilsson, A. Human meconium contains significant amounts of alkaline sphingomyelinase, neutral ceramidase, and sphingolipid metabolites. *Pediatr. Res.* **2007**, *61*, 61–66. [CrossRef]
124. Norris, G.H.; Jiang, C.; Ryan, J.; Porter, C.M.; Blesso, C.N. Milk sphingomyelin improves lipid metabolism and alters gut microbiota in high fat diet-fed mice. *J. Nutr. Biochem.* **2016**, *30*, 93–101. [CrossRef]
125. Miklavcic, J.J.; Schnabl, K.L.; Mazurak, V.C.; Thomson, A.B.; Clandinin, M.T. Dietary ganglioside reduces proinflammatory signaling in the intestine. *J. Nutr. Metab.* **2012**, *2012*, 280286. [CrossRef]
126. Schnabl, K.L.; Larsen, B.; Van Aerde, J.E.; Lees, G.; Evans, M.; Belosevic, M.; Field, C.; Thomson, A.B.; Clandinin, M.T. Gangliosides protect bowel in an infant model of necrotizing enterocolitis by suppressing proinflammatory signals. *J. Pediatr. Gastroenterol. Nutr.* **2009**, *49*, 382–392. [CrossRef] [PubMed]
127. Park, E.J.; Suh, M.; Thomson, B.; Thomson, A.B.; Ramanujam, K.S.; Clandinin, M.T. Dietary ganglioside decreases cholesterol content, caveolin expression and inflammatory mediators in rat intestinal microdomains. *Glycobiology* **2005**, *15*, 935–942. [CrossRef] [PubMed]
128. Park, E.J.; Suh, M.; Thomson, B.; Ma, D.W.; Ramanujam, K.; Thomson, A.B.; Clandinin, M.T. Dietary ganglioside inhibits acute inflammatory signals in intestinal mucosa and blood induced by systemic inflammation of Escherichia coli lipopolysaccharide. *Shock* **2007**, *28*, 112–117. [CrossRef]
129. Rueda, R.; Sabatel, J.L.; Maldonado, J.; Molina-Font, J.A.; Gil, A. Addition of gangliosides to an adapted milk formula modifies levels of fecal Escherichia coli in preterm newborn infants. *J. Pediatr.* **1998**, *133*, 90–94. [CrossRef]

130. Calder, P.C. Functional roles of fatty acids and their effects on human health. *JPEN J. Parenter. Enteral. Nutr.* **2015**, *39*, 18S–32S. [CrossRef]
131. Koletzko, B.; Bergmann, K.; Brenna, J.T.; Calder, P.C.; Campoy, C.; Clandinin, M.T.; Colombo, J.; Daly, M.; Decsi, T.; Demmelmair, H.; et al. Should formula for infants provide arachidonic acid along with DHA? A position paper of the European Academy of Paediatrics and the Child Health Foundation. *Am. J Clin. Nutr.* **2020**, *111*, 10–16. [CrossRef]

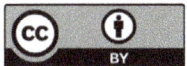

© 2020 by the authors. Licensee MDPI, Basel, Switzerland. This article is an open access article distributed under the terms and conditions of the Creative Commons Attribution (CC BY) license (http://creativecommons.org/licenses/by/4.0/).

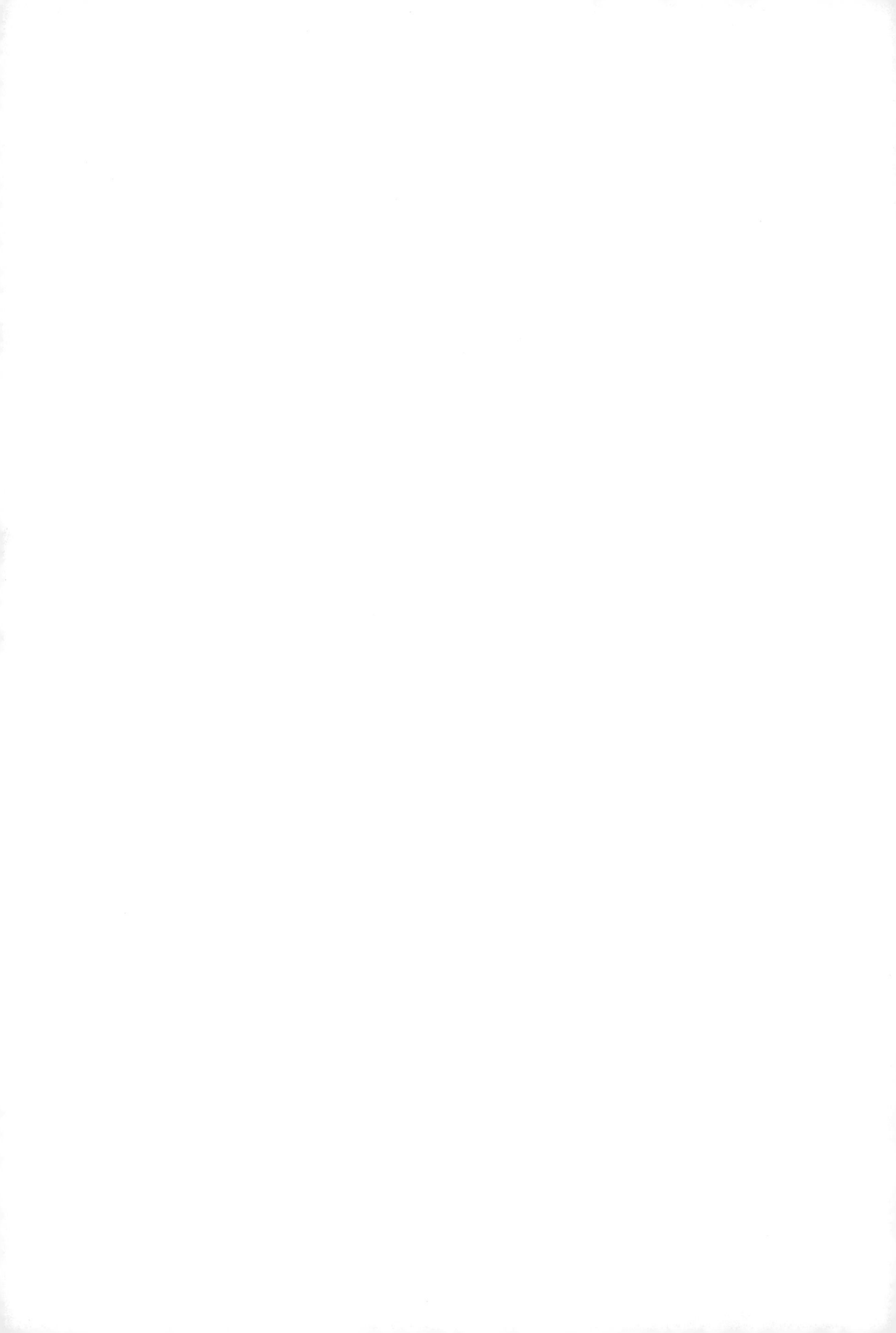

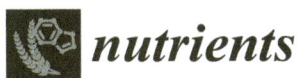 

Review

# The Role of Glycosaminoglycans in Protection from Neonatal Necrotizing Enterocolitis: A Narrative Review

Kathryn Burge, Erynn Bergner, Aarthi Gunasekaran, Jeffrey Eckert and Hala Chaaban *

Department of Pediatrics, Division of Neonatology, University of Oklahoma Health Sciences Center, 1200 North Everett Dr., ETNP7504, Oklahoma City, OK 73104, USA; Kathryn-Burge@ouhsc.edu (K.B.); Erynn-Bergner@ouhsc.edu (E.B.); Aarthi-Gunasekaran@ouhsc.edu (A.G.); Jeffrey-Eckert@ouhsc.edu (J.E.)
* Correspondence: Hala-Chaaban@ouhsc.edu; Tel.: +1-405-271-5215

Received: 21 January 2020; Accepted: 16 February 2020; Published: 20 February 2020

**Abstract:** Necrotizing enterocolitis, a potentially fatal intestinal inflammatory disorder affecting primarily premature infants, is a significant cause of morbidity and mortality in neonates. While the etiology of the disease is, as yet, unknown, a number of risk factors for the development of necrotizing enterocolitis have been identified. One such risk factor, formula feeding, has been shown to contribute to both increased incidence and severity of the disease. The protective influences afforded by breastfeeding are likely attributable to the unique composition of human milk, an extremely potent, biologically active fluid. This review brings together knowledge on the pathogenesis of necrotizing enterocolitis and current thinking on the instrumental role of one of the more prominent classes of bioactive components in human breast milk, glycosaminoglycans.

**Keywords:** necrotizing enterocolitis; inflammation; neonatal; intestine; prematurity; human milk; glycosaminoglycans

## 1. Introduction

Necrotizing enterocolitis (NEC) is a common intestinal inflammatory disorder developing during the neonatal period. The disease progresses rapidly from subtle abdominal distension to necrosis, intestinal perforation, multi-organ failure, and, in severe cases, death [1,2]. Because of better survivorship among the smallest premature infants [3], as well as a dearth of treatments for the disease [4], the incidence and health burden of NEC have only grown in recent decades [1]. Mortality rates often approach 30% in infants born less than 1500 g, and range higher in those babies requiring surgical intervention [1]. Infants surviving NEC often suffer from long-term morbidities related to both the disease and its treatment, including neurodevelopmental delays, retinopathy, and short-bowel syndrome [5,6].

Although the exact etiology of the disease is still unclear [7], a number of risk factors have been identified. These include, among others, prematurity and low birthweight status, developmental immaturity of both the intestine and immune system, inappropriate microbial colonization of the gut, and formula feeding [8]. What few advances have been made in NEC treatment recently revolve around the growing understanding of the importance of optimal infant nutrition, particularly that provided by human breast milk (HM), sourced either from the mother or a donor [5,9,10].

HM functions in several critical biological roles in neonates, including support for intestinal development and maturation, protection against pathogens, and basic dietary sustenance for growth [9,11]. In babies fed exclusively HM, enteric infections are reduced by approximately 50% compared to infants fed bovine-based formula [12,13]. In the preterm population specifically, infants fed exclusively HM, as opposed to at least partial bovine-based feedings, experience significant reductions in morbidity and mortality [14]. In very low birthweight (VLBW, <1500 g) infants, feedings composed of at least 50% HM in the first two weeks of life correlate with a six-fold decrease in the incidence of NEC [15]. Additional studies [16–18] have also indicated HM, particularly that sourced from the biological mother, reduces the incidence and severity of NEC in preterm infants. Donor milk, while arguably preferable to bovine-based formula [19], loses effectiveness through the pasteurization process, and is also not age-matched to the developmental stage of the infant to whom it is donated [20,21]. Thus, studies utilizing donor HM have shown mixed results when examining utility in protection against preterm pathogens, NEC, and mortality [22–24].

This narrative [25,26] review briefly summarizes what is known about the pathogenesis of NEC in premature infants, and expands upon the potential role of glycosaminoglycans, bioactive components of HM, in protection from NEC.

## 2. Pathogenesis of Necrotizing Enterocolitis

The pathogenesis of NEC appears to be highly complex and multifactorial. Data predominantly implicate developmental immaturity of the intestinal immune system [27], as well as an altered microbiome [28,29], in the development of a dysfunctional intestinal barrier [30] in necrotizing enterocolitis. While the sequence of events in NEC etiology remains unclear, the disease is likely initiated by an excessive stimulation of toll-like receptor 4 (TLR4) by Gram-negative bacteria [31] in the ileum of the premature infant. Activation of this receptor [32–38] leads to extensive inflammation, denoted by apoptosis of enterocytes along the luminal border, impaired replacement of these enterocytes, increased release of proinflammatory cytokines and chemokines, and, in total, breakdown of the intestinal barrier [39–41]. This impaired intestinal barrier allows for greater bacterial translocation [42], leading to increased inflammation via direct contact of pathogenic bacterial antigens with the mucosal immune system [43]. Neutrophil recruitment to the intestinal border and production of reactive oxygen species (ROS) further contributes to this inflammation [1,44,45]. TLR4 activation of the underlying endothelium initiates microvascular complications, including a reduction in endothelial nitric oxide synthase (eNOS), resulting in intestinal ischemia and necrosis [38,46,47]. Altogether, a positive feedback loop of inflammation is created, overwhelming any counterregulatory attempts by the host. Inflammation spreads systemically, leading to full-blown NEC and complications in organs as distant as the brain [48]. Our understanding of the clinical picture in NEC is muddied by a lack of appropriate animal models through which researchers can replicate most aspects of the human condition, and subsequent inability to translate findings in these animal models to the bedside. In particular, our limited understanding of the immature innate and adaptive immune systems and developing microbiome, and potential interplay of these two factors, hinders abilities to target effective treatments for NEC.

*2.1. Developmental Immaturity*

2.1.1. Innate Immune System

The innate immune system in the small intestine is comprised of both a physical barrier of intestinal epithelial cells (IECs) and their biochemical products, and an underlying and complementary immunological barrier [49]. The physical barrier is often considered to include intestinal alkaline phosphatase, a loose layer of mucus [50], tight junctions linking IECs, and antimicrobial proteins (AMPs) released by a specialized lineage of IECs, Paneth cells [51].

A number of developmental differences in IECs and the innate intestinal immune system have been associated with the pathogenesis of NEC. For example, goblet cell numbers and levels of their signature mucin, Muc2, are reduced in both mouse models and premature human infants with NEC [32], likely associated with developmental immaturity of the ileum [52]. Reductions in goblet cell numbers are thought to contribute to increased severity and incidence of NEC [52,53], potentially due to increased levels of bacterial translocation across an epithelium now inadequately guarded by mucus [53,54]. In addition, Paneth cells in premature infants are deficient both in number and function [55], altering the levels of lysozyme and defensins [56,57] and likely contributing to the development of NEC via associated changes in the microbiome [58].

Immune cells in the intestines of premature infants often appear to function differently than those of term neonates and adults, predisposing these infants to the development of NEC. Neutrophils, first responders to tissue injury, demonstrate impaired phagocytic ability, increased oxidative burst products, and variable cytokine production in premature infants compared to term babies [59]. Intestinal macrophages in preterm infants appear to be hyperreactive and produce excessive proinflammatory cytokines [60–62]. In addition, dendritic cell morphology and functionality in preterm neonates appears to differ from that of term babies [63], and in a mouse model of experimental NEC, the recruitment of dendritic cells to the luminal border directly disrupts intestinal barrier function [64].

Alterations in inflammatory signaling also predispose premature infants to the development of NEC by creating a host environment hyperreactive to both commensal and pathogenic organisms [33,65]. TLR4, specifically, is thought to play a crucial role in NEC [66] due to its abnormally increased expression in prematurity, both in mice and human infants [67,68]. Increased TLR4 expression appears to precede histological damage of the intestine in mouse NEC models, strongly implicating a role for TLR4 in the pathogenesis of the disease [65,69].

2.1.2. Adaptive Immune System

Adaptive immunity in the small intestine, thought to be less effective than innate immunity in a newborn [70], is dependent upon antigen-presenting cells (APC), primarily dendritic cells and IECs. A number of differences in adaptive immune function exist in infants with NEC, many of which are likely a developmental artifact of prematurity. Levels of secretory immunoglobulin A (sIgA), an antibody produced by lamina propia B cells and recognized for its ability to maintain the microbiome by neutralizing pathogenic bacteria [71], are reduced in premature infants compared to term babies [72,73], with clear implications for the development of NEC. Additionally, a significant role for T cells in the pathogenesis of NEC is becoming increasingly evident. For example, mice lacking functional T and B cells are less susceptible to NEC, but transfer of functional T cells to these animals increases susceptibility to the disease [34].

Intraepithelial lymphocytes (IELs), regulators and initiators of both innate and adaptive immune responses to bacterial invasion [74], are dispersed within the intestinal epithelium [41]. The γδ subset of IELs, created during embryogenesis, are more reactive in the neonate than in the adult [75], and preterm infants with NEC show significantly lower levels of these specialized T cells compared to healthy preterm babies [76]. Regulatory T cells (Tregs), T cells modulating the immune response and promoting tolerogenicity, are decreased in both experimental mouse [34] and human [77] NEC. In neonates, baseline levels of the Treg inhibitor STAT3 (signal transducer and activator of transcription 3) are increased compared to those of adults [34]. In a mouse model of NEC, when a STAT3 inhibitor is introduced, levels of Tregs increase and NEC severity is reduced [34].

Finally, T helper (Th) cell differentiation also appears to be dysregulated during NEC. In particular, Th17 cells, characterized by production of the inflammatory interleukin 17A (IL-17A) cytokine, have been shown to be upregulated in both murine and human NEC, and are thought to play a role in intestinal barrier dysfunction [34]. In an experimental model of NEC, mice treated with all-trans retinoic acid (ATRA), an inhibitor of Th17 differentiation [78], showed lower levels of Th17 cells, increased populations of Tregs, and reduced NEC severity [34,79]. Interestingly, retinoic acid is produced endogenously by IECs, but this production is thought to be largely dictated by luminal commensal bacteria [80].

2.2. Dysbiosis

Colonization of the infant intestine, previously thought to commence at birth, may originate in the placenta [81], where the fetus is possibly surrounded by non-sterile amniotic fluid [82], though this finding has been recently debated [83,84]. The main event responsible for infant intestinal colonization, however, is likely birth [85]. Vaginal delivery of term infants results in initial colonization with predominantly aerobic bacteria, including *Streptococcus*, *Staphylococcus*, and *Lactobacillus* [86]. As these aerobic bacteria consume oxygen, the microbiome shifts to reflect greater populations of facultative anaerobes, followed by strict anaerobes such as Clostridia and Bifidobacteria species [87,88]. These obligate anaerobes produce short-chain fatty acids (SCFAs), anti-inflammatory lipids known to regulate epithelial and immune cell development in the gut [89], and protect against the proliferation of pathogenic bacteria [90]. In preterm infants, the development of the intestinal microbiome following birth appears to follow a reasonably predictable progression from Bacilli to Gammaproteobacteria to Clostridia [91]. The resulting intestinal population in preterm infants is characterized by lower diversity, fewer species numbers, and a greater proportion of pathogenic bacteria, many of which could initiate the TLR4 signaling cascade via lipopolysaccharide (LPS), compared to that of infants born at term [92–95]. This errant microbiome in the premature infant, together with an immature intestinal immune system, presents a mechanism for hyperinflammation and deterioration of the critical intestinal barrier.

Dysbiosis can refer to improper proportions of microbial species, as well as a lack of diversity and richness of species overall [96]. A skewed microbiome can also result from the gain or loss of critical microbial populations, often negatively affecting the functionality of both the intestine and its interwoven immune system. An appropriate microbiome is thought to be indispensable in triggering the maturation of the mucosal immune system in the gut [97]. Support for the role of dysbiosis in NEC is largely derived from studies in germ-free animals, in which the disease cannot be reproduced [98–100]. Additionally, factors indirectly influencing microbial colonization in the infant, such as antibiotic use in the mother [67], can increase NEC development risk in the infant. While a single pathogen is not thought to induce NEC, a series of microbial shifts in the microbiome has been associated with development of the disease [28], and these changes usually precede diagnosis [101], implicating a potential role for dysbiosis in the pathogenesis of NEC. For example, infants with NEC often have reduced populations of Bifidobacteria, Bacteroidetes, and Firmicutes anaerobes, particularly Negativicutes, and increased levels of Proteobacteria and Actinobacteria [28,101–105]. This reduction in anaerobes in NEC leads to a decline in the production of protective SCFAs [7,103,104], a further complication of NEC-associated dysbiosis. Generally, the microbiome of infants developing NEC appears to be characterized by reductions in both species richness and diversity [95,106,107], though not all studies have noted these trends [101,105,108].

A number of factors beyond prematurity can influence the microbial colonization of the infant intestine. The use of antibiotics, rampant in the premature infant population [109,110], is known to increase the risk of NEC development, with risk correlating strongly to duration of treatment [111,112]. Antibiotic exposure in neonates may lead to increases in Proteobacteria, decreases in Actinobacteria, and, as with all antibiotic usage, inadvertent selection for antibiotic-resistant strains [85,113–115]. Mode of delivery also strongly influences the development of the infant microbiome. Babies born via caesarean section are often colonized by increased populations of *Clostridium* and *Staphylococcus* and decreased levels of *Bifidobacterium* and *Bacteroides* compared to infants born vaginally [102,116,117]. Antacid use, particularly histamine-2 ($H_2$) blockers, can disrupt the acid-base balance in the premature intestine [118], predisposing the infant to NEC [119,120] by favoring populations of Proteobacteria over those of Firmicutes [121,122]. Even endogenous factors may affect the relative proportions of intestinal colonizers. For example, Paneth cell lysozyme and defensin secretion patterns, altered in premature infants [56,57], can lead to irregular microbial colonization in infants [58,123]. Finally, mode of feeding can direct the development of the neonatal microbiome. HM contains a microbiome of its own [124], likely specialized for the infant with whom it is associated [125,126], and thus may be uniquely protective. While breastfeeding stimulates the expansion of *Bifidobacterium*, in particular, and inhibits the growth of pathogenic bacteria [127,128], formula feeding often leads to a slightly more diverse assemblage of Enterobacteriaceae, *Bacteroides*, *Lactobacillus*, *Prevotella*, and, especially, *Clostridium* [87,129–131]. A number of biological components of HM are thought to help shape the development of the infant microbiome, as well as prime intestinal immune development and maturation.

## 3. Glycosaminoglycans in Milk

HM is a complex mixture of biologically active molecules known to play a role in infant nutrition, protection from pathogens, and development and maturation of the intestinal immune system. The composition of HM is not static, changing over time to meet the needs of a growing infant. Colostrum, the first milk, is high in minerals, vitamins, hormones, and growth factors [132]. Transitional milk replaces colostrum at approximately one week postpartum, and is high in fat and lactose [133]. Finally, mature milk follows at two weeks postpartum, consisting largely of water and nutritional macronutrients necessary for infant growth [134]. All stages of HM, however, contain various compounds necessary for development of the microbiome and protection of the infant from pathogens. For example, oligosaccharides, commonly referred to as human milk oligosaccharides (HMOS), are found in large quantities in HM and are largely unabsorbed, serving as prebiotics for commensal gut bacteria [5], thereby bolstering and developing the innate immune system and microbiome in neonates [135,136]. HM also contains immunoglobulins, such as sIga, which potentially serve as prebiotics capable of assisting in the proper colonization of the newborn gut [137] while inhibiting growth of pathogenic bacteria [138]. Glycosaminoglycans (GAGs), a class of polysaccharides found in the extracellular matrix and outer surface of cells, are also prevalent in HM. Our understanding of the potential functions of this class of molecules is still evolving, but their elevated concentrations in early HM and a number of studies indicating protective capabilities of these molecules against pathogens may indicate importance in the prevention of NEC.

GAGs, molecules composed of repeating, often highly sulfated disaccharides, include heparin, heparan sulfate (HS), keratan sulfate (KS), hyaluronic acid (HA), chondroitin sulfate (CS), and dermatan sulfate (DS) [139]. In HM, these GAGs, with the exception of HA, are bound to a protein core and expressed as proteoglycans [140]. HA, uniquely, is neither sulfated nor assembled bound to a protein core [141]. Once in the small intestine, pancreatic enzymes digest the proteins, resulting in free GAGs (Figure 1a). Due to a lack of endogenous host enzymes in the small intestine capable of further breaking down free GAGs [142], these molecules remain largely undigested through the majority of the gastrointestinal tract [143], with eventual breakdown likely occurring in the cecum or colon [142]. In the case of HA, and potentially other GAGs, the resulting fragment sizes, whether created by endogenous breakdown of the parent molecule or intentional supplementation of a specific molecular weight, may differ vastly in function [144,145].

The composition of GAGs in milk differs greatly depending upon the source. In term HM, GAGs, in sum, are approximately seven times more prevalent than in bovine milk, the basis of most infant formulas [146]. Coppa et al. [146] determined, via a variety of methods, that large differences in GAG relative composition also exist between the two milks (Figure 1b). CS accounts for 55% of the term HM GAGs compared to only 21% of GAGs in bovine milk, but because of the reduced total quantity of GAGs in bovine milk, this amounts to nearly 23 times as much CS in term human compared to bovine milk. Term HM also has substantially higher levels of heparin (173 mg/L compared to 21 mg/L) and HA (5 mg/L compared to 2 mg/L) and lower levels of DS (7 mg/L compared to 24 mg/L) than bovine milk, though, interestingly, bovine milk is higher in HA by percentage (4.5% compared to 1.3%). Additionally, GAGs present in term HM appear to be generally less sulfated compared with those in bovine milk [146], though any impact of this difference on the infant has not been explored.

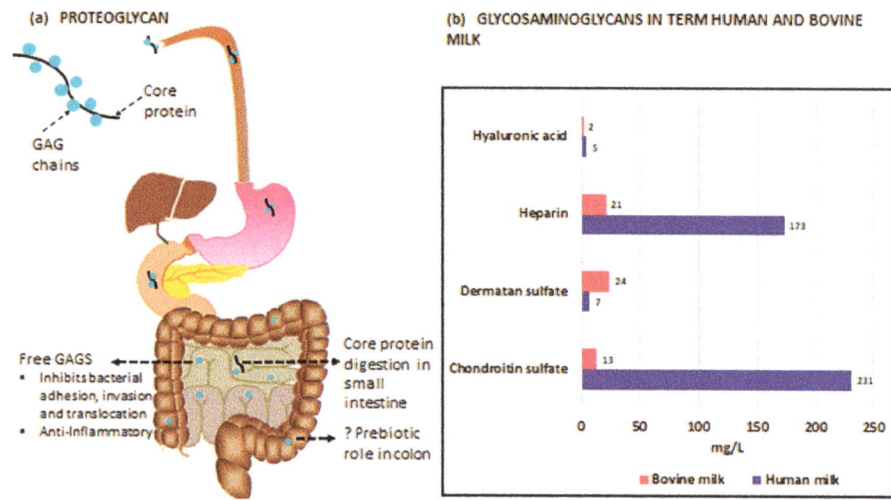

**Figure 1.** Glycosaminoglycans, found in much greater quantities in human breast milk (HM), traverse the intestines largely untouched: (**a**) Digestion and potential function of glycosaminoglycan-associated proteoglycans in milk. (**b**) Comparison of total glycosaminoglycan content of term human and bovine milk. GAG: glycosaminoglycan; GAGS: glycosaminoglycans.

A disparity in bioavailability also appears to exist between human and bovine milk. Maccari et al. [143] compared the residual GAG content of the feces of term infants fed either HM or formula, and noted significantly lower recovery of HM GAGs compared to those from formula, indicating a much greater utilization of the GAGs derived from HM. In addition, a greater proportion of highly sulfated GAGs, present at higher levels in bovine milk compared to HM, appeared in the feces of both groups, potentially suggesting an inability of distal intestinal bacteria to catabolize these compounds [147]. Differences in milk glycosaminoglycan composition, overall quantity, and bioavailability may underly some of the protective effects of breastfeeding with regard to NEC pathogenesis.

Notably, gestational age of the infant at birth and stage of lactation have prominent influences on the GAG composition of HM. Coppa et al. [148] demonstrated that while preterm and term HM have consistent proportions of the two foremost GAGs, chondroitin sulfate and heparin, the total GAG content is approximately three times higher in preterm milk. The respective percentages of CS and heparin are maintained as total GAG levels vary over the first month of lactation, with peak levels of GAGs on day 4 of colostrum (9.3 g/L and 3.8 g/L in preterm and term HM, respectively) and a subsequent decline to the end of the month (4.3 g/L and 0.4 g/L in preterm and term HM, respectively). Interestingly, 50% (preterm) and 73% (term) of this reduction in GAG content is noted to occur between days 4 and 10 [148]. Wang et al. [149] have established this progressive decrease of HM GAG content occurs through at least the first six months of lactation. Additionally, differences in the degree of sulfation occur during the lactation period, with HS sulfation increasing slightly over the first six months and CS sulfation peaking at day 43 before subsequently declining [149]. While the physiological rationale underlying GAG sulfation variability during the breastfeeding period has not yet been appreciated, these changes in sulfation patterns are likely functionally significant [150].

Maternal characteristics may also alter both the GAG composition of HM and the ability of the infant, indirectly, to break down those GAGs in the distal intestine. While Volpi et al. [151] did not find GAG compositional changes among milk samples from mothers of varying ethnicities, Mannello et al. [152] noted maternal health could directly influence GAG composition, as alterations in the structure and sulfation levels of CS in the milk of a breast affected by invasive carcinoma differed with those in the unaffected breast of the same mother. Finally, Cerdó et al. [153] have established that the microbiome of infants born to obese mothers is more capable of glycosaminoglycan degradation compared with that of infants born to mothers of normal weight, with unspecified effects on the risk of developing NEC. Further investigation into the potential impact of maternal obesity on GAG content of HM and the ability of infants born to obese mothers to utilize HM GAGs would be of interest.

The utility of donor milk as a suitable substitute for formula has often been questioned, particularly given the pasteurization process is known to reduce the bioactivity and concentration of critical immunoglobulins, growth factors, and digestive enzymes [19]. HM contains active glycosidases, enzymes capable of degrading glycoconjugates such as glycosaminoglycans in a time- and temperature-dependent manner; however, these enzymes are unlikely to significantly alter the composition of GAGs in donor milk, as little breakdown in glycoconjugates is seen with storage at 37 °C for up to 16 h [154]. Additionally, Coscia et al. [155] subjected donor milk samples to Holder pasteurization, a method often utilized by milk banks, and noted the concentration and proportions of HM GAGs are not significantly altered by the process. Thus, the current preference for donor milk over formula may be warranted in this context, especially in at-risk, preterm infants, as GAG concentrations and relative proportions remain largely unaffected by common storage and processing techniques.

## 4. Glycosaminoglycan Protection against NEC

In the small intestine, GAGs are believed to participate in a number of biological processes, including molecular trafficking, maturation, and differentiation of a variety of cell types, modulation of inflammatory events, structural support, and adhesion to bacteria in the intestinal lumen [156–159]. Importantly, GAG incorporation into the extracellular matrix and epithelial cell surface is thought to be essential to a functional intestinal barrier [160]. Inflammation, particularly driven by proinflammatory cytokine release, has been shown to disrupt endogenous production of sulfated GAGs [161]. In NEC, impaired distribution of intestinal GAGs appears to mirror the patchy, skip lesion nature of the disease [162]. While GAGs are not digested and incorporated into small intestinal tissue [143], their supplementation through HM or other means may still provide significant benefits to the neonatal small intestinal epithelium through their interaction with the epithelial surface or luminal contents [163], especially in the context of their potential loss during inflammation. These extracellular interactions of GAGs with IECs or luminal bacteria likely contribute substantially to the protective effects of HM against NEC. While the precise function of GAGs in HM is incompletely understood (Figure 2), studies attributing protective effects to individual GAGs, sourced either from HM extractions or biosynthetic preparations, are accumulating, with the large majority focusing on CS, HA, and heparin.

Generally, GAGs are believed to exhibit antiviral and antibacterial properties [164]. HA has been demonstrated to inhibit bacterial growth [165,166], and is a common matrix component of bioengineered orthopedic scaffolding because of this bacteriostatic property. HM GAGs may also influence the composition of the neonatal microbiome beyond growth constraints applied to certain microbial species, resulting in a wide variety of potential physiological effects. Recently, several species of human commensal bacteria, including strains associated with common probiotic formulas, have been shown to actively degrade host GAGs in the intestine [167], lending some credence to the idea that HM or formula-supplemented GAGs could act as prebiotics [168], promoting the growth of only those commensal species outfitted with the enzymes necessary to metabolize these compounds. While these prebiotic effects would be far more likely to affect the distal intestine as opposed to the ileum, the ramifications of this potential GAG influence on the microbiome in total may include changes in NEC susceptibility and require further investigation.

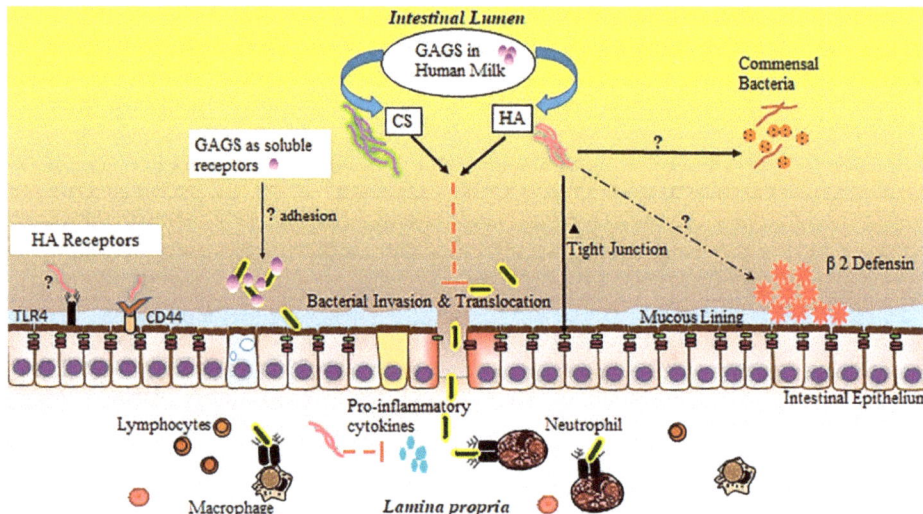

**Figure 2.** Schematic of potential glycosaminoglycan mechanisms of protection in necrotizing enterocolitis (NEC). CS: chondroitin sulfate; HA: hyaluronic acid; GAGS: glycosaminoglycans.

GAGs are also known to reduce microbial adhesion to IECs, often the initial step in infection. Sava et al. [169] pretreated Caco-2 colonocytes with a mixture of heparin, HS, and CS, reducing the capacity of Enterococci bacteria to adhere to the host cell surface. Hafez et al. [170] demonstrated similar findings with regard to Staphylococci adhesion to host epithelial cells in the presence of free GAGs. Treatment of HT-29 colorectal cells with heparin, a prominent GAG in HM, has also been shown to reduce internalization of a number of bacterial species via a reduction in cellular adhesion [171]. Antimicrobial characteristics of GAGs have also been shown to extend to those isolated directly from HM. For example, Newburg et al. [172] demonstrated CS or a CS-like compound extracted from HM can inhibit binding of the gp120 human immunodeficiency virus (HIV) envelope protein to its receptor, an essential early step in transmission of the virus. Coppa et al. [140] treated intestinal cell lines with GAGs extracted from HM and demonstrated a reduction in pathogenic bacterial binding of intestinal receptors, while Hill et al. [173] demonstrated the ability of HA 35 (biosynthetic HA of an intermediate 35 kDa size and with qualitatively similar effects to that of the inclusive HM HA fraction) to limit intestinal adhesion of *Salmonella* Typhimurium.

GAGs present in HM may also work synergistically with the host immune system to both upregulate endogenous defenses and tame the type of destructive, runaway inflammation characteristic of NEC [174]. HA fragments of varied sizes have been shown to have protective effects on the intestinal epithelium. Zheng et al. [175] noted exogenous administration of 750 kDa HA fragments ameliorated disease in a colitis mouse model through a TLR4- and cyclooxygenase-2 (COX-2)-dependent repair of the epithelium, while Riehl et al. [176] found similar protective effects in irradiated small intestinal tissue. HA of 900 kDa size has also been shown to protect the intestinal epithelium of immunocompromised mice through a reduction in inflammatory signaling [177]. Additionally, both HA 35 and a polydisperse HM HA extract upregulate the antimicrobial protein human β-defensin 2 (HβD2) in human intestinal epithelial cells and its ortholog in the murine large intestine [173,178].

Our group recently demonstrated the effectiveness of HA 35 in reducing the incidence and severity of disease in a mouse model of necrotizing enterocolitis. Gunasekaran et al. [179] treated mouse pups (age P14–16) with HA 35 (15 mg/kg or 30 mg/kg) once per day for three days prior to the initiation of NEC. NEC was induced using a two-hit model of intraperitoneal dithizone injection followed by oral administration of *Klebsiella pneumoniae* [55]. A stark reduction in proinflammatory cytokine release (tumor necrosis factor-alpha (TNF-α), GRO-α (growth-regulated oncogene-alpha), IL-12p70, and IL-6) was seen with HA 35 treatment (either dose) compared to untreated NEC. These changes, coupled with upregulation in tight junction proteins, likely led to the reduction in pathological intestinal permeability and associated bacteremia, ultimately resulting in significantly improved pathology of the ileum, substantially diminished disease severity, and significantly greater pup survival.

CS also exerts a number of well-documented effects on inflammation, including reductions in pro-inflammatory cytokine and NF-κB (nuclear factor kappa-light-chain-enhancer of activated B cells) levels [180], weakened COX-2 and NOS-2 (nitric oxide synthase-2) activities [181], and the upregulation of a variety of antioxidant enzymes [182]. CS has demonstrated positive impacts in intestinal bowel disease (IBD) [183,184], likely through anti-inflammatory effects [185] and increased epithelial and mucosal tissue repair [183]. The anti-inflammatory effects of heparin, including reductions in pro-inflammatory TNF-α and IL-6 signaling [186], have also been demonstrated in the context of intestinal inflammatory diseases. Often utilized as a first line of treatment in IBD [187], heparin, specifically low-molecular-weight or unfractionated heparin, has been shown to ameliorate disease activity through a combination of anti-inflammatory and anticoagulative effects [188], resulting in increased mucosal healing and improved intestinal barrier function [189].

Altogether, glycosaminoglycan-associated reduction in pathogen binding to host IECs, an upregulation in intestinal defenses by GAGs, and a reduction in excessive inflammatory signaling is likely to lead to an improvement in intestinal barrier function and a significant decline in bacterial invasion and translocation, critical events in the pathogenesis of NEC [190,191]. Hall et al. [192] established a line of goblet-like cells are more susceptible to invasion when bacteria are freely suspended in bovine-based formula compared to HM. Hill et al. [173] demonstrated a polydisperse HM HA extract is capable of protecting colonocytes from *Salmonella* infection in vitro. Mice treated with HA 35 are protected from *Citrobacter rodentium* infection via an upregulation in the critical tight junction protein, ZO-1 (zonula occludens-1), resulting in reduced intestinal permeability and inhibited bacterial translocation across colonic epithelium [193], similar to our findings in a murine NEC model [179].

Our group has also directly interrogated the ability of CS, the most common GAG in HM [146], to limit both bacterial invasion (Figure 3a) and translocation (Figure 3b) in T84 colonocyte monolayers, an in vitro model of the intestinal epithelium [194]. CS, at a concentration of 750 µg/mL given prophylactically for 48 h prior to bacterial challenge, reduces invasion and translocation of SCB34 *Escherichia coli*, an invasive, multi-drug resistant bacterial strain isolated from a neonatal early-onset sepsis case [195], by 75% compared to control. In this study, CS shows no effects on cell viability while also reducing, though not significantly, the production of the inflammatory chemokine, IL-8. Given the potent effects of GAGs on inflammation and prevention of infection, the availability of these compounds in HM, and potentially their supplementation in formula following further systematic review, may be critical to neonatal health in general, and specifically, in the prevention of NEC.

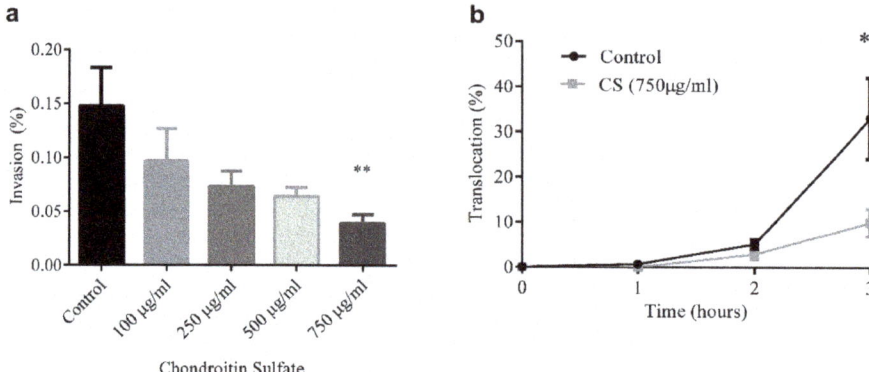

**Figure 3.** The effects of chondroitin sulfate on *E. coli* invasion and translocation of T84 colonocyte monolayers: (**a**) chondroitin sulfate (CS) was given prophylactically for 48 h prior to infection. A dose-dependent reduction in bacterial invasion occurred with CS (M ± SEM), with 750 µg/mL showing significantly lower bacterial invasion compared to control (** $p$ = 0.0071; eta-squared = 0.0944); (**b**) CS at 750 µg/mL was significantly protective by the third hour of inoculation (M ± SEM, ** $p$ = 0.0018). (Reprinted with permission of authors and SAGE Publishing [194]).

## 5. Conclusions

In this review, we assessed the GAG composition of sources of neonatal nutrition and relative changes across the duration of infant feeding, as well as summarized the potential protective effects of these GAGs against necrotizing enterocolitis. As common components of HM, GAGs are receiving increased attention because of their demonstrated antimicrobial and anti-inflammatory effects, and their potential to ameliorate intestinal inflammation and associated bacterial translocation of the epithelium. The protective effects on host barrier function, combined with beneficial interactions with, and positive influences on, luminal bacteria, likely serve to strengthen innate defenses against gastrointestinal infection in the neonate. Additional studies are needed to further characterize the effects of HM-derived GAGs on the intestinal epithelium, their interactions with specific bacteria, and their influence on the neonatal intestinal microbiome in full, particularly in the contexts of prematurity and NEC.

**Author Contributions:** All authors participated in the literature review. K.B. and E.B. wrote the manuscript. A.G. prepared the figures. J.E. and H.C. reviewed, edited, and revised the manuscript. All authors have read and agreed to the published version of the manuscript.

**Funding:** This research received funding from the National Institute of General Medical Sciences, grant number K08GM127308, provided to H.C.

**Acknowledgments:** The authors acknowledge support from the Division of Neonatology at the University of Oklahoma Health Sciences Center (OUHSC) and the National Institute of General Medical Sciences (K08GM127308).

**Conflicts of Interest:** The authors declare no conflict of interest. Funding played no role in the preparation of this manuscript.

## References

1. Neu, J.; Walker, W.A. Necrotizing Enterocolitis. *N. Engl. J. Med.* **2011**, *364*, 255–264. [CrossRef] [PubMed]
2. Tanner, S.M.; Berryhill, T.F.; Ellenburg, J.L.; Jilling, T.; Cleveland, D.S.; Lorenz, R.G.; Martin, C.A. Pathogenesis of necrotizing enterocolitis: Modeling the innate immune response. *Am. J. Pathol.* **2015**, *185*, 4–16. [CrossRef] [PubMed]
3. Victora, J.D.; Silveira, M.F.; Tonial, C.T.; Victora, C.G.; Barros, F.C.; Horta, B.L.; Santos, I.S.D.; Bassani, D.G.; Garcia, P.C.R.; Scheeren, M.; et al. Prevalence, mortality and risk factors associated with very low birth weight preterm infants: An analysis of 33 years. *J. Pediatr.* **2018**. [CrossRef] [PubMed]

4. Rich, B.S.; Dolgin, S.E. Necrotizing Enterocolitis. *Pediatr. Rev.* **2017**, *38*, 552–559. [CrossRef]
5. Bering, S.B. Human Milk Oligosaccharides to Prevent Gut Dysfunction and Necrotizing Enterocolitis in Preterm Neonates. *Nutrients* **2018**, *10*, 1461. [CrossRef]
6. Bhatia, J. Human milk and the premature infant. *Ann. Nutr. Metab.* **2013**, *62* (Suppl. 3), 8–14. [CrossRef]
7. Neu, J.; Pammi, M. Pathogenesis of NEC: Impact of an altered intestinal microbiome. *Semin. Perinatol.* **2017**, *41*, 29–35. [CrossRef]
8. Samuels, N.; van de Graaf, R.A.; de Jonge, R.C.J.; Reiss, I.K.M.; Vermeulen, M.J. Risk factors for necrotizing enterocolitis in neonates: A systematic review of prognostic studies. *BMC Pediatr.* **2017**, *17*, 105. [CrossRef]
9. Cacho, N.T.; Parker, L.A.; Neu, J. Necrotizing Enterocolitis and Human Milk Feeding: A Systematic Review. *Clin. Perinatol.* **2017**, *44*, 49–67. [CrossRef]
10. Miller, J.; Tonkin, E.; Damarell, R.A.; McPhee, A.J.; Suganuma, M.; Suganuma, H.; Middleton, P.F.; Makrides, M.; Collins, C.T. A Systematic Review and Meta-Analysis of Human Milk Feeding and Morbidity in Very Low Birth Weight Infants. *Nutrients* **2018**, *10*, 707. [CrossRef]
11. Andreas, N.J.; Kampmann, B.; Mehring Le-Doare, K. Human breast milk: A review on its composition and bioactivity. *Early Hum. Dev.* **2015**, *91*, 629–635. [CrossRef] [PubMed]
12. Grulee, C.G.; Sanford, H.N.; Herron, P.H. Breast and artificial feeding: Influence on morbidity and mortality of twenty thousand infants. *JAMA J. Am. Med. Assoc.* **1934**, *103*, 735–738. [CrossRef]
13. Howie, P.W.; Forsyth, J.S.; Ogston, S.A.; Clark, A.; Florey, C.D. Protective effect of breast feeding against infection. *BMJ* **1990**, *300*, 11–16. [CrossRef]
14. Abrams, S.A.; Schanler, R.J.; Lee, M.L.; Rechtman, D.J. Greater mortality and morbidity in extremely preterm infants fed a diet containing cow milk protein products. *Breastfeed. Med.* **2014**, *9*, 281–285. [CrossRef]
15. Sisk, P.M.; Lovelady, C.A.; Dillard, R.G.; Gruber, K.J.; O'Shea, T.M. Early human milk feeding is associated with a lower risk of necrotizing enterocolitis in very low birth weight infants. *J. Perinatol.* **2007**, *27*, 428–433. [CrossRef] [PubMed]
16. Lucas, A.; Cole, T.J. Breast milk and neonatal necrotising enterocolitis. *Lancet* **1990**, *336*, 1519–1523. [CrossRef]
17. Meinzen-Derr, J.; Poindexter, B.; Wrage, L.; Morrow, A.L.; Stoll, B.; Donovan, E.F. Role of human milk in extremely low birth weight infants' risk of necrotizing enterocolitis or death. *J. Perinatol.* **2009**, *29*, 57–62. [CrossRef] [PubMed]
18. Corpeleijn, W.E.; Kouwenhoven, S.M.; Paap, M.C.; van Vliet, I.; Scheerder, I.; Muizer, Y.; Helder, O.K.; van Goudoever, J.B.; Vermeulen, M.J. Intake of own mother's milk during the first days of life is associated with decreased morbidity and mortality in very low birth weight infants during the first 60 days of life. *Neonatology* **2012**, *102*, 276–281. [CrossRef]
19. Arslanoglu, S.; Corpeleijn, W.; Moro, G.; Braegger, C.; Campoy, C.; Colomb, V.; Decsi, T.; Domellof, M.; Fewtrell, M.; Hojsak, I.; et al. Donor human milk for preterm infants: Current evidence and research directions. *J. Pediatr. Gastroenterol. Nutr.* **2013**, *57*, 535–542. [CrossRef]
20. Li, Y.; Nguyen, D.N.; de Waard, M.; Christensen, L.; Zhou, P.; Jiang, P.; Sun, J.; Bojesen, A.M.; Lauridsen, C.; Lykkesfeldt, J.; et al. Pasteurization Procedures for Donor Human Milk Affect Body Growth, Intestinal Structure, and Resistance against Bacterial Infections in Preterm Pigs. *J. Nutr.* **2017**, *147*, 1121–1130. [CrossRef]
21. Aksu, T.; Atalay, Y.; Turkyilmaz, C.; Gulbahar, O.; Hirfanoglu, I.M.; Demirel, N.; Onal, E.; Ergenekon, E.; Koc, E. The effects of breast milk storage and freezing procedure on interleukine-10 levels and total antioxidant activity. *J. Matern. Fetal Neonatal Med.* **2015**, *28*, 1799–1802. [CrossRef] [PubMed]
22. Corpeleijn, W.E.; de Waard, M.; Christmann, V.; van Goudoever, J.B.; Jansen-van der Weide, M.C.; Kooi, E.M.; Koper, J.F.; Kouwenhoven, S.M.; Lafeber, H.N.; Mank, E.; et al. Effect of Donor Milk on Severe Infections and Mortality in Very-Low-Birth-Weight Infants: The Early Nutrition Study Randomized Clinical Trial. *JAMA Pediatr.* **2016**, *170*, 654–661. [CrossRef] [PubMed]
23. Canizo Vazquez, D.; Salas Garcia, S.; Izquierdo Renau, M.; Iglesias-Platas, I. Availability of Donor Milk for Very Preterm Infants Decreased the Risk of Necrotizing Enterocolitis without Adversely Impacting Growth or Rates of Breastfeeding. *Nutrients* **2019**, *11*, 1895. [CrossRef] [PubMed]
24. Ford, S.L.; Lohmann, P.; Preidis, G.A.; Gordon, P.S.; O'Donnell, A.; Hagan, J.; Venkatachalam, A.; Balderas, M.; Luna, R.A.; Hair, A.B. Improved feeding tolerance and growth are linked to increased gut microbial community diversity in very-low-birth-weight infants fed mother's own milk compared with donor breast milk. *Am. J. Clin. Nutr.* **2019**, *109*, 1088–1097. [CrossRef]

25. Baethge, C.; Goldbeck-Wood, S.; Mertens, S. SANRA-a scale for the quality assessment of narrative review articles. *Res. Integr. Peer Rev.* **2019**, *4*, 5. [CrossRef]
26. Ferrari, R. Writing narrative style literature reviews. *Med Writ.* **2015**, *24*, 230–235. [CrossRef]
27. Battersby, A.J.; Gibbons, D.L. The gut mucosal immune system in the neonatal period. *Pediatr. Allergy Immunol.* **2013**, *24*, 414–421. [CrossRef]
28. Pammi, M.; Cope, J.; Tarr, P.I.; Warner, B.B.; Morrow, A.L.; Mai, V.; Gregory, K.E.; Kroll, J.S.; McMurtry, V.; Ferris, M.J.; et al. Intestinal dysbiosis in preterm infants preceding necrotizing enterocolitis: A systematic review and meta-analysis. *Microbiome* **2017**, *5*, 31. [CrossRef]
29. Denning, N.L.; Prince, J.M. Neonatal intestinal dysbiosis in necrotizing enterocolitis. *Mol. Med.* **2018**, *24*, 4. [CrossRef]
30. Moore, S.A.; Nighot, P.; Reyes, C.; Rawat, M.; McKee, J.; Lemon, D.; Hanson, J.; Ma, T.Y. Intestinal barrier dysfunction in human necrotizing enterocolitis. *J. Pediatr. Surg.* **2016**, *51*, 1907–1913. [CrossRef]
31. Krappmann, D.; Wegener, E.; Sunami, Y.; Esen, M.; Thiel, A.; Mordmuller, B.; Scheidereit, C. The IkappaB kinase complex and NF-kappaB act as master regulators of lipopolysaccharide-induced gene expression and control subordinate activation of AP-1. *Mol. Cell. Biol.* **2004**, *24*, 6488–6500. [CrossRef] [PubMed]
32. Sodhi, C.P.; Neal, M.D.; Siggers, R.; Sho, S.; Ma, C.; Branca, M.F.; Prindle, T., Jr.; Russo, A.M.; Afrazi, A.; Good, M.; et al. Intestinal epithelial Toll-like receptor 4 regulates goblet cell development and is required for necrotizing enterocolitis in mice. *Gastroenterology* **2012**, *143*, 708–718. [CrossRef] [PubMed]
33. Leaphart, C.L.; Cavallo, J.; Gribar, S.C.; Cetin, S.; Li, J.; Branca, M.F.; Dubowski, T.D.; Sodhi, C.P.; Hackam, D.J. A critical role for TLR4 in the pathogenesis of necrotizing enterocolitis by modulating intestinal injury and repair. *J. Immunol.* **2007**, *179*, 4808–4820. [CrossRef] [PubMed]
34. Egan, C.E.; Sodhi, C.P.; Good, M.; Lin, J.; Jia, H.; Yamaguchi, Y.; Lu, P.; Ma, C.; Branca, M.F.; Weyandt, S.; et al. Toll-like receptor 4-mediated lymphocyte influx induces neonatal necrotizing enterocolitis. *J. Clin. Investig.* **2016**, *126*, 495–508. [CrossRef] [PubMed]
35. Good, M.; Siggers, R.H.; Sodhi, C.P.; Afrazi, A.; Alkhudari, F.; Egan, C.E.; Neal, M.D.; Yazji, I.; Jia, H.; Lin, J.; et al. Amniotic fluid inhibits Toll-like receptor 4 signaling in the fetal and neonatal intestinal epithelium. *Proc. Natl. Acad. Sci. USA* **2012**, *109*, 11330–11335. [CrossRef]
36. Good, M.; Sodhi, C.P.; Egan, C.E.; Afrazi, A.; Jia, H.; Yamaguchi, Y.; Lu, P.; Branca, M.F.; Ma, C.; Prindle, T., Jr.; et al. Breast milk protects against the development of necrotizing enterocolitis through inhibition of Toll-like receptor 4 in the intestinal epithelium via activation of the epidermal growth factor receptor. *Mucosal. Immunol.* **2015**, *8*, 1166–1179. [CrossRef]
37. Neal, M.D.; Jia, H.; Eyer, B.; Good, M.; Guerriero, C.J.; Sodhi, C.P.; Afrazi, A.; Prindle, T., Jr.; Ma, C.; Branca, M.; et al. Discovery and validation of a new class of small molecule Toll-like receptor 4 (TLR4) inhibitors. *PLoS ONE* **2013**, *8*, e65779. [CrossRef]
38. Good, M.; Sodhi, C.P.; Yamaguchi, Y.; Jia, H.; Lu, P.; Fulton, W.B.; Martin, L.Y.; Prindle, T.; Nino, D.F.; Zhou, Q.; et al. The human milk oligosaccharide 2′-fucosyllactose attenuates the severity of experimental necrotising enterocolitis by enhancing mesenteric perfusion in the neonatal intestine. *Br. J. Nutr.* **2016**, *116*, 1175–1187. [CrossRef]
39. Lu, P.; Sodhi, C.P.; Hackam, D.J. Toll-like receptor regulation of intestinal development and inflammation in the pathogenesis of necrotizing enterocolitis. *Pathophysiol. Off. J. Int. Soc. Pathophysiol.* **2014**, *21*, 81–93. [CrossRef]
40. Burge, K.; Gunasekaran, A.; Eckert, J.; Chaaban, H. Curcumin and Intestinal Inflammatory Diseases: Molecular Mechanisms of Protection. *Int. J. Mol. Sci.* **2019**, *20*, 1912. [CrossRef]
41. Mara, M.A.; Good, M.; Weitkamp, J.H. Innate and adaptive immunity in necrotizing enterocolitis. *Semin. Fetal Neonatal Med.* **2018**, *23*, 394–399. [CrossRef] [PubMed]
42. Udall, J.N.; Pang, K.; Fritze, L.; Kleinman, R.; Walker, W.A. Development of gastrointestinal mucosal barrier. I. The effect of age on intestinal permeability to macromolecules. *Pediatr. Res.* **1981**, *15*, 241–244. [CrossRef] [PubMed]
43. Managlia, E.; Liu, S.X.L.; Yan, X.; Tan, X.D.; Chou, P.M.; Barrett, T.A.; De Plaen, I.G. Blocking NF-kappaB Activation in Ly6c(+) Monocytes Attenuates Necrotizing Enterocolitis. *Am. J. Pathol.* **2019**, *189*, 604–618. [CrossRef]

44. De Plaen, I.G.; Liu, S.X.; Tian, R.; Neequaye, I.; May, M.J.; Han, X.B.; Hsueh, W.; Jilling, T.; Lu, J.; Caplan, M.S. Inhibition of nuclear factor-kappaB ameliorates bowel injury and prolongs survival in a neonatal rat model of necrotizing enterocolitis. *Pediatr. Res.* **2007**, *61*, 716–721. [CrossRef] [PubMed]
45. Markel, T.A.; Crisostomo, P.R.; Wairiuko, G.M.; Pitcher, J.; Tsai, B.M.; Meldrum, D.R. Cytokines in necrotizing enterocolitis. *Shock* **2006**, *25*, 329–337. [CrossRef] [PubMed]
46. Yazji, I.; Sodhi, C.P.; Lee, E.K.; Good, M.; Egan, C.E.; Afrazi, A.; Neal, M.D.; Jia, H.; Lin, J.; Ma, C.; et al. Endothelial TLR4 activation impairs intestinal microcirculatory perfusion in necrotizing enterocolitis via eNOS-NO-nitrite signaling. *Proc. Natl. Acad. Sci. USA* **2013**, *110*, 9451–9456. [CrossRef] [PubMed]
47. Watkins, D.J.; Besner, G.E. The role of the intestinal microcirculation in necrotizing enterocolitis. *Semin. Pediatr. Surg.* **2013**, *22*, 83–87. [CrossRef] [PubMed]
48. Thoma, C. Preventing brain damage in necrotizing enterocolitis. *Nat. Rev. Gastroenterol. Hepatol.* **2019**, *16*, 75. [CrossRef] [PubMed]
49. Bischoff, S.C.; Barbara, G.; Buurman, W.; Ockhuizen, T.; Schulzke, J.D.; Serino, M.; Tilg, H.; Watson, A.; Wells, J.M. Intestinal permeability–a new target for disease prevention and therapy. *BMC Gastroenterol.* **2014**, *14*, 189. [CrossRef] [PubMed]
50. Schroeder, B.O. Fight them or feed them: How the intestinal mucus layer manages the gut microbiota. *Gastroenterol. Rep.* **2019**, *7*, 3–12. [CrossRef]
51. Wang, J.; Ghosh, S.S.; Ghosh, S. Curcumin improves intestinal barrier function: Modulation of intracellular signaling, and organization of tight junctions. *Am. J. Physiol. Gastrointest. Liver Physiol.* **2017**, *312*, C438–C445. [CrossRef]
52. Martin, N.A.; Mount Patrick, S.K.; Estrada, T.E.; Frisk, H.A.; Rogan, D.T.; Dvorak, B.; Halpern, M.D. Active transport of bile acids decreases mucin 2 in neonatal ileum: Implications for development of necrotizing enterocolitis. *PLoS ONE* **2011**, *6*, e27191. [CrossRef] [PubMed]
53. Clark, J.A.; Doelle, S.M.; Halpern, M.D.; Saunders, T.A.; Holubec, H.; Dvorak, K.; Boitano, S.A.; Dvorak, B. Intestinal barrier failure during experimental necrotizing enterocolitis: Protective effect of EGF treatment. *Am. J. Physiol. Gastrointest. Liver Physiol.* **2006**, *291*, G938–G949. [CrossRef]
54. McElroy, S.J.; Prince, L.S.; Weitkamp, J.H.; Reese, J.; Slaughter, J.C.; Polk, D.B. Tumor necrosis factor receptor 1-dependent depletion of mucus in immature small intestine: A potential role in neonatal necrotizing enterocolitis. *Am. J. Physiol. Gastrointest. Liver Physiol.* **2011**, *301*, G656–G666. [CrossRef] [PubMed]
55. Zhang, C.; Sherman, M.P.; Prince, L.S.; Bader, D.; Weitkamp, J.H.; Slaughter, J.C.; McElroy, S.J. Paneth cell ablation in the presence of Klebsiella pneumoniae induces necrotizing enterocolitis (NEC)-like injury in the small intestine of immature mice. *Dis. Models Mech.* **2012**, *5*, 522–532. [CrossRef] [PubMed]
56. Markasz, L.; Wanders, A.; Szekely, L.; Lilja, H.E. Diminished DEFA6 Expression in Paneth Cells Is Associated with Necrotizing Enterocolitis. *Gastroenterol Res Pract.* **2018**, *2018*, 7345426. [CrossRef] [PubMed]
57. Coutinho, H.B.; da Mota, H.C.; Coutinho, V.B.; Robalinho, T.I.; Furtado, A.F.; Walker, E.; King, G.; Mahida, Y.R.; Sewell, H.F.; Wakelin, D. Absence of lysozyme (muramidase) in the intestinal Paneth cells of newborn infants with necrotising enterocolitis. *J. Clin. Pathol.* **1998**, *51*, 512–514. [CrossRef]
58. Salzman, N.H.; Bevins, C.L. Dysbiosis–a consequence of Paneth cell dysfunction. *Semin. Immunol.* **2013**, *25*, 334–341. [CrossRef]
59. Strunk, T.; Temming, P.; Gembruch, U.; Reiss, I.; Bucsky, P.; Schultz, C. Differential maturation of the innate immune response in human fetuses. *Pediatr. Res.* **2004**, *56*, 219–226. [CrossRef]
60. Maheshwari, A.; Kelly, D.R.; Nicola, T.; Ambalavanan, N.; Jain, S.K.; Murphy-Ullrich, J.; Athar, M.; Shimamura, M.; Bhandari, V.; Aprahamian, C.; et al. TGF-beta2 suppresses macrophage cytokine production and mucosal inflammatory responses in the developing intestine. *Gastroenterology* **2011**, *140*, 242–253. [CrossRef]
61. MohanKumar, K.; Namachivayam, K.; Chapalamadugu, K.C.; Garzon, S.A.; Premkumar, M.H.; Tipparaju, S.M.; Maheshwari, A. Smad7 interrupts TGF-beta signaling in intestinal macrophages and promotes inflammatory activation of these cells during necrotizing enterocolitis. *Pediatr. Res.* **2016**, *79*, 951–961. [CrossRef] [PubMed]
62. Namachivayam, K.; Blanco, C.L.; MohanKumar, K.; Jagadeeswaran, R.; Vasquez, M.; McGill-Vargas, L.; Garzon, S.A.; Jain, S.K.; Gill, R.K.; Freitag, N.E.; et al. Smad7 inhibits autocrine expression of TGF-beta2 in intestinal epithelial cells in baboon necrotizing enterocolitis. *Am. J. Physiol. Gastrointest. Liver Physiol.* **2013**, *304*, G167–G180. [CrossRef] [PubMed]

63. Schuller, S.S.; Sadeghi, K.; Wisgrill, L.; Dangl, A.; Diesner, S.C.; Prusa, A.R.; Klebermasz-Schrehof, K.; Greber-Platzer, S.; Neumuller, J.; Helmer, H.; et al. Preterm neonates display altered plasmacytoid dendritic cell function and morphology. *J. Leukoc. Biol.* **2013**, *93*, 781–788. [CrossRef] [PubMed]
64. Emami, C.N.; Mittal, R.; Wang, L.; Ford, H.R.; Prasadarao, N.V. Recruitment of dendritic cells is responsible for intestinal epithelial damage in the pathogenesis of necrotizing enterocolitis by Cronobacter sakazakii. *J. Immunol.* **2011**, *186*, 7067–7079. [CrossRef]
65. Jilling, T.; Simon, D.; Lu, J.; Meng, F.J.; Li, D.; Schy, R.; Thomson, R.B.; Soliman, A.; Arditi, M.; Caplan, M.S. The roles of bacteria and TLR4 in rat and murine models of necrotizing enterocolitis. *J. Immunol.* **2006**, *177*, 3273–3282. [CrossRef]
66. Le Mandat Schultz, A.; Bonnard, A.; Barreau, F.; Aigrain, Y.; Pierre-Louis, C.; Berrebi, D.; Peuchmaur, M. Expression of TLR-2, TLR-4, NOD2 and pNF-kappaB in a neonatal rat model of necrotizing enterocolitis. *PLoS ONE* **2007**, *2*, e1102. [CrossRef]
67. Dimmitt, R.A.; Staley, E.M.; Chuang, G.; Tanner, S.M.; Soltau, T.D.; Lorenz, R.G. Role of postnatal acquisition of the intestinal microbiome in the early development of immune function. *J. Pediatr. Gastroenterol. Nutr.* **2010**, *51*, 262–273. [CrossRef]
68. Nanthakumar, N.; Meng, D.; Goldstein, A.M.; Zhu, W.; Lu, L.; Uauy, R.; Llanos, A.; Claud, E.C.; Walker, W.A. The mechanism of excessive intestinal inflammation in necrotizing enterocolitis: An immature innate immune response. *PLoS ONE* **2011**, *6*, e17776. [CrossRef]
69. Liu, Y.; Zhu, L.; Fatheree, N.Y.; Liu, X.; Pacheco, S.E.; Tatevian, N.; Rhoads, J.M. Changes in intestinal Toll-like receptors and cytokines precede histological injury in a rat model of necrotizing enterocolitis. *Am. J. Physiol. Gastrointest. Liver Physiol.* **2009**, *297*, G442–G450. [CrossRef]
70. Dowling, D.J.; Levy, O. Ontogeny of early life immunity. *Trends Immunol.* **2014**, *35*, 299–310. [CrossRef]
71. Gutzeit, C.; Magri, G.; Cerutti, A. Intestinal IgA production and its role in host-microbe interaction. *Immunol. Rev.* **2014**, *260*, 76–85. [CrossRef] [PubMed]
72. Borges, M.C.; Sesso, M.L.; Roberti, L.R.; de Menezes Oliveira, M.A.; Nogueira, R.D.; Geraldo-Martins, V.R.; Ferriani, V.P. Salivary antibody response to streptococci in preterm and fullterm children: A prospective study. *Arch. Oral Biol.* **2015**, *60*, 116–125. [CrossRef] [PubMed]
73. Nogueira, R.D.; Sesso, M.L.; Borges, M.C.; Mattos-Graner, R.O.; Smith, D.J.; Ferriani, V.P. Salivary IgA antibody responses to Streptococcus mitis and Streptococcus mutans in preterm and fullterm newborn children. *Arch. Oral Biol.* **2012**, *57*, 647–653. [CrossRef] [PubMed]
74. Ismail, A.S.; Behrendt, C.L.; Hooper, L.V. Reciprocal interactions between commensal bacteria and gamma delta intraepithelial lymphocytes during mucosal injury. *J. Immunol.* **2009**, *182*, 3047–3054. [CrossRef] [PubMed]
75. Gibbons, D.L.; Haque, S.F.; Silberzahn, T.; Hamilton, K.; Langford, C.; Ellis, P.; Carr, R.; Hayday, A.C. Neonates harbour highly active gammadelta T cells with selective impairments in preterm infants. *Eur. J. Immunol.* **2009**, *39*, 1794–1806. [CrossRef] [PubMed]
76. Weitkamp, J.H.; Rosen, M.J.; Zhao, Z.; Koyama, T.; Geem, D.; Denning, T.L.; Rock, M.T.; Moore, D.J.; Halpern, M.D.; Matta, P.; et al. Small intestinal intraepithelial TCRgammadelta+ T lymphocytes are present in the premature intestine but selectively reduced in surgical necrotizing enterocolitis. *PLoS ONE* **2014**, *9*, e99042. [CrossRef] [PubMed]
77. Weitkamp, J.H.; Koyama, T.; Rock, M.T.; Correa, H.; Goettel, J.A.; Matta, P.; Oswald-Richter, K.; Rosen, M.J.; Engelhardt, B.G.; Moore, D.J.; et al. Necrotising enterocolitis is characterised by disrupted immune regulation and diminished mucosal regulatory (FOXP3)/effector (CD4, CD8) T cell ratios. *Gut* **2013**, *62*, 73–82. [CrossRef]
78. Elias, K.M.; Laurence, A.; Davidson, T.S.; Stephens, G.; Kanno, Y.; Shevach, E.M.; O'Shea, J.J. Retinoic acid inhibits Th17 polarization and enhances FoxP3 expression through a Stat-3/Stat-5 independent signaling pathway. *Blood* **2008**, *111*, 1013–1020. [CrossRef]
79. Nino, D.F.; Sodhi, C.P.; Egan, C.E.; Zhou, Q.; Lin, J.; Lu, P.; Yamaguchi, Y.; Jia, H.; Martin, L.Y.; Good, M.; et al. Retinoic Acid Improves Incidence and Severity of Necrotizing Enterocolitis by Lymphocyte Balance Restitution and Repopulation of LGR5+ Intestinal Stem Cells. *Shock* **2017**, *47*, 22–32. [CrossRef]
80. Grizotte-Lake, M.; Zhong, G.; Duncan, K.; Kirkwood, J.; Iyer, N.; Smolenski, I.; Isoherranen, N.; Vaishnava, S. Commensals Suppress Intestinal Epithelial Cell Retinoic Acid Synthesis to Regulate Interleukin-22 Activity and Prevent Microbial Dysbiosis. *Immunity* **2018**, *49*, 1103–1115. [CrossRef]

81. Aagaard, K.; Ma, J.; Antony, K.M.; Ganu, R.; Petrosino, J.; Versalovic, J. The placenta harbors a unique microbiome. *Sci. Transl. Med.* **2014**, *6*, 237ra265. [CrossRef] [PubMed]
82. Stinson, L.F.; Boyce, M.C.; Payne, M.S.; Keelan, J.A. The Not-so-Sterile Womb: Evidence That the Human Fetus Is Exposed to Bacteria Prior to Birth. *Front. Microbiol.* **2019**, *10*, 1124. [CrossRef] [PubMed]
83. Leiby, J.S.; McCormick, K.; Sherrill-Mix, S.; Clarke, E.L.; Kessler, L.R.; Taylor, L.J.; Hofstaedter, C.E.; Roche, A.M.; Mattei, L.M.; Bittinger, K.; et al. Lack of detection of a human placenta microbiome in samples from preterm and term deliveries. *Microbiome* **2018**, *6*, 196. [CrossRef] [PubMed]
84. de Goffau, M.C.; Lager, S.; Sovio, U.; Gaccioli, F.; Cook, E.; Peacock, S.J.; Parkhill, J.; Charnock-Jones, D.S.; Smith, G.C.S. Human placenta has no microbiome but can contain potential pathogens. *Nature* **2019**, *572*, 329–334. [CrossRef]
85. Patel, R.M.; Denning, P.W. Intestinal microbiota and its relationship with necrotizing enterocolitis. *Pediatr. Res.* **2015**, *78*, 232–238. [CrossRef]
86. Palmer, C.; Bik, E.M.; DiGiulio, D.B.; Relman, D.A.; Brown, P.O. Development of the human infant intestinal microbiota. *PLoS Biol.* **2007**, *5*, e177. [CrossRef]
87. Jost, T.; Lacroix, C.; Braegger, C.P.; Chassard, C. New insights in gut microbiota establishment in healthy breast fed neonates. *PLoS ONE* **2012**, *7*, e44595. [CrossRef]
88. Elgin, T.G.; Kern, S.L.; McElroy, S.J. Development of the Neonatal Intestinal Microbiome and Its Association with Necrotizing Enterocolitis. *Clin. Ther.* **2016**, *38*, 706–715. [CrossRef]
89. Parada Venegas, D.; De la Fuente, M.K.; Landskron, G.; Gonzalez, M.J.; Quera, R.; Dijkstra, G.; Harmsen, H.J.M.; Faber, K.N.; Hermoso, M.A. Short Chain Fatty Acids (SCFAs)-Mediated Gut Epithelial and Immune Regulation and Its Relevance for Inflammatory Bowel Diseases. *Front. Immunol.* **2019**, *10*, 277. [CrossRef]
90. Byndloss, M.X.; Olsan, E.E.; Rivera-Chavez, F.; Tiffany, C.R.; Cevallos, S.A.; Lokken, K.L.; Torres, T.P.; Byndloss, A.J.; Faber, F.; Gao, Y.; et al. Microbiota-activated PPAR-gamma signaling inhibits dysbiotic Enterobacteriaceae expansion. *Science* **2017**, *357*, 570–575. [CrossRef]
91. La Rosa, P.S.; Warner, B.B.; Zhou, Y.; Weinstock, G.M.; Sodergren, E.; Hall-Moore, C.M.; Stevens, H.J.; Bennett, W.E., Jr.; Shaikh, N.; Linneman, L.A.; et al. Patterned progression of bacterial populations in the premature infant gut. *Proc. Natl. Acad. Sci. USA* **2014**, *111*, 12522–12527. [CrossRef] [PubMed]
92. Gibson, M.K.; Wang, B.; Ahmadi, S.; Burnham, C.A.; Tarr, P.I.; Warner, B.B.; Dantas, G. Developmental dynamics of the preterm infant gut microbiota and antibiotic resistome. *Nat. Microbiol.* **2016**, *1*, 16024. [CrossRef] [PubMed]
93. Ward, D.V.; Scholz, M.; Zolfo, M.; Taft, D.H.; Schibler, K.R.; Tett, A.; Segata, N.; Morrow, A.L. Metagenomic Sequencing with Strain-Level Resolution Implicates Uropathogenic *E. coli* in Necrotizing Enterocolitis and Mortality in Preterm Infants. *Cell Rep.* **2016**, *14*, 2912–2924. [CrossRef] [PubMed]
94. Carlisle, E.M.; Morowitz, M.J. The intestinal microbiome and necrotizing enterocolitis. *Curr. Opin. Pediatr.* **2013**, *25*, 382–387. [CrossRef]
95. Wang, Y.; Hoenig, J.D.; Malin, K.J.; Qamar, S.; Petrof, E.O.; Sun, J.; Antonopoulos, D.A.; Chang, E.B.; Claud, E.C. 16S rRNA gene-based analysis of fecal microbiota from preterm infants with and without necrotizing enterocolitis. *ISME J.* **2009**, *3*, 944–954. [CrossRef]
96. Levy, M.; Kolodziejczyk, A.A.; Thaiss, C.A.; Elinav, E. Dysbiosis and the immune system. *Nat. Rev. Immunol.* **2017**, *17*, 219–232. [CrossRef]
97. Shi, N.; Li, N.; Duan, X.; Niu, H. Interaction between the gut microbiome and mucosal immune system. *Mil. Med. Res.* **2017**, *4*, 14. [CrossRef]
98. Afrazi, A.; Sodhi, C.P.; Richardson, W.; Neal, M.; Good, M.; Siggers, R.; Hackam, D.J. New insights into the pathogenesis and treatment of necrotizing enterocolitis: Toll-like receptors and beyond. *Pediatr. Res.* **2011**, *69*, 183–188. [CrossRef]
99. Musemeche, C.A.; Kosloske, A.M.; Bartow, S.A.; Umland, E.T. Comparative effects of ischemia, bacteria, and substrate on the pathogenesis of intestinal necrosis. *J. Pediatr. Surg.* **1986**, *21*, 536–538. [CrossRef]
100. Morowitz, M.J.; Poroyko, V.; Caplan, M.; Alverdy, J.; Liu, D.C. Redefining the role of intestinal microbes in the pathogenesis of necrotizing enterocolitis. *Pediatrics* **2010**, *125*, 777–785. [CrossRef]
101. Mai, V.; Young, C.M.; Ukhanova, M.; Wang, X.; Sun, Y.; Casella, G.; Theriaque, D.; Li, N.; Sharma, R.; Hudak, M.; et al. Fecal microbiota in premature infants prior to necrotizing enterocolitis. *PLoS ONE* **2011**, *6*, e20647. [CrossRef] [PubMed]

102. Torrazza, R.M.; Neu, J. The altered gut microbiome and necrotizing enterocolitis. *Clin. Perinatol.* **2013**, *40*, 93–108. [CrossRef] [PubMed]
103. Warner, B.B.; Deych, E.; Zhou, Y.; Hall-Moore, C.; Weinstock, G.M.; Sodergren, E.; Shaikh, N.; Hoffmann, J.A.; Linneman, L.A.; Hamvas, A.; et al. Gut bacteria dysbiosis and necrotising enterocolitis in very low birthweight infants: A prospective case-control study. *Lancet* **2016**, *387*, 1928–1936. [CrossRef]
104. Neu, J.; Pammi, M. Necrotizing enterocolitis: The intestinal microbiome, metabolome and inflammatory mediators. *Semin. Fetal Neonatal Med.* **2018**, *23*, 400–405. [CrossRef]
105. Torrazza, R.M.; Ukhanova, M.; Wang, X.; Sharma, R.; Hudak, M.L.; Neu, J.; Mai, V. Intestinal microbial ecology and environmental factors affecting necrotizing enterocolitis. *PLoS ONE* **2013**, *8*, e83304. [CrossRef] [PubMed]
106. Dobbler, P.T.; Procianoy, R.S.; Mai, V.; Silveira, R.C.; Corso, A.L.; Rojas, B.S.; Roesch, L.F.W. Low Microbial Diversity and Abnormal Microbial Succession Is Associated with Necrotizing Enterocolitis in Preterm Infants. *Front. Microbiol.* **2017**, *8*, 2243. [CrossRef]
107. Gopalakrishna, K.P.; Macadangdang, B.R.; Rogers, M.B.; Tometich, J.T.; Firek, B.A.; Baker, R.; Ji, J.; Burr, A.H.P.; Ma, C.; Good, M.; et al. Maternal IgA protects against the development of necrotizing enterocolitis in preterm infants. *Nat. Med.* **2019**, *25*, 1110–1115. [CrossRef]
108. Morrow, A.L.; Lagomarcino, A.J.; Schibler, K.R.; Taft, D.H.; Yu, Z.; Wang, B.; Altaye, M.; Wagner, M.; Gevers, D.; Ward, D.V.; et al. Early microbial and metabolomic signatures predict later onset of necrotizing enterocolitis in preterm infants. *Microbiome* **2013**, *1*, 13. [CrossRef]
109. Bizzarro, M.J. Avoiding Unnecessary Antibiotic Exposure in Premature Infants: Understanding When (Not) to Start and When to Stop. *JAMA Netw. Open* **2018**, *1*, e180165. [CrossRef]
110. Greenberg, R.G.; Chowdhury, D.; Hansen, N.I.; Smith, P.B.; Stoll, B.J.; Sanchez, P.J.; Das, A.; Puopolo, K.M.; Mukhopadhyay, S.; Higgins, R.D.; et al. Prolonged duration of early antibiotic therapy in extremely premature infants. *Pediatr. Res.* **2019**, *85*, 994–1000. [CrossRef]
111. Cotten, C.M. Adverse consequences of neonatal antibiotic exposure. *Curr. Opin. Pediatr.* **2016**, *28*, 141–149. [CrossRef] [PubMed]
112. Alexander, V.N.; Northrup, V.; Bizzarro, M.J. Antibiotic exposure in the newborn intensive care unit and the risk of necrotizing enterocolitis. *J. Pediatr.* **2011**, *159*, 392–397. [CrossRef] [PubMed]
113. Fouhy, F.; Guinane, C.M.; Hussey, S.; Wall, R.; Ryan, C.A.; Dempsey, E.M.; Murphy, B.; Ross, R.P.; Fitzgerald, G.F.; Stanton, C.; et al. High-throughput sequencing reveals the incomplete, short-term recovery of infant gut microbiota following parenteral antibiotic treatment with ampicillin and gentamicin. *Antimicrob. Agents Chemother.* **2012**, *56*, 5811–5820. [CrossRef] [PubMed]
114. Tanaka, S.; Kobayashi, T.; Songjinda, P.; Tateyama, A.; Tsubouchi, M.; Kiyohara, C.; Shirakawa, T.; Sonomoto, K.; Nakayama, J. Influence of antibiotic exposure in the early postnatal period on the development of intestinal microbiota. *FEMS Immunol. Med. Microbiol.* **2009**, *56*, 80–87. [CrossRef]
115. Greenwood, C.; Morrow, A.L.; Lagomarcino, A.J.; Altaye, M.; Taft, D.H.; Yu, Z.; Newburg, D.S.; Ward, D.V.; Schibler, K.R. Early empiric antibiotic use in preterm infants is associated with lower bacterial diversity and higher relative abundance of Enterobacter. *J. Pediatr.* **2014**, *165*, 23–29. [CrossRef] [PubMed]
116. Dominguez-Bello, M.G.; Costello, E.K.; Contreras, M.; Magris, M.; Hidalgo, G.; Fierer, N.; Knight, R. Delivery mode shapes the acquisition and structure of the initial microbiota across multiple body habitats in newborns. *Proc. Natl. Acad. Sci. USA* **2010**, *107*, 11971–11975. [CrossRef]
117. Biasucci, G.; Rubini, M.; Riboni, S.; Morelli, L.; Bessi, E.; Retetangos, C. Mode of delivery affects the bacterial community in the newborn gut. *Early Hum. Dev.* **2010**, *86* (Suppl. 1), 13–15. [CrossRef]
118. Singh, N.; Dhayade, A.; Mohamed, A.L.; Chaudhari, T.V. Morbidity and Mortality in Preterm Infants following Antacid Use: A Retrospective Audit. *Int. J. Pediatr.* **2016**, *2016*, 9649162. [CrossRef]
119. Terrin, G.; Passariello, A.; De Curtis, M.; Manguso, F.; Salvia, G.; Lega, L.; Messina, F.; Paludetto, R.; Canani, R.B. Ranitidine is associated with infections, necrotizing enterocolitis, and fatal outcome in newborns. *Pediatrics* **2012**, *129*, e40–e45. [CrossRef]
120. Bilali, A.; Galanis, P.; Bartsocas, C.; Sparos, L.; Velonakis, E. H2-blocker therapy and incidence of necrotizing enterocolitis in preterm infants: A case-control study. *Pediatr. Neonatol.* **2013**, *54*, 141–142. [CrossRef]
121. Gupta, R.W.; Tran, L.; Norori, J.; Ferris, M.J.; Eren, A.M.; Taylor, C.M.; Dowd, S.E.; Penn, D. Histamine-2 receptor blockers alter the fecal microbiota in premature infants. *J. Pediatr. Gastroenterol. Nutr.* **2013**, *56*, 397–400. [CrossRef] [PubMed]

122. Shin, N.R.; Whon, T.W.; Bae, J.W. Proteobacteria: Microbial signature of dysbiosis in gut microbiota. *Trends Biotechnol.* **2015**, *33*, 496–503. [CrossRef] [PubMed]
123. Lueschow, S.R.; Stumphy, J.; Gong, H.; Kern, S.L.; Elgin, T.G.; Underwood, M.A.; Kalanetra, K.M.; Mills, D.A.; Wong, M.H.; Meyerholz, D.K.; et al. Loss of murine Paneth cell function alters the immature intestinal microbiome and mimics changes seen in neonatal necrotizing enterocolitis. *PLoS ONE* **2018**, *13*, e0204967. [CrossRef] [PubMed]
124. Pannaraj, P.S.; Li, F.; Cerini, C.; Bender, J.M.; Yang, S.; Rollie, A.; Adisetiyo, H.; Zabih, S.; Lincez, P.J.; Bittinger, K.; et al. Association Between Breast Milk Bacterial Communities and Establishment and Development of the Infant Gut Microbiome. *JAMA Pediatr.* **2017**, *171*, 647–654. [CrossRef] [PubMed]
125. Hunt, K.M.; Foster, J.A.; Forney, L.J.; Schutte, U.M.; Beck, D.L.; Abdo, Z.; Fox, L.K.; Williams, J.E.; McGuire, M.K.; McGuire, M.A. Characterization of the diversity and temporal stability of bacterial communities in human milk. *PLoS ONE* **2011**, *6*, e21313. [CrossRef] [PubMed]
126. Lewis, Z.T.; Totten, S.M.; Smilowitz, J.T.; Popovic, M.; Parker, E.; Lemay, D.G.; Van Tassell, M.L.; Miller, M.J.; Jin, Y.S.; German, J.B.; et al. Maternal fucosyltransferase 2 status affects the gut bifidobacterial communities of breastfed infants. *Microbiome* **2015**, *3*, 13. [CrossRef]
127. Putignani, L.; Del Chierico, F.; Petrucca, A.; Vernocchi, P.; Dallapiccola, B. The human gut microbiota: A dynamic interplay with the host from birth to senescence settled during childhood. *Pediatr. Res.* **2014**, *76*, 2–10. [CrossRef]
128. Oozeer, R.; van Limpt, K.; Ludwig, T.; Ben Amor, K.; Martin, R.; Wind, R.D.; Boehm, G.; Knol, J. Intestinal microbiology in early life: Specific prebiotics can have similar functionalities as human-milk oligosaccharides. *Am. J. Clin. Nutr.* **2013**, *98*, 561s–571s. [CrossRef]
129. Gomez-Llorente, C.; Plaza-Diaz, J.; Aguilera, M.; Munoz-Quezada, S.; Bermudez-Brito, M.; Peso-Echarri, P.; Martinez-Silla, R.; Vasallo-Morillas, M.I.; Campana-Martin, L.; Vives-Pinera, I.; et al. Three main factors define changes in fecal microbiota associated with feeding modality in infants. *J. Pediatr. Gastroenterol. Nutr.* **2013**, *57*, 461–466. [CrossRef]
130. Penders, J.; Thijs, C.; Vink, C.; Stelma, F.F.; Snijders, B.; Kummeling, I.; van den Brandt, P.A.; Stobberingh, E.E. Factors influencing the composition of the intestinal microbiota in early infancy. *Pediatrics* **2006**, *118*, 511–521. [CrossRef]
131. Penders, J.; Vink, C.; Driessen, C.; London, N.; Thijs, C.; Stobberingh, E.E. Quantification of Bifidobacterium spp.; Escherichia coli and Clostridium difficile in faecal samples of breast-fed and formula-fed infants by real-time PCR. *FEMS Microbiol. Lett.* **2005**, *243*, 141–147. [CrossRef] [PubMed]
132. Aydin, S.; Aydin, S.; Ozkan, Y.; Kumru, S. Ghrelin is present in human colostrum, transitional and mature milk. *Peptides* **2006**, *27*, 878–882. [CrossRef] [PubMed]
133. Michalski, M.C.; Briard, V.; Michel, F.; Tasson, F.; Poulain, P. Size distribution of fat globules in human colostrum, breast milk, and infant formula. *J. Dairy Sci.* **2005**, *88*, 1927–1940. [CrossRef]
134. Ballard, O.; Morrow, A.L. Human milk composition: Nutrients and bioactive factors. *Pediatr. Clin. N. Am.* **2013**, *60*, 49–74. [CrossRef]
135. Coppa, G.V.; Gabrielli, O.; Zampini, L.; Galeazzi, T.; Ficcadenti, A.; Padella, L.; Santoro, L.; Soldi, S.; Carlucci, A.; Bertino, E.; et al. Oligosaccharides in 4 different milk groups, Bifidobacteria, and Ruminococcus obeum. *J. Pediatr. Gastroenterol. Nutr.* **2011**, *53*, 80–87. [CrossRef]
136. Morrow, A.L.; Ruiz-Palacios, G.M.; Altaye, M.; Jiang, X.; Guerrero, M.L.; Meinzen-Derr, J.K.; Farkas, T.; Chaturvedi, P.; Pickering, L.K.; Newburg, D.S. Human milk oligosaccharides are associated with protection against diarrhea in breast-fed infants. *J. Pediatr.* **2004**, *145*, 297–303. [CrossRef]
137. Goldman, A.S. Modulation of the gastrointestinal tract of infants by human milk. Interfaces and interactions. An evolutionary perspective. *J. Nutr.* **2000**, *130*, 426s–431s. [CrossRef]
138. Santaolalla, R.; Fukata, M.; Abreu, M.T. Innate immunity in the small intestine. *Curr. Opin. Gastroenterol.* **2011**, *27*, 125–131. [CrossRef]
139. Ricard-Blum, S. Glycosaminoglycans: Major biological players. *Glycoconj. J.* **2017**, *34*, 275–276. [CrossRef]
140. Coppa, G.V.; Facinelli, B.; Magi, G.; Marini, E.; Zampini, L.; Mantovani, V.; Galeazzi, T.; Padella, L.; Marchesiello, R.L.; Santoro, L.; et al. Human milk glycosaminoglycans inhibit in vitro the adhesion of Escherichia coli and Salmonella fyris to human intestinal cells. *Pediatr. Res.* **2016**, *79*, 603–607. [CrossRef]
141. Stern, R.; Asari, A.A.; Sugahara, K.N. Hyaluronan fragments: An information-rich system. *Eur. J. Cell Biol.* **2006**, *85*, 699–715. [CrossRef] [PubMed]

142. Barthe, L.; Woodley, J.; Lavit, M.; Przybylski, C.; Philibert, C.; Houin, G. In vitro intestinal degradation and absorption of chondroitin sulfate, a glycosaminoglycan drug. *Arzneimittelforschung* **2004**, *54*, 286–292. [CrossRef] [PubMed]
143. Maccari, F.; Mantovani, V.; Gabrielli, O.; Carlucci, A.; Zampini, L.; Galeazzi, T.; Galeotti, F.; Coppa, G.V.; Volpi, N. Metabolic fate of milk glycosaminoglycans in breastfed and formula fed newborns. *Glycoconj. J.* **2016**, *33*, 181–188. [CrossRef] [PubMed]
144. Fallacara, A.; Baldini, E.; Manfredini, S.; Vertuani, S. Hyaluronic Acid in the Third Millennium. *Polymers* **2018**, *10*, 701. [CrossRef]
145. Lee-Sayer, S.S.; Dong, Y.; Arif, A.A.; Olsson, M.; Brown, K.L.; Johnson, P. The where, when, how, and why of hyaluronan binding by immune cells. *Front. Immunol.* **2015**, *6*, 150. [CrossRef]
146. Coppa, G.V.; Gabrielli, O.; Buzzega, D.; Zampini, L.; Galeazzi, T.; Maccari, F.; Bertino, E.; Volpi, N. Composition and structure elucidation of human milk glycosaminoglycans. *Glycobiology* **2011**, *21*, 295–303. [CrossRef]
147. Volpi, N.; Gabrielli, O.; Carlucci, A.; Zampini, L.; Santoro, L.; Padella, L.; Marchesello, R.L.; Maccari, F.; Coppa, G.V. Human milk glycosaminoglycans in feces of breastfed newborns: Preliminary structural elucidation and possible biological role. *Breastfeed. Med. Off. J. Acad. Breastfeed. Med.* **2014**, *9*, 105–106. [CrossRef]
148. Coppa, G.V.; Gabrielli, O.; Zampini, L.; Galeazzi, T.; Maccari, F.; Buzzega, D.; Galeotti, F.; Bertino, E.; Volpi, N. Glycosaminoglycan content in term and preterm milk during the first month of lactation. *Neonatology* **2012**, *101*, 74–76. [CrossRef]
149. Wang, C.; Lang, Y.; Li, Q.; Jin, X.; Li, G.; Yu, G. Glycosaminoglycanomic profiling of human milk in different stages of lactation by liquid chromatography-tandem mass spectrometry. *Food Chem.* **2018**, *258*, 231–236. [CrossRef]
150. Soares da Costa, D.; Reis, R.L.; Pashkuleva, I. Sulfation of Glycosaminoglycans and Its Implications in Human Health and Disorders. *Annu. Rev. Biomed. Eng.* **2017**, *19*, 1–26. [CrossRef]
151. Volpi, N.; Maccari, F.; Galeotti, F.; Peila, C.; Coscia, A.; Zampini, L.; Monachesi, C.; Gabrielli, O.; Coppa, G. Human milk glycosaminoglycan composition from women of different countries: A pilot study. *J. Matern. Fetal Neonatal Med.* **2018**. [CrossRef] [PubMed]
152. Mannello, F.; Maccari, F.; Santinelli, A.; Volpi, N. Chondroitin sulfate structure is modified in human milk produced by breast affected by invasive carcinoma. *Breast* **2011**, *20*, 586–587. [CrossRef] [PubMed]
153. Cerdo, T.; Ruiz, A.; Jauregui, R.; Azaryah, H.; Torres-Espinola, F.J.; Garcia-Valdes, L.; Teresa Segura, M.; Suarez, A.; Campoy, C. Maternal obesity is associated with gut microbial metabolic potential in offspring during infancy. *J. Physiol. Biochem.* **2018**, *74*, 159–169. [CrossRef] [PubMed]
154. Wiederschain, G.Y.; Newburg, D.S. Glycoconjugate stability in human milk: Glycosidase activities and sugar release. *J. Nutr. Biochem.* **2001**, *12*, 559–564. [CrossRef]
155. Coscia, A.; Peila, C.; Bertino, E.; Coppa, G.V.; Moro, G.E.; Gabrielli, O.; Zampini, L.; Galeazzi, T.; Maccari, F.; Volpi, N. Effect of holder pasteurisation on human milk glycosaminoglycans. *J. Pediatr. Gastroenterol. Nutr.* **2015**, *60*, 127–130. [CrossRef] [PubMed]
156. Cartmell, A.; Lowe, E.C.; Basle, A.; Firbank, S.J.; Ndeh, D.A.; Murray, H.; Terrapon, N.; Lombard, V.; Henrissat, B.; Turnbull, J.E.; et al. How members of the human gut microbiota overcome the sulfation problem posed by glycosaminoglycans. *Proc. Natl. Acad. Sci. USA* **2017**, *114*, 7037–7042. [CrossRef] [PubMed]
157. Wang, M.; Liu, X.; Lyu, Z.; Gu, H.; Li, D.; Chen, H. Glycosaminoglycans (GAGs) and GAG mimetics regulate the behavior of stem cell differentiation. *Colloids Surf. B Biointerfaces* **2017**, *150*, 175–182. [CrossRef]
158. Poterucha, T.J.; Libby, P.; Goldhaber, S.Z. More than an anticoagulant: Do heparins have direct anti-inflammatory effects? *Thromb. Haemost.* **2017**, *117*, 437–444. [CrossRef]
159. Pomin, V.H. Sulfated glycans in inflammation. *Eur. J. Med. Chem.* **2015**, *92*, 353–369. [CrossRef]
160. Bode, L.; Salvestrini, C.; Park, P.W.; Li, J.-P.; Esko, J.D.; Yamaguchi, Y.; Murch, S.; Freeze, H.H. Heparan sulfate and syndecan-1 are essential in maintaining murine and human intestinal epithelial barrier function. *J. Clin. Investig.* **2008**, *118*, 229–238. [CrossRef]
161. Klein, N.J.; Shennan, G.I.; Heyderman, R.S.; Levin, M. Alteration in glycosaminoglycan metabolism and surface charge on human umbilical vein endothelial cells induced by cytokines, endotoxin and neutrophils. *J. Cell Sci.* **1992**, *102*, 821–832. [PubMed]

162. Ade-Ajayi, N.; Spitz, L.; Kiely, E.; Drake, D.; Klein, N. Intestinal glycosaminoglycans in neonatal necrotizing enterocolitis. *Br. J. Surg.* **1996**, *83*, 415–418. [CrossRef] [PubMed]
163. Yamamoto, S.; Nakase, H.; Matsuura, M.; Honzawa, Y.; Matsumura, K.; Uza, N.; Yamaguchi, Y.; Mizoguchi, E.; Chiba, T. Heparan sulfate on intestinal epithelial cells plays a critical role in intestinal crypt homeostasis via Wnt/beta-catenin signaling. *Am. J. Physiol. Gastrointest. Liver Physiol.* **2013**, *305*, G241–G249. [CrossRef] [PubMed]
164. Rozin, A.P.; Goldstein, M.; Sprecher, H. Antibacterial activity of glucosamine sulfate and chondroitine sulfate? *Clin. Exp. Rheumatol.* **2008**, *26*, 509–510.
165. Carlson, G.A.; Dragoo, J.L.; Samimi, B.; Bruckner, D.A.; Bernard, G.W.; Hedrick, M.; Benhaim, P. Bacteriostatic properties of biomatrices against common orthopaedic pathogens. *Biochem. Biophys. Res. Commun.* **2004**, *321*, 472–478. [CrossRef] [PubMed]
166. Pirnazar, P.; Wolinsky, L.; Nachnani, S.; Haake, S.; Pilloni, A.; Bernard, G.W. Bacteriostatic effects of hyaluronic acid. *J. Periodontol.* **1999**, *70*, 370–374. [CrossRef] [PubMed]
167. Kawai, K.; Kamochi, R.; Oiki, S.; Murata, K.; Hashimoto, W. Probiotics in human gut microbiota can degrade host glycosaminoglycans. *Sci. Rep.* **2018**, *8*, 10674. [CrossRef]
168. Zuniga, M.; Monedero, V.; Yebra, M.J. Utilization of Host-Derived Glycans by Intestinal Lactobacillus and Bifidobacterium Species. *Front. Microbiol.* **2018**, *9*, 1917. [CrossRef]
169. Sava, I.G.; Zhang, F.; Toma, I.; Theilacker, C.; Li, B.; Baumert, T.F.; Holst, O.; Linhardt, R.J.; Huebner, J. Novel interactions of glycosaminoglycans and bacterial glycolipids mediate binding of enterococci to human cells. *J. Biol. Chem.* **2009**, *284*, 18194–18201. [CrossRef]
170. Hafez, M.M.; Aboulwafa, M.M.; Yassien, M.A.; Hassouna, N.A. Role of different classes of mammalian cell surface molecules in adherence of coagulase positive and coagulase negative staphylococci. *J. Basic Microbiol.* **2008**, *48*, 353–362. [CrossRef]
171. Henry-Stanley, M.J.; Hess, D.J.; Erlandsen, S.L.; Wells, C.L. Ability of the heparan sulfate proteoglycan syndecan-1 to participate in bacterial translocation across the intestinal epithelial barrier. *Shock* **2005**, *24*, 571–576. [CrossRef] [PubMed]
172. Newburg, D.S.; Linhardt, R.J.; Ampofo, S.A.; Yolken, R.H. Human milk glycosaminoglycans inhibit HIV glycoprotein gp120 binding to its host cell CD4 receptor. *J. Nutr.* **1995**, *125*, 419–424. [CrossRef] [PubMed]
173. Hill, D.R.; Rho, H.K.; Kessler, S.P.; Amin, R.; Homer, C.R.; McDonald, C.; Cowman, M.K.; de la Motte, C.A. Human milk hyaluronan enhances innate defense of the intestinal epithelium. *J. Biol. Chem.* **2013**, *288*, 29090–29104. [CrossRef] [PubMed]
174. De Plaen, I.G. Inflammatory signaling in necrotizing enterocolitis. *Clin. Perinatol.* **2013**, *40*, 109–124. [CrossRef]
175. Zheng, L.; Riehl, T.E.; Stenson, W.F. Regulation of colonic epithelial repair in mice by Toll-like receptors and hyaluronic acid. *Gastroenterology* **2009**, *137*, 2041–2051. [CrossRef]
176. Riehl, T.E.; Foster, L.; Stenson, W.F. Hyaluronic acid is radioprotective in the intestine through a TLR4 and COX-2-mediated mechanism. *Am. J. Physiol. Gastrointest. Liver Physiol.* **2012**, *302*, G309–G316. [CrossRef]
177. Asari, A.; Kanemitsu, T.; Kurihara, H. Oral administration of high molecular weight hyaluronan (900 kDa) controls immune system via Toll-like receptor 4 in the intestinal epithelium. *J. Biol. Chem.* **2010**, *285*, 24751–24758. [CrossRef]
178. Hill, D.R.; Kessler, S.P.; Rho, H.K.; Cowman, M.K.; de la Motte, C.A. Specific-sized hyaluronan fragments promote expression of human beta-defensin 2 in intestinal epithelium. *J. Biol. Chem.* **2012**, *287*, 30610–30624. [CrossRef]
179. Gunasekaran, A.; Eckert, J.; Burge, K.; Zheng, W.; Yu, Z.; Kessler, S.; de la Motte, C.; Chaaban, H. Hyaluronan 35 kDa enhances epithelial barrier function and protects against the development of murine necrotizing enterocolitis. *Pediatr. Res.* **2019**. [CrossRef]
180. Stabler, T.V.; Huang, Z.; Montell, E.; Verges, J.; Kraus, V.B. Chondroitin sulphate inhibits NF-kappaB activity induced by interaction of pathogenic and damage associated molecules. *Osteoarthr. Cartil.* **2017**, *25*, 166–174. [CrossRef]
181. du Souich, P.; Garcia, A.G.; Verges, J.; Montell, E. Immunomodulatory and anti-inflammatory effects of chondroitin sulphate. *J. Cell Mol. Med.* **2009**, *13*, 1451–1463. [CrossRef] [PubMed]
182. Egea, J.; Garcia, A.G.; Verges, J.; Montell, E.; Lopez, M.G. Antioxidant, antiinflammatory and neuroprotective actions of chondroitin sulfate and proteoglycans. *Osteoarthr. Cartil.* **2010**, *18* (Suppl. 1), S24–S27. [CrossRef]

183. Linares, P.M.; Chaparro, M.; Algaba, A.; Roman, M.; Moreno Arza, I.; Abad Santos, F.; Ochoa, D.; Guerra, I.; Bermejo, F.; Gisbert, J.P. Effect of Chondroitin Sulphate on Pro-Inflammatory Mediators and Disease Activity in Patients with Inflammatory Bowel Disease. *Digestion* **2015**, *92*, 203–210. [CrossRef] [PubMed]
184. Hori, Y.; Hoshino, J.; Yamazaki, C.; Sekiguchi, T.; Miyauchi, S.; Horie, K. Effects of chondroitin sulfate on colitis induced by dextran sulfate sodium in rats. *Jpn. J. Pharm.* **2001**, *85*, 155–160. [CrossRef] [PubMed]
185. Segarra, S.; Martinez-Subiela, S.; Cerda-Cuellar, M.; Martinez-Puig, D.; Munoz-Prieto, A.; Rodriguez-Franco, F.; Rodriguez-Bertos, A.; Allenspach, K.; Velasco, A.; Ceron, J. Oral chondroitin sulfate and prebiotics for the treatment of canine Inflammatory Bowel Disease: A randomized, controlled clinical trial. *BMC Vet. Res* **2016**, *12*, 49. [CrossRef]
186. Luo, J.; Cao, J.; Jiang, X.; Cui, H. Effect of low molecular weight heparin rectal suppository on experimental ulcerative colitis in mice. *Biomed. Pharm.* **2010**, *64*, 441–445. [CrossRef]
187. Zezos, P.; Kouklakis, G.; Saibil, F. Inflammatory bowel disease and thromboembolism. *World J. Gastroenterol.* **2014**, *20*, 13863–13878. [CrossRef]
188. Mousavi, S.; Moradi, M.; Khorshidahmad, T.; Motamedi, M. Anti-Inflammatory Effects of Heparin and Its Derivatives: A Systematic Review. *Adv. Pharm. Sci.* **2015**, *2015*, 507151. [CrossRef]
189. Lean, Q.Y.; Gueven, N.; Eri, R.D.; Bhatia, R.; Sohal, S.S.; Stewart, N.; Peterson, G.M.; Patel, R.P. Heparins in ulcerative colitis: Proposed mechanisms of action and potential reasons for inconsistent clinical outcomes. *Exp. Rev. Clin. Pharm.* **2015**, *8*, 795–811. [CrossRef]
190. Remon, J.I.; Amin, S.C.; Mehendale, S.R.; Rao, R.; Luciano, A.A.; Garzon, S.A.; Maheshwari, A. Depth of bacterial invasion in resected intestinal tissue predicts mortality in surgical necrotizing enterocolitis. *J. Perinatol.* **2015**, *35*, 755–762. [CrossRef]
191. Heida, F.H.; Harmsen, H.J.; Timmer, A.; Kooi, E.M.; Bos, A.F.; Hulscher, J.B. Identification of bacterial invasion in necrotizing enterocolitis specimens using fluorescent in situ hybridization. *J. Perinatol.* **2017**, *37*, 67–72. [CrossRef] [PubMed]
192. Hall, T.; Dymock, D.; Corfield, A.P.; Weaver, G.; Woodward, M.; Berry, M. Bacterial invasion of HT29-MTX-E12 monolayers: Effects of human breast milk. *J. Pediatr. Surg.* **2013**, *48*, 353–357, discussion 357–358. [CrossRef] [PubMed]
193. Kim, Y.; Kessler, S.P.; Obery, D.R.; Homer, C.R.; McDonald, C.; de la Motte, C.A. Hyaluronan 35 kDa treatment protects mice from Citrobacter rodentium infection and induces epithelial tight junction protein ZO-1 in vivo. *Matrix Biol.* **2017**, *62*, 28–39. [CrossRef] [PubMed]
194. Burge, K.Y.; Hannah, L.; Eckert, J.V.; Gunasekaran, A.; Chaaban, H. The Protective Influence of Chondroitin Sulfate, a Component of Human Milk, on Intestinal Bacterial Invasion and Translocation. *J. Hum. Lact.* **2019**, *35*, 538–549. [CrossRef] [PubMed]
195. Chavez-Bueno, S.; Day, M.W.; Toby, I.T.; Akins, D.R.; Dyer, D.W. Genome Sequence of SCB34, a Sequence Type 131 Multidrug-Resistant Escherichia coli Isolate Causing Neonatal Early-Onset Sepsis. *Genome Announc.* **2014**, *2*. [CrossRef]

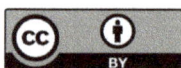 © 2020 by the authors. Licensee MDPI, Basel, Switzerland. This article is an open access article distributed under the terms and conditions of the Creative Commons Attribution (CC BY) license (http://creativecommons.org/licenses/by/4.0/).

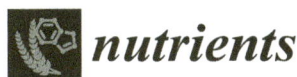 

*Review*

# The Therapeutic Potential of Breast Milk-Derived Extracellular Vesicles

Jeffrey D. Galley and Gail E. Besner *

Center for Perinatal Research, The Research Institute at Nationwide Children's Hospital, Department of Pediatric Surgery, Nationwide Children's Hospital, Columbus, OH 43205, USA; jeffrey.galley@nationwidechildrens.org
* Correspondence: gail.besner@nationwidechildrens.org; Tel.: +1-614-722-3900

Received: 9 January 2020; Accepted: 8 March 2020; Published: 11 March 2020

**Abstract:** In the past few decades, interest in the therapeutic benefits of exosomes and extracellular vesicles (EVs) has grown exponentially. Exosomes/EVs are small particles which are produced and exocytosed by cells throughout the body. They are loaded with active regulatory and stimulatory molecules from the parent cell including miRNAs and enzymes, making them prime targets in therapeutics and diagnostics. Breast milk, known for years to have beneficial health effects, contains a population of EVs which may mediate its therapeutic effects. This review offers an update on the therapeutic potential of exosomes/EVs in disease, with a focus on EVs present in human breast milk and their remedial effect in the gastrointestinal disease necrotizing enterocolitis. Additionally, the relationship between EV miRNAs, health, and disease will be examined, along with the potential for EVs and their miRNAs to be engineered for targeted treatments.

**Keywords:** extracellular vesicle; exosome; necrotizing enterocolitis; breast milk

## 1. Exosomes

Since secreted extracellular vesicles (EVs) were first discovered over 30 years ago [1,2], their involvement in the interrelated fields of physiology [3,4], immunology [5–7], and metabolism [8–10] has been the subject of extensive research. EVs are nanosized particles, between 30 and 2000 nanometers in size, that can be grouped based on their range of sizes. EVs between 30 and 150 nm are termed exosomes, while larger particles between 150 and 1000 nm are known as microvesicles [11]. The mechanism of formation for exosomes and microvesicles differ, in that exosomes are initially intraluminal vesicles, located in intracellular multivesicular bodies. As these bodies directly fuse with the parent cellular membrane, the smaller vesicles are exocytosed into the luminal space [12]. Microvesicles, the larger of the two, can fuse with the cellular membrane and directly bud from the cell [13]. Both exosomes and microvesicles are packaged with an assortment of molecules from the parent cell, including proteins, lipids, messenger RNA, and microRNAs [14,15]. The mechanism of formation of EVs as a whole is mediated by numerous proteins that eventually become part of the EV structure. These proteins, which embed in the EV bilipid layer, have been established as positive markers in EV confirmatory analysis, including tetraspanins such as CD63 and CD81 [16], vesicular fusion proteins such as flotillin [17], and the vesicular formation protein Alix [18].

EVs are released from multiple cell types throughout the body and participate in intercellular communication by fusing with recipient cell membranes and delivering the parent cell molecular cargo to the recipient target cell [19]. The functional outputs that occur as a result of EV-mediated shuttling of cargo are expansive. EVs can increase the proliferation and survivability of disparate cell types, including cartilage and endothelial cells, through modulation of AKT/ERK proliferative transcription pathways [20,21]. EVs can also influence innate and adaptive immunity, as demonstrated by their ability to modulate the NF-kB inflammatory signal transduction pathway, as well as T-cell priming and activation [22–24]. The source of the EVs has a major influence on their function. For example, stem cell (SC)-derived EVs have notable beneficial properties, including the ability to reduce the incidence of the severe intestinal disease necrotizing enterocolitis (NEC) in rat pups [25]. SC-EVs can also increase contractility and reduce diastolic pressure in murine hearts, accelerate mouse bone fracture healing, and increase neural growth—all hallmarks of beneficial health outcomes [3,26,27]. Additionally, EV cargo function is often analogous to the function of the parent cell from which the cargo originated. For example, EVs that are derived from immune cells such as dendritic cells are associated with regulation of the immune system [22], while EVs of cardiac origin mediate cardiac-related outcomes including anti-apoptosis of cardiomyocytes [28,29]. The cross-cell communicable functionality of EVs is also wide-ranging, with as many recipient cell types as there are cellular origins of EVs [30–32].

## 2. The Therapeutic Potential of Exosomes

The identification of EVs, and particularly of exosomes, as intercellular communicators that have far-reaching effects on human health has opened the door to a surfeit of potential uses for these nanoparticles. One common thread throughout exosomal and EV research is their therapeutic potential, and how they might be able to improve health outcomes systemically. The diverse molecules that compose EV cargo are the primary effectors of these therapeutic functions, and they can be surface-bound or found within the vesicle itself. Surface-bound bioactive molecules include antibodies, which can ameliorate complement-mediated cytotoxicity [33], and e-cadherin, a molecule involved in adhesion that can be bound to exosomes and utilized in tumor angiogenesis [34].

The internal cargo of EVs, including enzymes and miRNAs, impart therapeutic function on recipient cells upon delivery from the EV [35,36]. miRNAs, which are 18–22 nucleotide non-coding RNAs, have been identified as a primary player in EV therapeutic function by regulating gene expression post-transcriptionally [37]. The miRNAs form the RNA-induced silencing complex (RISC) in combination with the Argonaute silencing protein [38]. miRNAs have a specific seed sequence that targets a complementary sequence on the 3'-untranslated region of target mRNA [39]. At this point, the Argonaute protein represses translation by blocking formation of the translational protein complex or by actually degrading the mRNA [40]. Given the wide breadth of genes regulated by miRNAs in this manner [41], it is not surprising that exosomal/EV miRNAs have multiple natural therapeutic effects on health. For example, miRNAs delivered by secreted exosomes/EVs can enhance T-cell antigenic tolerance to contact sensitivity [42], increase neurite growth [43], and modulate the integrity of the brain vasculature by induction of endothelial cadherin [44], which maintains endothelial tight junctions. These miRNAs have also proven therapeutic in models of hepatitis, sepsis, and heart disease [45–47]. EV-derived miRNAs can have broad targeting effects on protein levels. Pro-inflammatory miRNAs, like miR-155, can increase pro-inflammatory IL6 protein levels in response to LPS when delivered via exosomes, while exosomal anti-inflammatory miR-146 reduce IL6 and IL12 protein levels while increasing the immunomodulatory cytokine, IL10 [48]. Innovations in exosome biology have allowed researchers to engineer exosomes/EVs for delivery of specific miRNA cargo [49,50]. Exosomes and miRNAs are highly stable and can withstand the stresses of the GI tract and the bloodstream, strengthening their case as a potentially tunable therapeutic system [51–53]. This can be done through transfection of a parent cell with an miRNA-mimic to over-produce a particular miRNA, or by transfecting exosomes/EVs directly, leading to an increase in miRNAs packaged within exosomes [35,49,50,54]. Electroporation, commonly used in the transformation or transfection of bacterial and mammalian genomes respectively, is often utilized to introduce over-expression of miRNA constructs into exosomes/EVs [49,50]. Upon in vitro synthesis, the exosomes can then be extracted, purified, and delivered therapeutically. In a study by Qu et al., adipose-derived mesenchymal stem cells were engineered to over-express miRNA-181-5p. Exosomes released from these stem cells were able to abrogate fibrosis in a liver disease model by increasing autophagy and inhibiting cell survival pathways [55]. A different study showed that over-expressed exosomal miRNA-181 reduced cardiac infarction and resultant inflammatory readouts including the IL-6 cytokine [56]. This can extend to other miRNAs, such as miR-134, which reduced breast cancer cell migration when over-expressed and released by EVs [57].

## 3. Disease and Exosomal miRNAs

Exosomes/EVs are not always associated with therapeutic outcomes. They have also been associated with disease states which has led to their cargo, especially miRNAs, being utilized as disease biomarkers for inflammatory diseases [58], neural disorders such as Alzheimer's disease [59], and cancers such as leukemia and colon cancer [60,61]. Exosomal/EV miRNAs can also confer disease phenotypes, including transferring cancer drug resistance between cancer cells [62]. One such study demonstrated that sensitivity to tyrosine kinase inhibitors, a drug used against chronic myeloid leukemia, can be reduced by the export of miR-365 from resistant cells to sensitive cells [63]. Similar findings were reported by Wei et al., wherein exosomal release of miR-221/222 conveyed tamoxifen resistance to breast cancer cells [62]. Other studies have shown that exosomal miRNA-155 is inflammogenic through IL6 and IL8 upregulation [64], while exosomal miRNA-214-3p can inhibit bone development by interfering with osteogenic transcription factors [36], highlighting the wide range of deleterious health effects that exosomal/EV miRNAs are capable of mediating. Angiogenesis is associated with both negative health outcomes (e.g., tumor growth) and beneficial outcomes (e.g., wound healing and the resolution of cardiovascular disease), and EVs are capable of increasing angiogenesis [65–67]. Specifically, the transfer of miRNAs from exosomes/EVs has been associated with elevations in angiogenesis. miR-30b is one such miR that is transported via stem cell exosomes and can increase vessel branching via the inhibitory binding of DLL4, an anti-angiogenesis transcription factor [65].

In an extension of synthetically increasing miRNA expression as detailed above, researchers can also inhibit disease-associated miRNAs with anti-miR oligonucleotides, which are complementary to specific miRNAs and can bind and block their regulatory activity [36,68,69]. In one example, anti-miR-9 was constructed, and mesenchymal stem cells were seeded with the engineered anti-miRs. The authors showed that anti-miRs derived from these stem cells were able to inhibit miR-9-mediated resistance to the chemotherapeutic drug temozolomide, by increasing caspase activity [70]. Engineering elevations in miRNA production can also increase disease pathology. Over-expression of miRNA-212/132 increased the leakiness of the blood–brain barrier, while anti-miRs were able to abrogate these changes [71].

Pre-term birth is associated with multiple disease and adverse health outcomes, including necrotizing enterocolitis. Work is underway to examine how exosome/EVs and their miRNA cargo are involved in pre-term birth. One such study demonstrated considerable changes in the plasma-derived exosomal-miRNA profile of human mothers that delivered pre-term compared to those that delivered at term. Increased among the pre-term exosomal miRNA populations were miRNAs involved in glucocorticoid signaling, which is often elevated before labor progression [72]. Even non-EV-derived circulating miRNAs isolated as early as the first trimester can predict pre-term birth [73,74]. In mice, exosomal cargo composition shifts based on gestational age of the dam were observed, and proteomic analyses demonstrated that exosomes isolated from E18 dams were highest in inflammatory mediators. The authors of this paper surmised that this could be for cervical relaxation prior to birth. The importance of gestational age on exosomal composition was further established by the observation that E18 exosomes were capable of inducing pre-term birth, indicating that exosomes may be instrumental in the birthing process [75]. These studies offer compelling evidence for the wide-ranging effects that EV-miRNAs can have, acting as compositional biomarkers for pre-term labor and also being closely involved in the process of labor, pre-term or otherwise.

## 4. Breast Milk as a Therapeutic Bio-Fluid

Historically, the importance of breast milk (BM) in neonatal and infant health is unquestioned. The inherent benefits of BM are many and well-documented, including aiding in the development of the neonatal immune system through the delivery of antibodies like secretory immunoglobulin A [76], seeding and normalizing the infant microbiota as the BM is rich in beneficial bacterial species including

Lactobacillus and Bifidobacterium [77], and reducing infant mortality in NEC and sudden infant death syndrome [78,79]. The reason for the multitudinous benefits of BM are due primarily to its composition. BM has a high quantity of proteins, many of which have immunological functions, including lactoferrin, immunoglobulin A, and cytokines [80]. Breast milk also contains milk oligosaccharides that are involved in infant immunity by strengthening gut barrier integrity [81], assisting in modeling health-associated microbiota [82], and activating production of the anti-inflammatory cytokine IL-10 [83]. Clinical reports also suggest that human milk oligosaccharide, whether supplemented in breast milk or formula, is protective against bronchitis and other lower respiratory tract infections [84].

Fatty acids (FAs) within breast milk are also impactful on neonate health, and their levels are differentially associated with disease prevalence. FAs are generally distributed between the saturated and unsaturated categories, and in total, make up nearly half of the energy supply for a breastfed infant. The major FA constituents of breast milk are of the polyunsaturated variety, including linoleic acid and its derivatives, arachidonic acid (ARA), and docosahexaenoic acid (DHA). FAs have been associated closely with cognitive neurodevelopment and motor development. Breast milk is also a major source of vitamins for the newborn infant, with considerable concentrations of vitamins B, C, A, and D, as well as niacin and riboflavin [85]. While the mother's diet is a major determinant of the levels of these vitamins, their prevalence in BM further establishes BM as an acutely important foundation of any infant's diet.

## 5. Breast Milk Exosomes

In the search for exosomes/EVs that have a higher propensity for therapeutic effects, while also having the potential to be easily administered clinically, BM-derived exosomes have become a key player. Recently, there has been a spike in interest of the potential beneficial effects of BM exosomes [86,87]. These effects are spread across numerous mammals, including humans, bovines, camels, and pigeons [86–89]. A particular focus is being paid to the effect that BM exosomes have on the gastrointestinal (GI) tract, given recent studies that have shown that these human BM exosomes are resilient to digestion and can be endocytosed by intestinal epithelial cells, indicating that BM exosomes have the ideal qualities of a potential therapeutic. Resilience to digestion extends to BM EV-derived miRNAs [51,53,90]. In a study by Hock et al., rat BM-derived exosomes increased intestinal cell proliferation through the activation of stem cell marker, Lgr5 [87]. Similar findings were reported in a hydrogen peroxide model of oxidative stress. H2O2 increased cell death in the rat IEC-6 intestinal cell line. The addition of human BM-derived exosomes abrogated H2O2-induced increase in cell death, while significantly elevating cell viability over control [91].

The composition of BM-EVs is an open question. In a recent study, Wang et al. performed peptidomic analysis of BM exosomes, comparing mother's milk from term pregnancies to mother's milk from preterm pregnancies [92]. The authors discovered that preterm and term milk exosomes had altered peptide compositions comparatively. Cells treated with pre-term BM exosomes exhibited increased proliferation which was potentially associated with lactotransferrin and lactadherin, peptides that were up-regulated in the pre-term group [92]. Milk oligosaccharide has also been identified as a beneficial component in BM. In one study, the human milk oligosaccharide 2'-fucosyllactose protected against intestinal disease by increasing eNOS production. The elevated eNOS modulates mesenteric perfusion within the gut, a process that combats necrotic pathology [93].

Work is also underway to characterize the BM-EV miRNA profile, with miR-30d-5p, let-7b-5p, and let-7a-5p amongst the most abundant [94]. EV-miR-30d mediates the expression of genes involved in embryonic development, and let-7b is a well-known regulator of inflammation that mediates Toll-like receptor 4 activation, which can stimulate inflammation [95,96]. The composition of highly abundant EV-miRNAs is similar between term and pre-term milk, and both can be internalized by intestinal epithelial cells [51,90]. These miRNAs can then alter gene transcription within the cells. For example, internalized miR-148a reduces DNTM1 expression [97], while miR-22-3p, a highly expressed human BM-EV miRNA [51], downregulates NF-kB, a pro-inflammatory transcription factor [98]. As with protein composition, researchers have investigated how the "age" of the BM affects miRNA composition. One study reported that early milk in pandas, such as colostrum, contained miRNAs more closely associated with immune regulation and response, while later mature milk had more of a development and metabolism profile [99]. Interestingly, milk collected within the first week of a baby's birth has a higher concentration of exosomes compared to milk collected by the baby's second month of life [100].

As detailed above, breastfeeding has numerous beneficial effects, and in offspring it is negatively associated with obesity as well as reductions in exacerbations of asthma [101,102]. Given the correlation between BM-EV miRNA compositions and specific physiological functions including inflammation modulation and metabolism, it comes as no surprise that BM-EV miRNAs are likely to play a major role in preventing offspring disease prevalence. However, while these specific connections have not yet been made, it is generally known that exosomes derived from BM have broad immunomodulatory function, including reducing IL-2 and TNF-α production and inducing T-regulatory cell activation [103,104]. While deeper analysis tying BM-EV miRNAs to reduced risk of obesity or asthma development is necessary to draw conclusions, the breadth of beneficial outcomes mediated by BM-EVs gives credence to the hypothesis that BM-EV miRNAs are likely key mediators in most breastfeeding-associated outcomes.

The effect mediated by BM-derived exosomes can also be deleterious. Human BM exosomes are capable of inducing epithelial to mesenchymal transition (EMT), a phenomenon in which epithelial cells can lose their normal polarity and become increasingly migratory as the basement membrane breaks down [105]. This is often associated with the development of cancer, and cells that undergo this transition are generally invasive [106]. Additionally, mothers with Type-1 diabetes have an altered BM-EV miRNA profile, of which some of the differentially-expressed miRNAs are capable of inducing pro-inflammatory cytokine expression [107].

## 6. Breast Milk Extracellular Vesicles and Necrotizing Enterocolitis

BM-EVs have been targeted as a compelling therapeutic for NEC, a disease that affects premature infants, particularly in the low birth weight subset [108]. Early NEC symptomology includes abdominal distension, feeding intolerance, and ileus. In moderate cases, clinicians treat the disease with antibiotics, withholding of enteral feeds, and administration of total parenteral nutrition [109]. In severe cases, babies develop fulminant intestinal inflammation and eventual necrosis of the intestinal tissue. Mortality rates are as high as 40%–50% [108,110], and survivors can suffer from developmental disorders later in life, including memory deficits [111]. Infants that have undergone surgery may also have short bowel syndrome later in life, due to the reduction in overall intestinal length [109]. With these abundant issues associated with NEC, it is incumbent upon researchers to develop targeted, specific treatments for the disease. BM components, such as human milk saccharides (i.e., oligosaccharides like 2′-fucosyllactose and glycosaminoglycans like hyaluronan) and anti-microbial peptides (i.e., lactoferrin), have proven to have some efficacy in the treatment of NEC [93,112,113].

There is much interest in BM-EV therapeutic development for NEC. NEC animal models are widely used by research labs, including rat, mouse, and pig models [25,114–117]. Using the well-characterized rat NEC model, we have demonstrated that human BM-derived EVs reduce the incidence of NEC in rat pups when delivered orally with formula feeds. Orally delivered BM-EVs had improved efficacy compared to BM-EVs delivered intraperitoneally, which may be related to the stability of the BM-EVs trafficking through the digestive tract [51,86,90]. Human BM-EVs had pro-proliferative and anti-apoptotic effects in both rat (IEC-6) and human (FHS74) intestinal cell culture models, suggesting that the therapeutic properties of BM-EVs are mediated through a protective effect on intestinal epithelial cells [86]. These results corroborated other research demonstrating that BM-EVs have similar protective effects on cellular proliferation and growth [87]. We have also demonstrated that stem cell-derived EVs released from multiple sources, including amniotic fluid-derived mesenchymal stem cells (MSCs), bone marrow-derived MSCs, and amniotic fluid-derived neural SCs, also have therapeutic effects in NEC, significantly reducing overall NEC incidence in rat pups [25,115]. Both SC-derived EVs and SCs alone were associated with improved gut barrier function, abrogating the gut leakiness often associated with NEC, though the mechanistic involvement of SC-EVs in this process is presently unknown [115,118]. Protein production is likely one of the primary targets in EV/exosome-mediated therapeutics. BM-derived exosomes were able to mediate the expression of multiple proteins to reduce NEC severity, including reducing myeloperoxidase, a pro-inflammatory molecule released by neutrophils that is elevated in a mouse model of NEC, while increasing MUC2 and GRP94, which are expressed by goblet cells and are major components in the intact gut barrier [119]. In a murine LPS model, exosome administration reduced LPS-induced elevations in pro-inflammatory cytokine protein levels (e.g. IL-1, IL-6, TNF-α) [120]. In the same model, exosomes reduced pro-apoptotic caspase-3, as well as components of the pro-inflammatory signal transduction proteins, TLR4 and MyD88. Exosomes were also able to reduce LPS-induced phosphorylation of the NFκB pathway. Many of these anti-apoptotic and anti-inflammatory effects were mediated by exosomal miRNAs. Given previous studies that have demonstrated the tunable nature of EV miRNAs [35,36], BM-derived EVs continue to be a strong candidate in disease therapeutics.

## 7. Future Directions of EV Therapy for NEC

Going forward, there is a crucial need for a better understanding of: (1) NEC pathophysiology, (2) NEC etiology, and (3) NEC inflammatory mechanisms. This knowledge will allow more stringent focusing of therapeutic EV cargos. As numerous studies have shown, NEC incidence and severity, as well as intestinal injury in commonly used in vitro models of gut disease, can be ameliorated through EV treatment [25,86,87]. The reductions in NEC injury severity by EVs may be mediated through EV-miRNAs, given their well-known ability to mediate disease outcomes [57]. Targeted treatments for these pathways, particularly through fine-tuning of EV-miRNA cargos, may prove to be an especially valuable avenue to pursue. Additionally, continued study on synthetically-produced EVs with specific pre-loaded cargos will provide members of the medical community an improved tool with proven ability to traffic to specific sites where their cargo can be unloaded.

## 8. Conclusions

This review has summarized recent research breakthroughs in the functionality of exosomes/EVs, particularly those derived from BM, as therapeutics in disease treatment. The fact that these EVs can store and transport stimulatory and regulatory elements, including miRNAs and enzymes, forms the basis for these nanoparticles to act as intercellular communicators as well as potential remedies for, or disseminators of, disease. Nearly every cell produces and exocytoses exosomes/EVs, including breast cells. BM is rife with exosomes/EVs, and given that the beneficial qualities of BM are well documented, it is of considerable interest to examine the extent to which these nanoparticles may mediate its positive effects. Herein, we have reviewed many of the recent studies that have investigated this very question, and we conclude that the evidence conveys strongly that BM-EVs are closely involved in health mediation. This is particularly observed in the treatment of necrotizing enterocolitis [86,119]. The use of BM-exosomes/EVs has proven to be a promising treatment in animal models of NEC, through pro-cellular proliferation and anti-apoptosis mechanisms [86]. However, further investigation is necessary prior to delivering these therapies clinically.

Researchers have discovered methods of amplifying or ablating EV miRNA composition, using silencing or over-expression vectors, and have demonstrated that such changes can have either deleterious or beneficial health effects [35,36,56,69]. These studies show promise for what can be performed with these particles and their cargos synthetically. The knowledge regarding the ability of these nanoparticles to be administered, to traffic to sites of disease, and to deliver their cargo, in combination with the capability to manipulate, tune, and improve their efficacy, creates a truly exciting opportunity in disease therapeutics.

**Author Contributions:** Literature review, J.D.G. and G.E.B.; writing—original draft preparation, J.D.G.; writing—review and editing, G.E.B. and J.D.G.; supervision, G.E.B. All authors have read and agreed to the published version of the manuscript.

**Funding:** This work was funded by R01GM113236 (GEB).

**Conflicts of Interest:** The authors declare no conflict of interest.

## References

1. Pan, B.T.; Johnstone, R.M. Fate of the transferrin receptor during maturation of sheep reticulocytes in vitro: Selective externalization of the receptor. *Cell* **1983**, *33*, 967–978. [CrossRef]
2. Harding, C.; Stahl, P. Transferrin recycling in reticulocytes: pH and iron are important determinants of ligand binding and processing. *Biochem. Biophys. Res. Commun.* **1983**, *113*, 650–658. [CrossRef]
3. Arslan, F.; Lai, R.C.; Smeets, M.B.; Akeroyd, L.; Choo, A.; Aguor, E.N.; Timmers, L.; van Rijen, H.V.; Doevendans, P.A.; Pasterkamp, G.; et al. Mesenchymal stem cell-derived exosomes increase ATP levels, decrease oxidative stress and activate PI3K/Akt pathway to enhance myocardial viability and prevent adverse remodeling after myocardial ischemia/reperfusion injury. *Stem Cell Res.* **2013**, *10*, 301–312. [CrossRef] [PubMed]
4. Greco, V.; Hannus, M.; Eaton, S. Argosomes: A potential vehicle for the spread of morphogens through epithelia. *Cell* **2001**, *106*, 633–645. [CrossRef]
5. Chen, X.; Song, C.H.; Feng, B.S.; Li, T.L.; Li, P.; Zheng, P.Y.; Chen, X.M.; Xing, Z.; Yang, P.C. Intestinal epithelial cell-derived integrin alphabeta6 plays an important role in the induction of regulatory T cells and inhibits an antigen-specific Th2 response. *J. Leukoc. Biol.* **2011**, *90*, 751–759. [CrossRef]
6. Brown, M.; Johnson, L.A.; Leone, D.A.; Majek, P.; Vaahtomeri, K.; Senfter, D.; Bukosza, N.; Schachner, H.; Asfour, G.; Langer, B.; et al. Lymphatic exosomes promote dendritic cell migration along guidance cues. *J. Cell Biol.* **2018**, *217*, 2205–2221. [CrossRef]
7. Majumdar, R.; Tavakoli Tameh, A.; Parent, C.A. Exosomes Mediate LTB4 Release during Neutrophil Chemotaxis. *PLoS Biol.* **2016**, *14*, e1002336. [CrossRef]
8. Kranendonk, M.E.; Visseren, F.L.; van Herwaarden, J.A.; Nolte-'t Hoen, E.N.; de Jager, W.; Wauben, M.H.; Kalkhoven, E. Effect of extracellular vesicles of human adipose tissue on insulin signaling in liver and muscle cells. *Obesity* **2014**, *22*, 2216–2223. [CrossRef]
9. Zhao, H.; Shang, Q.; Pan, Z.; Bai, Y.; Li, Z.; Zhang, H.; Zhang, Q.; Guo, C.; Zhang, L.; Wang, Q. Exosomes From Adipose-Derived Stem Cells Attenuate Adipose Inflammation and Obesity Through Polarizing M2 Macrophages and Beiging in White Adipose Tissue. *Diabetes* **2018**, *67*, 235–247. [CrossRef]
10. Garcia, N.A.; Moncayo-Arlandi, J.; Sepulveda, P.; Diez-Juan, A. Cardiomyocyte exosomes regulate glycolytic flux in endothelium by direct transfer of GLUT transporters and glycolytic enzymes. *Cardiovasc. Res.* **2016**, *109*, 397–408. [CrossRef]
11. Colombo, M.; Raposo, G.; Thery, C. Biogenesis, secretion, and intercellular interactions of exosomes and other extracellular vesicles. *Annu. Rev. Cell Dev. Biol.* **2014**, *30*, 255–289. [CrossRef] [PubMed]
12. Pan, B.T.; Teng, K.; Wu, C.; Adam, M.; Johnstone, R.M. Electron microscopic evidence for externalization of the transferrin receptor in vesicular form in sheep reticulocytes. *J. Cell Biol.* **1985**, *101*, 942–948. [CrossRef] [PubMed]
13. Heijnen, H.F.; Schiel, A.E.; Fijnheer, R.; Geuze, H.J.; Sixma, J.J. Activated platelets release two types of membrane vesicles: Microvesicles by surface shedding and exosomes derived from exocytosis of multivesicular bodies and alpha-granules. *Blood* **1999**, *94*, 3791–3799. [CrossRef] [PubMed]
14. Haraszti, R.A.; Didiot, M.C.; Sapp, E.; Leszyk, J.; Shaffer, S.A.; Rockwell, H.E.; Gao, F.; Narain, N.R.; DiFiglia, M.; Kiebish, M.A.; et al. High-resolution proteomic and lipidomic analysis of exosomes and microvesicles from different cell sources. *J. Extracell. Vesicles* **2016**, *5*, 32570. [CrossRef]
15. Waldenstrom, A.; Genneback, N.; Hellman, U.; Ronquist, G. Cardiomyocyte microvesicles contain DNA/RNA and convey biological messages to target cells. *PLoS ONE* **2012**, *7*, e34653. [CrossRef]
16. Escola, J.M.; Kleijmeer, M.J.; Stoorvogel, W.; Griffith, J.M.; Yoshie, O.; Geuze, H.J. Selective enrichment of tetraspan proteins on the internal vesicles of multivesicular endosomes and on exosomes secreted by human B-lymphocytes. *J. Biol. Chem.* **1998**, *273*, 20121–20127. [CrossRef]
17. Kowal, J.; Arras, G.; Colombo, M.; Jouve, M.; Morath, J.P.; Primdal-Bengtson, B.; Dingli, F.; Loew, D.; Tkach, M.; Thery, C. Proteomic comparison defines novel markers to characterize heterogeneous populations of extracellular vesicle subtypes. *Proc. Natl. Acad. Sci. USA* **2016**, *113*, E968–E977. [CrossRef]

18. Willms, E.; Johansson, H.J.; Mager, I.; Lee, Y.; Blomberg, K.E.; Sadik, M.; Alaarg, A.; Smith, C.I.; Lehtio, J.; El Andaloussi, S.; et al. Cells release subpopulations of exosomes with distinct molecular and biological properties. *Sci. Rep.* **2016**, *6*, 22519. [CrossRef]
19. Montecalvo, A.; Larregina, A.T.; Shufesky, W.J.; Stolz, D.B.; Sullivan, M.L.; Karlsson, J.M.; Baty, C.J.; Gibson, G.A.; Erdos, G.; Wang, Z.; et al. Mechanism of transfer of functional microRNAs between mouse dendritic cells via exosomes. *Blood* **2012**, *119*, 756–766. [CrossRef]
20. Ren, S.; Chen, J.; Duscher, D.; Liu, Y.; Guo, G.; Kang, Y.; Xiong, H.; Zhan, P.; Wang, Y.; Wang, C.; et al. Microvesicles from human adipose stem cells promote wound healing by optimizing cellular functions via AKT and ERK signaling pathways. *Stem Cell Res.* **2019**, *10*, 47. [CrossRef]
21. Zhang, S.; Chuah, S.J.; Lai, R.C.; Hui, J.H.P.; Lim, S.K.; Toh, W.S. MSC exosomes mediate cartilage repair by enhancing proliferation, attenuating apoptosis and modulating immune reactivity. *Biomaterials* **2018**, *156*, 16–27. [CrossRef] [PubMed]
22. Segura, E.; Nicco, C.; Lombard, B.; Veron, P.; Raposo, G.; Batteux, F.; Amigorena, S.; Thery, C. ICAM-1 on exosomes from mature dendritic cells is critical for efficient naive T-cell priming. *Blood* **2005**, *106*, 216–223. [CrossRef] [PubMed]
23. Wang, Y.; Zheng, F.; Gao, G.; Yan, S.; Zhang, L.; Wang, L.; Cai, X.; Wang, X.; Xu, D.; Wang, J. MiR-548a-3p regulates inflammatory response via TLR4/NF-kappaB signaling pathway in rheumatoid arthritis. *J. Cell Biochem.* **2018**. [CrossRef]
24. Tkach, M.; Kowal, J.; Zucchetti, A.E.; Enserink, L.; Jouve, M.; Lankar, D.; Saitakis, M.; Martin-Jaular, L.; Thery, C. Qualitative differences in T-cell activation by dendritic cell-derived extracellular vesicle subtypes. *Embo J.* **2017**, *36*, 3012–3028. [CrossRef] [PubMed]
25. McCulloh, C.J.; Olson, J.K.; Wang, Y.; Zhou, Y.; Tengberg, N.H.; Deshpande, S.; Besner, G.E. Treatment of experimental necrotizing enterocolitis with stem cell-derived exosomes. *J. Pediatr Surg* **2018**, *53*, 1215–1220. [CrossRef] [PubMed]
26. Furuta, T.; Miyaki, S.; Ishitobi, H.; Ogura, T.; Kato, Y.; Kamei, N.; Miyado, K.; Higashi, Y.; Ochi, M. Mesenchymal Stem Cell-Derived Exosomes Promote Fracture Healing in a Mouse Model. *Stem Cells Transl. Med.* **2016**, *5*, 1620–1630. [CrossRef]
27. Lopez-Verrilli, M.A.; Caviedes, A.; Cabrera, A.; Sandoval, S.; Wyneken, U.; Khoury, M. Mesenchymal stem cell-derived exosomes from different sources selectively promote neuritic outgrowth. *Neuroscience* **2016**, *320*, 129–139. [CrossRef]
28. Xiao, J.; Pan, Y.; Li, X.H.; Yang, X.Y.; Feng, Y.L.; Tan, H.H.; Jiang, L.; Feng, J.; Yu, X.Y. Cardiac progenitor cell-derived exosomes prevent cardiomyocytes apoptosis through exosomal miR-21 by targeting PDCD4. *Cell Death Dis.* **2016**, *7*, e2277. [CrossRef]
29. Mol, E.A.; Goumans, M.J.; Sluijter, J.P.G. Cardiac Progenitor-Cell Derived Exosomes as Cell-Free Therapeutic for Cardiac Repair. *Adv. Exp. Med. Biol.* **2017**, *998*, 207–219.
30. Shelke, G.V.; Yin, Y.; Jang, S.C.; Lasser, C.; Wennmalm, S.; Hoffmann, H.J.; Li, L.; Gho, Y.S.; Nilsson, J.A.; Lotvall, J. Endosomal signalling via exosome surface TGFbeta-1. *J. Extracell. Vesicles* **2019**, *8*, 1650458. [CrossRef]
31. Li, J.; Liu, K.; Liu, Y.; Xu, Y.; Zhang, F.; Yang, H.; Liu, J.; Pan, T.; Chen, J.; Wu, M.; et al. Exosomes mediate the cell-to-cell transmission of IFN-alpha-induced antiviral activity. *Nat. Immunol.* **2013**, *14*, 793–803. [CrossRef] [PubMed]
32. Horibe, S.; Tanahashi, T.; Kawauchi, S.; Murakami, Y.; Rikitake, Y. Mechanism of recipient cell-dependent differences in exosome uptake. *BMC Cancer* **2018**, *18*, 47. [CrossRef] [PubMed]
33. Capello, M.; Vykoukal, J.V.; Katayama, H.; Bantis, L.E.; Wang, H.; Kundnani, D.L.; Aguilar-Bonavides, C.; Aguilar, M.; Tripathi, S.C.; Dhillon, D.S.; et al. Exosomes harbor B cell targets in pancreatic adenocarcinoma and exert decoy function against complement-mediated cytotoxicity. *Nat. Commun.* **2019**, *10*, 254. [CrossRef] [PubMed]
34. Tang, M.K.S.; Yue, P.Y.K.; Ip, P.P.; Huang, R.L.; Lai, H.C.; Cheung, A.N.Y.; Tse, K.Y.; Ngan, H.Y.S.; Wong, A.S.T. Soluble E-cadherin promotes tumor angiogenesis and localizes to exosome surface. *Nat. Commun.* **2018**, *9*, 2270. [CrossRef]
35. Che, Y.; Shi, X.; Shi, Y.; Jiang, X.; Ai, Q.; Shi, Y.; Gong, F.; Jiang, W. Exosomes Derived from miR-143-Overexpressing MSCs Inhibit Cell Migration and Invasion in Human Prostate Cancer by Downregulating TFF3. *Mol. Nucleic Acids* **2019**, *18*, 232–244. [CrossRef]

36. Li, D.; Liu, J.; Guo, B.; Liang, C.; Dang, L.; Lu, C.; He, X.; Cheung, H.Y.; Xu, L.; Lu, C.; et al. Osteoclast-derived exosomal miR-214-3p inhibits osteoblastic bone formation. *Nat. Commun.* **2016**, *7*, 10872. [CrossRef]
37. Shivdasani, R.A. MicroRNAs: Regulators of gene expression and cell differentiation. *Blood* **2006**, *108*, 3646–3653. [CrossRef]
38. Meister, G. Argonaute proteins: Functional insights and emerging roles. *Nat. Rev. Genet.* **2013**, *14*, 447–459. [CrossRef]
39. Bartel, D.P. MicroRNAs: Target recognition and regulatory functions. *Cell* **2009**, *136*, 215–233. [CrossRef]
40. Iwasaki, S.; Kawamata, T.; Tomari, Y. Drosophila argonaute1 and argonaute2 employ distinct mechanisms for translational repression. *Mol. Cell* **2009**, *34*, 58–67. [CrossRef]
41. Lewis, B.P.; Burge, C.B.; Bartel, D.P. Conserved seed pairing, often flanked by adenosines, indicates that thousands of human genes are microRNA targets. *Cell* **2005**, *120*, 15–20. [CrossRef] [PubMed]
42. Bryniarski, K.; Ptak, W.; Jayakumar, A.; Pullmann, K.; Caplan, M.J.; Chairoungdua, A.; Lu, J.; Adams, B.D.; Sikora, E.; Nazimek, K.; et al. Antigen-specific, antibody-coated, exosome-like nanovesicles deliver suppressor T-cell microRNA-150 to effector T cells to inhibit contact sensitivity. *J. Allergy Clin. Immunol.* **2013**, *132*, 170–181. [CrossRef] [PubMed]
43. Xin, H.; Li, Y.; Buller, B.; Katakowski, M.; Zhang, Y.; Wang, X.; Shang, X.; Zhang, Z.G.; Chopp, M. Exosome-mediated transfer of miR-133b from multipotent mesenchymal stromal cells to neural cells contributes to neurite outgrowth. *Stem Cells* **2012**, *30*, 1556–1564. [CrossRef] [PubMed]
44. Xu, B.; Zhang, Y.; Du, X.F.; Li, J.; Zi, H.X.; Bu, J.W.; Yan, Y.; Han, H.; Du, J.L. Neurons secrete miR-132-containing exosomes to regulate brain vascular integrity. *Cell Res.* **2017**, *27*, 882–897. [CrossRef]
45. Zhou, Y.; Li, P.; Goodwin, A.J.; Cook, J.A.; Halushka, P.V.; Chang, E.; Fan, H. Exosomes from Endothelial Progenitor Cells Improve the Outcome of a Murine Model of Sepsis. *Mol.* **2018**, *26*, 1375–1384. [CrossRef]
46. Qian, X.; Xu, C.; Fang, S.; Zhao, P.; Wang, Y.; Liu, H.; Yuan, W.; Qi, Z. Exosomal MicroRNAs Derived From Umbilical Mesenchymal Stem Cells Inhibit Hepatitis C Virus Infection. *Stem Cells Transl. Med.* **2016**, *5*, 1190–1203. [CrossRef]
47. Zhu, J.; Lu, K.; Zhang, N.; Zhao, Y.; Ma, Q.; Shen, J.; Lin, Y.; Xiang, P.; Tang, Y.; Hu, X.; et al. Myocardial reparative functions of exosomes from mesenchymal stem cells are enhanced by hypoxia treatment of the cells via transferring microRNA-210 in an nSMase2-dependent way. *Artif. Cells Nanomed. Biotechnol.* **2018**, *46*, 1659–1670. [CrossRef]
48. Alexander, M.; Hu, R.; Runtsch, M.C.; Kagele, D.A.; Mosbruger, T.L.; Tolmachova, T.; Seabra, M.C.; Round, J.L.; Ward, D.M.; O'Connell, R.M. Exosome-delivered microRNAs modulate the inflammatory response to endotoxin. *Nat. Commun.* **2015**, *6*, 7321. [CrossRef]
49. Lamichhane, T.N.; Jay, S.M. Production of Extracellular Vesicles Loaded with Therapeutic Cargo. *Methods Mol. Biol.* **2018**, *1831*, 37–47.
50. Pomatto, M.A.C.; Bussolati, B.; D'Antico, S.; Ghiotto, S.; Tetta, C.; Brizzi, M.F.; Camussi, G. Improved Loading of Plasma-Derived Extracellular Vesicles to Encapsulate Antitumor miRNAs. *Mol. Methods Clin. Dev.* **2019**, *13*, 133–144. [CrossRef]
51. Liao, Y.; Du, X.; Li, J.; Lonnerdal, B. Human milk exosomes and their microRNAs survive digestion in vitro and are taken up by human intestinal cells. *Mol. Nutr. Food Res.* **2017**, *61*, 1700082. [CrossRef] [PubMed]
52. Sanz-Rubio, D.; Martin-Burriel, I.; Gil, A.; Cubero, P.; Forner, M.; Khalyfa, A.; Marin, J.M. Stability of Circulating Exosomal miRNAs in Healthy Subjects. *Sci. Rep.* **2018**, *8*, 10306. [CrossRef] [PubMed]
53. Benmoussa, A.; Lee, C.H.; Laffont, B.; Savard, P.; Laugier, J.; Boilard, E.; Gilbert, C.; Fliss, I.; Provost, P. Commercial Dairy Cow Milk microRNAs Resist Digestion under Simulated Gastrointestinal Tract Conditions. *J. Nutr.* **2016**, *146*, 2206–2215. [CrossRef] [PubMed]
54. Liu, L.; Zhao, X.; Zhu, X.; Zhong, Z.; Xu, R.; Wang, Z.; Cao, J.; Hou, Y. Decreased expression of miR-430 promotes the development of bladder cancer via the upregulation of CXCR7. *Mol. Med. Rep.* **2013**, *8*, 140–146. [CrossRef] [PubMed]
55. Qu, Y.; Zhang, Q.; Cai, X.; Li, F.; Ma, Z.; Xu, M.; Lu, L. Exosomes derived from miR-181-5p-modified adipose-derived mesenchymal stem cells prevent liver fibrosis via autophagy activation. *J. Cell Mol. Med.* **2017**, *21*, 2491–2502. [CrossRef] [PubMed]
56. Wei, Z.; Qiao, S.; Zhao, J.; Liu, Y.; Li, Q.; Wei, Z.; Dai, Q.; Kang, L.; Xu, B. miRNA-181a over-expression in mesenchymal stem cell-derived exosomes influenced inflammatory response after myocardial ischemia-reperfusion injury. *Life Sci.* **2019**, *232*, 116632. [CrossRef] [PubMed]

57. O'Brien, K.; Lowry, M.C.; Corcoran, C.; Martinez, V.G.; Daly, M.; Rani, S.; Gallagher, W.M.; Radomski, M.W.; MacLeod, R.A.; O'Driscoll, L. miR-134 in extracellular vesicles reduces triple-negative breast cancer aggression and increases drug sensitivity. *Oncotarget* **2015**, *6*, 32774–32789. [CrossRef]
58. Ebrahimkhani, S.; Vafaee, F.; Young, P.E.; Hur, S.S.J.; Hawke, S.; Devenney, E.; Beadnall, H.; Barnett, M.H.; Suter, C.M.; Buckland, M.E. Exosomal microRNA signatures in multiple sclerosis reflect disease status. *Sci. Rep.* **2017**, *7*, 14293. [CrossRef]
59. Yang, T.T.; Liu, C.G.; Gao, S.C.; Zhang, Y.; Wang, P.C. The Serum Exosome Derived MicroRNA-135a, -193b, and -384 Were Potential Alzheimer's Disease Biomarkers. *Biomed. Environ. Sci.* **2018**, *31*, 87–96.
60. Hornick, N.I.; Huan, J.; Doron, B.; Goloviznina, N.A.; Lapidus, J.; Chang, B.H.; Kurre, P. Serum Exosome MicroRNA as a Minimally-Invasive Early Biomarker of AML. *Sci. Rep.* **2015**, *5*, 11295. [CrossRef]
61. Ogata-Kawata, H.; Izumiya, M.; Kurioka, D.; Honma, Y.; Yamada, Y.; Furuta, K.; Gunji, T.; Ohta, H.; Okamoto, H.; Sonoda, H.; et al. Circulating exosomal microRNAs as biomarkers of colon cancer. *PLoS ONE* **2014**, *9*, e92921. [CrossRef] [PubMed]
62. Wei, Y.; Lai, X.; Yu, S.; Chen, S.; Ma, Y.; Zhang, Y.; Li, H.; Zhu, X.; Yao, L.; Zhang, J. Exosomal miR-221/222 enhances tamoxifen resistance in recipient ER-positive breast cancer cells. *Breast Cancer Res. Treat.* **2014**, *147*, 423–431. [CrossRef] [PubMed]
63. Min, Q.H.; Wang, X.Z.; Zhang, J.; Chen, Q.G.; Li, S.Q.; Liu, X.Q.; Li, J.; Liu, J.; Yang, W.M.; Jiang, Y.H.; et al. Exosomes derived from imatinib-resistant chronic myeloid leukemia cells mediate a horizontal transfer of drug-resistant trait by delivering miR-365. *Exp. Cell Res.* **2018**, *362*, 386–393. [CrossRef] [PubMed]
64. Chen, C.; Luo, F.; Liu, X.; Lu, L.; Xu, H.; Yang, Q.; Xue, J.; Shi, L.; Li, J.; Zhang, A.; et al. NF-kB-regulated exosomal miR-155 promotes the inflammation associated with arsenite carcinogenesis. *Cancer Lett.* **2017**, *388*, 21–33. [CrossRef] [PubMed]
65. Gong, M.; Yu, B.; Wang, J.; Wang, Y.; Liu, M.; Paul, C.; Millard, R.W.; Xiao, D.S.; Ashraf, M.; Xu, M. Mesenchymal stem cells release exosomes that transfer miRNAs to endothelial cells and promote angiogenesis. *Oncotarget* **2017**, *8*, 45200–45212. [CrossRef] [PubMed]
66. Lin, X.J.; Fang, J.H.; Yang, X.J.; Zhang, C.; Yuan, Y.; Zheng, L.; Zhuang, S.M. Hepatocellular Carcinoma Cell-Secreted Exosomal MicroRNA-210 Promotes Angiogenesis In Vitro and In Vivo. *Mol. Nucleic Acids* **2018**, *11*, 243–252. [CrossRef]
67. Wang, N.; Chen, C.; Yang, D.; Liao, Q.; Luo, H.; Wang, X.; Zhou, F.; Yang, X.; Yang, J.; Zeng, C.; et al. Mesenchymal stem cells-derived extracellular vesicles, via miR-210, improve infarcted cardiac function by promotion of angiogenesis. *Biochim. Biophys. Acta Mol. Basis Dis.* **2017**, *1863*, 2085–2092. [CrossRef]
68. Hu, Y.; Tao, X.; Han, X.; Xu, L.; Yin, L.; Sun, H.; Qi, Y.; Xu, Y.; Peng, J. MicroRNA-351-5p aggravates intestinal ischaemia/reperfusion injury through the targeting of MAPK13 and Sirtuin-6. *Br. J. Pharm.* **2018**, *175*, 3594–3609. [CrossRef]
69. Pakravan, G.; Foroughmand, A.M.; Peymani, M.; Ghaedi, K.; Hashemi, M.S.; Hajjari, M.; Nasr-Esfahani, M.H. Downregulation of miR-130a, antagonized doxorubicin-induced cardiotoxicity via increasing the PPARgamma expression in mESCs-derived cardiac cells. *Cell Death Dis.* **2018**, *9*, 758. [CrossRef]
70. Munoz, J.L.; Bliss, S.A.; Greco, S.J.; Ramkissoon, S.H.; Ligon, K.L.; Rameshwar, P. Delivery of Functional Anti-miR-9 by Mesenchymal Stem Cell-derived Exosomes to Glioblastoma Multiforme Cells Conferred Chemosensitivity. *Mol. Nucleic Acids* **2013**, *2*, e126. [CrossRef]
71. Burek, M.; Konig, A.; Lang, M.; Fiedler, J.; Oerter, S.; Roewer, N.; Bohnert, M.; Thal, S.C.; Blecharz-Lang, K.G.; Woitzik, J.; et al. Hypoxia-Induced MicroRNA-212/132 Alter Blood-Brain Barrier Integrity Through Inhibition of Tight Junction-Associated Proteins in Human and Mouse Brain Microvascular Endothelial Cells. *Transl. Stroke Res.* **2019**, *10*, 672–683. [CrossRef] [PubMed]
72. Menon, R.; Debnath, C.; Lai, A.; Guanzon, D.; Bhatnagar, S.; Kshetrapal, P.K.; Sheller-Miller, S.; Salomon, C.; Garbhini Study, T. Circulating Exosomal miRNA Profile During Term and Preterm Birth Pregnancies: A Longitudinal Study. *Endocrinology* **2019**, *160*, 249–275. [CrossRef] [PubMed]
73. Cook, J.; Bennett, P.R.; Kim, S.H.; Teoh, T.G.; Sykes, L.; Kindinger, L.M.; Garrett, A.; Binkhamis, R.; MacIntyre, D.A.; Terzidou, V. First Trimester Circulating MicroRNA Biomarkers Predictive of Subsequent Preterm Delivery and Cervical Shortening. *Sci. Rep.* **2019**, *9*, 5861. [CrossRef] [PubMed]
74. Winger, E.E.; Reed, J.L.; Ji, X. Early first trimester peripheral blood cell microRNA predicts risk of preterm delivery in pregnant women: Proof of concept. *PLoS ONE* **2017**, *12*, e0180124. [CrossRef] [PubMed]

75. Sheller-Miller, S.; Trivedi, J.; Yellon, S.M.; Menon, R. Exosomes Cause Preterm Birth in Mice: Evidence for Paracrine Signaling in Pregnancy. *Sci. Rep.* **2019**, *9*, 608. [CrossRef] [PubMed]
76. Rogier, E.W.; Frantz, A.L.; Bruno, M.E.; Wedlund, L.; Cohen, D.A.; Stromberg, A.J.; Kaetzel, C.S. Secretory antibodies in breast milk promote long-term intestinal homeostasis by regulating the gut microbiota and host gene expression. *Proc. Natl. Acad. Sci. USA* **2014**, *111*, 3074–3079. [CrossRef] [PubMed]
77. Martin, V.; Maldonado-Barragan, A.; Moles, L.; Rodriguez-Banos, M.; Campo, R.D.; Fernandez, L.; Rodriguez, J.M.; Jimenez, E. Sharing of bacterial strains between breast milk and infant feces. *J. Hum. Lact.* **2012**, *28*, 36–44. [CrossRef]
78. Sullivan, S.; Schanler, R.J.; Kim, J.H.; Patel, A.L.; Trawoger, R.; Kiechl-Kohlendorfer, U.; Chan, G.M.; Blanco, C.L.; Abrams, S.; Cotten, C.M.; et al. An exclusively human milk-based diet is associated with a lower rate of necrotizing enterocolitis than a diet of human milk and bovine milk-based products. *J. Pediatr.* **2010**, *156*, 562–567. [CrossRef]
79. Ip, S.; Chung, M.; Raman, G.; Chew, P.; Magula, N.; DeVine, D.; Trikalinos, T.; Lau, J. Breastfeeding and maternal and infant health outcomes in developed countries. *Evid. Rep. Technol. Assess.* **2007**, *153*, 1–186.
80. Ballard, O.; Morrow, A.L. Human milk composition: Nutrients and bioactive factors. *Pediatr. Clin. North. Am.* **2013**, *60*, 49–74. [CrossRef]
81. Kong, C.; Elderman, M.; Cheng, L.; de Haan, B.J.; Nauta, A.; de Vos, P. Modulation of Intestinal Epithelial Glycocalyx Development by Human Milk Oligosaccharides and Non-Digestible Carbohydrates. *Mol. Nutr. Food Res.* **2019**, *63*, e1900303. [CrossRef] [PubMed]
82. Marcobal, A.; Barboza, M.; Sonnenburg, E.D.; Pudlo, N.; Martens, E.C.; Desai, P.; Lebrilla, C.B.; Weimer, B.C.; Mills, D.A.; German, J.B.; et al. Bacteroides in the infant gut consume milk oligosaccharides via mucus-utilization pathways. *Cell Host Microbe* **2011**, *10*, 507–514. [CrossRef] [PubMed]
83. Comstock, S.S.; Wang, M.; Hester, S.N.; Li, M.; Donovan, S.M. Select human milk oligosaccharides directly modulate peripheral blood mononuclear cells isolated from 10-d-old pigs. *Br. J. Nutr.* **2014**, *111*, 819–828. [CrossRef] [PubMed]
84. Puccio, G.; Alliet, P.; Cajozzo, C.; Janssens, E.; Corsello, G.; Sprenger, N.; Wernimont, S.; Egli, D.; Gosoniu, L.; Steenhout, P. Effects of Infant Formula With Human Milk Oligosaccharides on Growth and Morbidity: A Randomized Multicenter Trial. *J. Pediatr. Gastroenterol. Nutr.* **2017**, *64*, 624–631. [CrossRef] [PubMed]
85. Bates, C.J.; Prentice, A. Breast milk as a source of vitamins, essential minerals and trace elements. *Pharmacol. Ther.* **1994**, *62*, 193–220. [CrossRef]
86. Pisano, C.; Galley, J.; Elbahrawy, M.; Wang, Y.; Farrell, A.; Brigstock, D.; Besner, G.E. Human Breast Milk-Derived Extracellular Vesicles in the Protection Against Experimental Necrotizing Enterocolitis. *J. Pediatr. Surg.* **2019**, in press. [CrossRef]
87. Hock, A.; Miyake, H.; Li, B.; Lee, C.; Ermini, L.; Koike, Y.; Chen, Y.; Maattanen, P.; Zani, A.; Pierro, A. Breast milk-derived exosomes promote intestinal epithelial cell growth. *J. Pediatr. Surg.* **2017**, *52*, 755–759. [CrossRef]
88. Badawy, A.A.; El-Magd, M.A.; AlSadrah, S.A. Therapeutic Effect of Camel Milk and Its Exosomes on MCF7 Cells In Vitro and In Vivo. *Integr. Cancer* **2018**, *17*, 1235–1246. [CrossRef]
89. Ma, Y.; Feng, S.; Wang, X.; Qazi, I.H.; Long, K.; Luo, Y.; Li, G.; Ning, C.; Wang, Y.; Hu, S.; et al. Exploration of exosomal microRNA expression profiles in pigeon 'Milk' during the lactation period. *BMC Genom.* **2018**, *19*, 828. [CrossRef]
90. Kahn, S.; Liao, Y.; Du, X.; Xu, W.; Li, J.; Lonnerdal, B. Exosomal MicroRNAs in Milk from Mothers Delivering Preterm Infants Survive in Vitro Digestion and Are Taken Up by Human Intestinal Cells. *Mol. Nutr. Food Res.* **2018**, *62*, e1701050. [CrossRef]
91. Martin, C.; Patel, M.; Williams, S.; Arora, H.; Brawner, K.; Sims, B. Human breast milk-derived exosomes attenuate cell death in intestinal epithelial cells. *Innate Immun.* **2018**, *24*, 278–284. [CrossRef] [PubMed]
92. Wang, X.; Yan, X.; Zhang, L.; Cai, J.; Zhou, Y.; Liu, H.; Hu, Y.; Chen, W.; Xu, S.; Liu, P.; et al. Identification and Peptidomic Profiling of Exosomes in Preterm Human Milk: Insights Into Necrotizing Enterocolitis Prevention. *Mol. Nutr. Food Res.* **2019**, e1801247. [CrossRef] [PubMed]
93. Good, M.; Sodhi, C.P.; Yamaguchi, Y.; Jia, H.; Lu, P.; Fulton, W.B.; Martin, L.Y.; Prindle, T.; Nino, D.F.; Zhou, Q.; et al. The human milk oligosaccharide 2'-fucosyllactose attenuates the severity of experimental necrotising enterocolitis by enhancing mesenteric perfusion in the neonatal intestine. *Br. J. Nutr.* **2016**, *116*, 1175–1187. [CrossRef] [PubMed]

94. van Herwijnen, M.J.C.; Driedonks, T.A.P.; Snoek, B.L.; Kroon, A.M.T.; Kleinjan, M.; Jorritsma, R.; Pieterse, C.M.J.; Hoen, E.; Wauben, M.H.M. Abundantly Present miRNAs in Milk-Derived Extracellular Vesicles Are Conserved Between Mammals. *Front. Nutr.* **2018**, *5*, 81. [CrossRef]
95. Guo, Z.; Cai, X.; Guo, X.; Xu, Y.; Gong, J.; Li, Y.; Zhu, W. Let-7b ameliorates Crohn's disease-associated adherent-invasive E coli induced intestinal inflammation via modulating Toll-Like Receptor 4 expression in intestinal epithelial cells. *Biochem. Pharm.* **2018**, *156*, 196–203. [CrossRef]
96. Vilella, F.; Moreno-Moya, J.M.; Balaguer, N.; Grasso, A.; Herrero, M.; Martinez, S.; Marcilla, A.; Simon, C. Hsa-miR-30d, secreted by the human endometrium, is taken up by the pre-implantation embryo and might modify its transcriptome. *Development* **2015**, *142*, 3210–3221. [CrossRef]
97. Golan-Gerstl, R.; Elbaum Shiff, Y.; Moshayoff, V.; Schecter, D.; Leshkowitz, D.; Reif, S. Characterization and biological function of milk-derived miRNAs. *Mol. Nutr. Food Res.* **2017**, *61*, 1700009. [CrossRef]
98. Takata, A.; Otsuka, M.; Kojima, K.; Yoshikawa, T.; Kishikawa, T.; Yoshida, H.; Koike, K. MicroRNA-22 and microRNA-140 suppress NF-kappaB activity by regulating the expression of NF-kappaB coactivators. *Biochem. Biophys. Res. Commun.* **2011**, *411*, 826–831. [CrossRef]
99. Ma, J.; Wang, C.; Long, K.; Zhang, H.; Zhang, J.; Jin, L.; Tang, Q.; Jiang, A.; Wang, X.; Tian, S.; et al. Exosomal microRNAs in giant panda (Ailuropoda melanoleuca) breast milk: Potential maternal regulators for the development of newborn cubs. *Sci. Rep.* **2017**, *7*, 3507. [CrossRef]
100. Torregrosa Paredes, P.; Gutzeit, C.; Johansson, S.; Admyre, C.; Stenius, F.; Alm, J.; Scheynius, A.; Gabrielsson, S. Differences in exosome populations in human breast milk in relation to allergic sensitization and lifestyle. *Allergy* **2014**, *69*, 463–471. [CrossRef]
101. Yan, J.; Liu, L.; Zhu, Y.; Huang, G.; Wang, P.P. The association between breastfeeding and childhood obesity: A meta-analysis. *BMC Public Health* **2014**, *14*, 1267. [CrossRef] [PubMed]
102. Ahmadizar, F.; Vijverberg, S.J.H.; Arets, H.G.M.; de Boer, A.; Garssen, J.; Kraneveld, A.D.; Maitland-van der Zee, A.H. Breastfeeding is associated with a decreased risk of childhood asthma exacerbations later in life. *Pediatr. Allergy Immunol.* **2017**, *28*, 649–654. [CrossRef] [PubMed]
103. Admyre, C.; Johansson, S.M.; Qazi, K.R.; Filen, J.J.; Lahesmaa, R.; Norman, M.; Neve, E.P.; Scheynius, A.; Gabrielsson, S. Exosomes with immune modulatory features are present in human breast milk. *J. Immunol.* **2007**, *179*, 1969–1978. [CrossRef] [PubMed]
104. Gu, Y.; Li, M.; Wang, T.; Liang, Y.; Zhong, Z.; Wang, X.; Zhou, Q.; Chen, L.; Lang, Q.; He, Z.; et al. Lactation-related microRNA expression profiles of porcine breast milk exosomes. *PLoS ONE* **2012**, *7*, e43691. [CrossRef] [PubMed]
105. Qin, W.; Tsukasaki, Y.; Dasgupta, S.; Mukhopadhyay, N.; Ikebe, M.; Sauter, E.R. Exosomes in Human Breast Milk Promote EMT. *Clin. Cancer Res.* **2016**, *22*, 4517–4524. [CrossRef] [PubMed]
106. Trimboli, A.J.; Fukino, K.; de Bruin, A.; Wei, G.; Shen, L.; Tanner, S.M.; Creasap, N.; Rosol, T.J.; Robinson, M.L.; Eng, C.; et al. Direct evidence for epithelial-mesenchymal transitions in breast cancer. *Cancer Res.* **2008**, *68*, 937–945. [CrossRef]
107. Mirza, A.H.; Kaur, S.; Nielsen, L.B.; Storling, J.; Yarani, R.; Roursgaard, M.; Mathiesen, E.R.; Damm, P.; Svare, J.; Mortensen, H.B.; et al. Breast Milk-Derived Extracellular Vesicles Enriched in Exosomes From Mothers With Type 1 Diabetes Contain Aberrant Levels of microRNAs. *Front. Immunol.* **2019**, *10*, 2543. [CrossRef]
108. Fitzgibbons, S.C.; Ching, Y.; Yu, D.; Carpenter, J.; Kenny, M.; Weldon, C.; Lillehei, C.; Valim, C.; Horbar, J.D.; Jaksic, T. Mortality of necrotizing enterocolitis expressed by birth weight categories. *J. Pediatr. Surg.* **2009**, *44*, 1072–1075. [CrossRef]
109. Rich, B.S.; Dolgin, S.E. Necrotizing Enterocolitis. *Pediatr. Rev.* **2017**, *38*, 552–559. [CrossRef]
110. Allin, B.S.R.; Long, A.M.; Gupta, A.; Lakhoo, K.; Knight, M. One-year outcomes following surgery for necrotising enterocolitis: A UK-wide cohort study. *Arch. Dis. Child. Fetal Neonatal Ed.* **2018**, *103*, F461–F466. [CrossRef]
111. Rees, C.M.; Pierro, A.; Eaton, S. Neurodevelopmental outcomes of neonates with medically and surgically treated necrotizing enterocolitis. *Arch. Dis. Child. Fetal Neonatal Ed.* **2007**, *92*, F193–F198. [CrossRef] [PubMed]
112. Pammi, M.; Suresh, G. Enteral lactoferrin supplementation for prevention of sepsis and necrotizing enterocolitis in preterm infants. *Cochrane Database Syst. Rev.* **2017**, *6*, CD007137. [CrossRef] [PubMed]

113. Gunasekaran, A.; Eckert, J.; Burge, K.; Zheng, W.; Yu, Z.; Kessler, S.; de la Motte, C.; Chaaban, H. Hyaluronan 35 kDa enhances epithelial barrier function and protects against the development of murine necrotizing enterocolitis. *Pediatr. Res.* **2019**. [CrossRef] [PubMed]
114. Olson, J.K.; Navarro, J.B.; Allen, J.M.; McCulloh, C.J.; Mashburn-Warren, L.; Wang, Y.; Varaljay, V.A.; Bailey, M.T.; Goodman, S.D.; Besner, G.E. An enhanced Lactobacillus reuteri biofilm formulation that increases protection against experimental necrotizing enterocolitis. *Am. J. Physiol. Gastrointest. Liver Physiol.* **2018**, *315*, G408–G419. [CrossRef]
115. Rager, T.M.; Olson, J.K.; Zhou, Y.; Wang, Y.; Besner, G.E. Exosomes secreted from bone marrow-derived mesenchymal stem cells protect the intestines from experimental necrotizing enterocolitis. *J. Pediatr. Surg.* **2016**, *51*, 942–947. [CrossRef]
116. Egan, C.E.; Sodhi, C.P.; Good, M.; Lin, J.; Jia, H.; Yamaguchi, Y.; Lu, P.; Ma, C.; Branca, M.F.; Weyandt, S.; et al. Toll-like receptor 4-mediated lymphocyte influx induces neonatal necrotizing enterocolitis. *J. Clin. Investig.* **2016**, *126*, 495–508. [CrossRef]
117. Robinson, J.L.; Smith, V.A.; Stoll, B.; Agarwal, U.; Premkumar, M.H.; Lau, P.; Cruz, S.M.; Manjarin, R.; Olutoye, O.; Burrin, D.G.; et al. Prematurity reduces citrulline-arginine-nitric oxide production and precedes the onset of necrotizing enterocolitis in piglets. *Am. J. Physiol. Gastrointest. Liver Physiol.* **2018**, *315*, G638–G649. [CrossRef]
118. McCulloh, C.J.; Olson, J.K.; Wang, Y.; Vu, J.; Gartner, S.; Besner, G.E. Evaluating the efficacy of different types of stem cells in preserving gut barrier function in necrotizing enterocolitis. *J. Surg. Res.* **2017**, *214*, 278–285. [CrossRef]
119. Li, B.; Hock, A.; Wu, R.Y.; Minich, A.; Botts, S.R.; Lee, C.; Antounians, L.; Miyake, H.; Koike, Y.; Chen, Y.; et al. Bovine milk-derived exosomes enhance goblet cell activity and prevent the development of experimental necrotizing enterocolitis. *PLoS ONE* **2019**, *14*, e0211431. [CrossRef]
120. Xie, M.Y.; Hou, L.J.; Sun, J.J.; Zeng, B.; Xi, Q.Y.; Luo, J.Y.; Chen, T.; Zhang, Y.L. Porcine Milk Exosome MiRNAs Attenuate LPS-Induced Apoptosis through Inhibiting TLR4/NF-kappaB and p53 Pathways in Intestinal Epithelial Cells. *J. Agric. Food Chem.* **2019**, *67*, 9477–9491. [CrossRef]

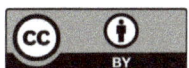

© 2020 by the authors. Licensee MDPI, Basel, Switzerland. This article is an open access article distributed under the terms and conditions of the Creative Commons Attribution (CC BY) license (http://creativecommons.org/licenses/by/4.0/).

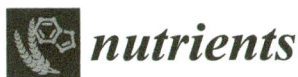 

Article

# Feeding Formula Eliminates the Necessity of Bacterial Dysbiosis and Induces Inflammation and Injury in the Paneth Cell Disruption Murine NEC Model in an Osmolality-Dependent Manner

Shiloh R Lueschow [1], Stacy L Kern [2], Huiyu Gong [2], Justin L Grobe [3], Jeffrey L Segar [4], Susan J Carlson [2] and Steven J McElroy [1,2,*]

[1] Department of Microbiology and Immunology, University of Iowa, Iowa City, IA 52242, USA; shiloh-lueschow@uiowa.edu
[2] Stead Family Department of Pediatrics, University of Iowa, Iowa City, IA 52242, USA; denn0122@umn.edu (S.L.K.); huiyu-gong@uiowa.edu (H.G.); susan-carlson@uiowa.edu (S.J.C.)
[3] Department of Physiology, Medical Coll5ge of Wisconsin, Milwaukee, WI 53226, USA; jgrobe@mcw.edu
[4] Department of Pediatrics, Medical College of Wisconsin, Milwaukee, WI 53226, USA; jsegar@mcw.edu
* Correspondence: steven-mcelroy@uiowa.edu; Tel.: +319-335-3100

Received: 26 February 2020; Accepted: 24 March 2020; Published: 26 March 2020

**Abstract:** Necrotizing enterocolitis (NEC) remains a significant cause of morbidity and mortality in preterm infants. Formula feeding is a risk factor for NEC and osmolality, which is increased by the fortification that is required for adequate growth of the infant, has been suggested as a potential cause. Our laboratory has shown that Paneth cell disruption followed by induction of dysbiosis can induce NEC-like pathology in the absence of feeds. We hypothesized adding formula feeds to the model would exacerbate intestinal injury and inflammation in an osmolality-dependent manner. NEC-like injury was induced in 14–16 day-old C57Bl/6J mice by Paneth cell disruption with dithizone or diphtheria toxin, followed by feeding rodent milk substitute with varying osmolality (250–1491 mOsm/kg $H_2O$). Animal weight, serum cytokines and osmolality, small intestinal injury, and cecal microbial composition were quantified. Paneth cell-disrupted mice fed formula had significant NEC scores compared to controls and no longer required induction of bacterial dysbiosis. Significant increases in serum inflammatory markers, small intestinal damage, and overall mortality were osmolality-dependent and not related to microbial changes. Overall, formula feeding in combination with Paneth cell disruption induced NEC-like injury in an osmolality-dependent manner, emphasizing the importance of vigilance in designing preterm infant feeds.

**Keywords:** necrotizing enterocolitis; immature intestine; formula; osmolality; inflammation; microbiome

## 1. Introduction

Necrotizing enterocolitis (NEC) remains the leading cause of gastrointestinal morbidity and mortality of premature infants, leading to the death of 1/3 to $\frac{1}{2}$ of the infants who develop disease [1,2]. Although the pathophysiology of NEC is still unknown, it is postulated to be the result of bacterial translocation across the immature epithelial barrier leading to tissue invasion, subsequent inflammation, and ultimately destruction [3,4]. In general, NEC onset is preceded by a bloom in Enterobacteriaceae species, although there has been no specific microorganism determined to be causative [5–11]. Studies have linked bacterial dysbiosis or microbiome disruption with NEC development and many murine NEC models capitalize on this fact by inducing bacterial dysbiosis, disruption of the microbiome, or utilizing lipopolysaccharide (LPS), particularly in young mice [12–16]. Formula feeding has been associated with increased risk for development of NEC [17] and in rat models has been shown to induce an inflammatory response in the immature intestine [18]. As an inflammatory milieu can induce dysbiosis in the immature intestine [6], it is reasonable to think that formula-induced inflammation may be one cause of the dysbiosis seen prior to development of NEC.

Our prior work has shown that NEC-like injury can be induced in 14–16 day-old mice (intestinally equivalent to a 22–24 week infant [19,20]) by disrupting Paneth cell biology followed by creation of an intestinal bacterial dysbiosis [21–24]. This model has direct relevance to human biology as multiple investigators have found a decrease in Paneth cells or their granular components following development of NEC [25–28] and an association with NEC and genetic disturbances in Paneth cell biology [29]. We mimic this Paneth cell disruption in wild type mice with dithizone treatment, or in genetically susceptible mice by exposure to diphtheria toxin [21–24,30,31]. Dithizone is a heavy metal chelator that disrupts zinc-rich Paneth cells by leading to an upregulation in autophagy pathways [31]. In contrast, our *PC-DTR* strain of mice has a human diphtheria toxin receptor bound to the Paneth cell-specific cryptdin 2 promoter [30–32], and exposure of these mice to diphtheria toxin induces Paneth cell-specific apoptosis. Following either method of Paneth cell disruption, enteral exposure of *Klebsiella pneumoniae* at a concentration of $1 \times 10^{11}$ colony forming units (CFU)/kilogram body weight to induce bacterial dysbiosis leads to consistent and rapid intestinal pathology that mimics human NEC [26]. Although this model represents two risk factors for NEC (intestinal immaturity and microbial dysbiosis) injury is induced while the mice are not fed.

Infants fed formula are at significantly more risk for NEC than those fed human milk [17,33–35]; however, the mechanism behind this discrepancy is unknown. Human breast milk contains many unique components including nutrients, immunoglobulins, growth factors, hormones, sugars, and proteins that nurture and help to immunologically protect the developing infant. In this fashion, human breast milk is tailored to feed term infants and has everything needed for these infants to grow and succeed [36,37]. However, the caloric requirements necessary to maintain the fetal growth trajectory after birth in preterm infants cannot be achieved by breast milk alone and thus requires fortification from an external source [38,39]. Providing adequate nutrition to preterm infants is critical as there is considerable evidence to support a relationship between poor post-natal growth and later development of neuro-developmental sequelae [40–42].

One side effect of breast milk fortification is a significant increase in osmolality [43]. Osmolality is a measure of the osmoles of solute per kilogram of solvent, with osmoles being defined as a unit of osmotic pressure equivalent to the amount of solute that dissociates in solution to form one mole of particle [44]. The osmolality of infant formula is important as it has been suggested that ingestion of hyperosmolar feeds may lead to NEC [45–47]. While this suggestion was first proposed almost 50 years ago, the understanding of the effect that osmolality has on the immature intestine remains limited. Two recent studies have shown that formula feeding induces changes in intestinal microcirculation and that the associated injury is not osmolality-dependent [48,49]. However, these studies used five- to nine-day-old mice which have not yet developed Paneth cells [20,50] and thus could represent a more immature intestinal epithelium than what is seen in infants who are most susceptible to developing NEC [2,51,52]. To help clarify these gaps in knowledge, we set out to examine the effect of adding formula feeding to our NEC model and to understand if formula induced injury was osmolality dependent. Our novel data show that the addition of formula feeding to either dithizone- or diphtheria toxin-induced Paneth cell disruption eliminated the need to induce dysbiosis to cause NEC-like injury. We additionally show that intestinal injury and markers of inflammation were osmolality-dependent, but not necessarily microbiome dependent. Furthermore, the effects observed were dependent on the method of increasing osmolality. These data expand our understanding of how formula feeding may increase the risk of developing NEC in the preterm infant.

## 2. Methods

### 2.1. Animals and Feeding Protocols

C57BL/6 mice were bred at the University of Iowa under standard conditions according to protocols approved by the Institutional Animal Care and Use Committee (Protocol #8041401) which was approved on 06/11/2018. Original founders were purchased from Jackson Laboratories (Bar Harbor, ME, USA). All mice were dam fed prior to experiments and, unless otherwise indicated, experiments were conducted with P14–P16 mice. All animals were dam fed prior to experimentation. On the day of experimentation, animals were separated from their mothers and maintained in a temperature and humidity-controlled chamber for the duration of the experiment. Formula feeds [23,53] were prepared and homogenized as previously described from their elemental components. Osmolality was measured using an OsmoPro Multi-Sample Micro-Osmometer (Advanced Instruments, Norwood, MA, USA). High osmolality formulas were achieved by adding Mannitol (MAN; Sigma-Aldrich, St. Louis, MO, USA), or by tripling the salt concentration of rodent milk substitution formula (RMS). Sham animals were given equal volumes of saline (Sigma-Aldrich, St. Louis, MO, USA). All prepared formulas and feeding solutions were given via a 24 × 1 W/1-1/4 blunt animal feeding needle (Cadence, Inc.) and a BD one ml Tuberculin syringe (Becton, Dickinson and Company, Franklin Lakes, NJ, USA). Mice were gavage fed 250 µL every three hours × four feeds with one of the following formulations: saline alone; RMS, MAN in saline, NaCl in saline (SALT), RMS$^{MAN}$ added, or RMS$^{SALT}$ (Table 1). Mice were weighed prior to the first feed and following the last feed. Mice were monitored for 3 hours after the final feed and were then euthanized for tissue harvesting. All experiments were performed on at least two separate occasions using at least two different litters. All controls were littermates from experimental animals.

**Table 1.** Definitions of the abbreviations for the feeds used in this paper along with the associated osmolality of each feed type.

| Feeding Type/Abbreviation | Formulation | Osmolality (mOsm/kg H$_2$O) |
|---|---|---|
| Control | Saline | 250 |
| RMS | Rodent milk substitute | 721 |
| Dam | Ad libitum dam feeding | 300 |
| Saline | Saline | 273 |
| MAN | 10% Mannitol in saline | 873 |
| SALT | Saline + 0.7 g NaCl | 581 |
| RMS$_{MAN}$ | RMS + 10% mannitol | 1491 |
| RMS$_{SALT}$ | RMS + 0.7 g NaCl | 982 |

### 2.2. Formula NEC Models

NEC was induced in postnatal day P14–P16 C57Bl/6J mice by giving an intraperitoneal injection of 75 mg/kg body weight dithizone (Sigma) dissolved in 25 mM LiCO$_3$, or an equivalent volume of LiCO$_3$ buffer alone. Depending on the group being considered, 250 µL of RMS (regular formula NEC), RMS$^{SALT}$ (high osmolality formula NEC), or saline (control animals) was fed through oral gavage one hour prior to injecting with dithizone and every three hours for a total of four feeds. Mice were sacrificed and tissues were harvested thirteen hours after the first RMS/saline gavage. NEC was induced in P14–P16 *PC-DTR* mice by giving an intraperitoneal injection of diphtheria toxin at a concentration of 40 ng/g body weight and oral gavage of saline (control animals) or RMS (formula NEC) one hour prior to injection as well as every three hours for a total of four feeds. Mice were sacrificed at sixteen hours after the first oral gavage and tissues were harvested. Similar to above, all experiments were performed on at least two separate occasions using at least two different litters and all controls were littermates from experimental animals.

*2.3. Serum and Cytokine Analysis*

Blood was obtained from the facial vein at the time of euthanasia and serum was processed as previously described [24,54]. Serum samples were used for cytokine (KC-GRO (mouse ortholog to IL-8), TNF-α, IL-6, IL-1β, and IL-10) quantification using a Meso-Scale Discovery V-Plex assay (Meso-Scale, Gaithersburg, MD) on a Mesoscale Sector Imager 2400. Serum osmolality was quantified using an OsmoPro Multi-Sample Micro-Osmometer (Advanced Instruments, Norwood, MA, USA).

*2.4. Microbiota Analysis*

Mice were sacrificed according to institutional guidelines at the University of Iowa and ceca were harvested for DNA extraction using the Zymo Fecal/Soil Microbe MiniPrep kit (Zymo Research, Irvine, CA, USA) as previously described [55,56]. Amplification and sequencing were performed on the 16s rRNA V4 domain using a barcoded forward primer 515F (5'-NNNNNNNNGTGTGCCAFCMGCCGCCGCGGTAA-3') and the reverse primer R806 (5'-GGACTACHVGGGTWTCTAAT-3'). The master mix for amplification of the DNA was made with 1x GoTaq Green Master Mix (Promega, Madison, WI, USA); 1 mM MgCl2; 200 nM 806R reverse primer; 200 nM 515F forward primer with barcode; nuclease free H20; and DNA. The thermocycler parameters for the PCR reaction were as follows: 94 °C for three minutes; 25 cycles of 94 °C for 45 s, 50 °C for 60 s, and 72 °C for 90 s, followed by 72 °C for 10 min and a 4 °C hold period indefinitely. PCR amplicons were run via gel electrophoresis to confirm amplification and then were pooled to relatively equal amplification intensities. The pooled amplicons were then resuspended in 2X the volume of Binding Buffer NTI from the Nucleospin PCR and Gel Purification Kit (Macherey-Nagel, Düren, Germany). The Nucleospin PCR Purification protocol was followed according to the manufacturer instructions (Macherey-Nagel, Düren, Germany). The purified pools were then quantitated using QuantIT dsDNA High Sensitivity Assay (Invitrogen, Carlsbad, CA, USA). Libraries were then submitted to the UC Davis DNA Technologies Center for 2 × 300 paired end Illumina MiSeq sequencing. Sequence data was analyzed using QIIME 1 (University of Colorado, Boulder, CO, USA, version 1.9.1) [57]. Sequences were first quality filtered and demultiplexed. Then, UCLUST (drive5.com, Tiburon, CA, USA) was used to assign operational taxonomic units (OTUs) based on a 97% pairwise identity. The OTUs went through a secondary filtration for low abundance OTUs at a 0.005% threshold. After both filtrations, the Ribosomal Database Project database (Michigan State University, East Lansing, MI, USA) was used to taxonomically classify the OTUs and compare with a representative set of the Greengenes 16s rRNA database (Second Genome, South San Francisco, CA, USA, gg_13_5 release). PyNAST (University of Colorado, Boulder, CO, USA) was used to align the OTU sequences and construct a phylogenetic tree for further β diversity analysis. Unweighted and abundance weighted UniFrac distance was used to calculate the β diversity. Samples were clustered based according to distances between samples.

*2.5. Injury Scoring*

Ileal samples were stained with hematoxylin and eosin to determine injury scores. For NEC models, injury was scored based on a standardized scale as we have described previously [22–24,31] from zero (healthy intestine) to four (full thickness necrosis). Scores of two or greater (separation from the basement membrane and disruption of the villus core) were considered significant for NEC. General non-NEC intestinal injury was assessed by two separate blinded investigators on a three-point scale evaluating villus integrity and separation from the basement membrane as previously described [55,58]. A score of zero was used to describe normal mucosa. Mild injury (score of one) encompassed the development of subepithelial Gruenhagen's space, vacuolization or subepithelial lifting limited to the lamina propria or tips of villi. Severe injury (score of two) involved epithelial lifting and vacuolization greater than half of the villi, villi distortion, or mucosal ulceration and disintegration of the lamina propria.

## 2.6. Statistical Analysis

All experiments were performed in at least triplicate and all experiments used animals from at least 2 separate litters. Specific sample sizes are denoted in the Figure legends. ANOVA and non-parametric Kruskal-Wallis testing was performed to determine statistical significance using Graph Pad Prism v8. Significance was set as $p < 0.05$ for all experiments.

## 3. Results

### 3.1. Formula Feeding in Combination with Dithizone Treatment Results in Inflammation and Removes the Requirement for Bacterial Exposure to Induce NEC-Like Injury in the Immature Murine Intestine

Our previous studies have shown that induction of Paneth cell dysfunction followed by exposure to an enteral bacterial challenge induces NEC-like injury [22,24,54]; however, as opposed to several other common models of NEC [13,59,60], our model does not include formula feeding as a required component. To understand the effect of adding formula exposure to the Paneth cell-disruption model of NEC, we fed a separate group of mice 250 µL of prepared rodent milk substitute (RMS) [23,53,56] every three hours for four feeds prior to and during injury induction and compared them to controls. NEC-like injury was scored as previously described [21–24,31]. Interestingly, animals fed RMS no longer needed additional bacterial exposure to induce significant levels of intestinal injury (Figure 1A). Rather, exposure to enteral RMS feeds, in addition to induction of Paneth cell disruption alone, was enough to induce NEC-like injury equivalent to mice that were exposed to both Paneth cell disruption and *Klebsiella*-induced dysbiosis. Representative histology of all treatments can be seen in Figure 1B. To determine if RMS feeds were inducing inflammation, serum samples were collected at the end of the experiment and measured for Infγ, IL-10, IL-1β, IL-6, KC-GRO (murine homologue of IL-8), and TNF, which are cytokines often associated with intestinal injury and human NEC [61]. Exposure to RMS significantly increased serum levels of all cytokines ($n > 7$ for all groups, $p < 0.001$ for all cytokines measured) (Figure 1C).

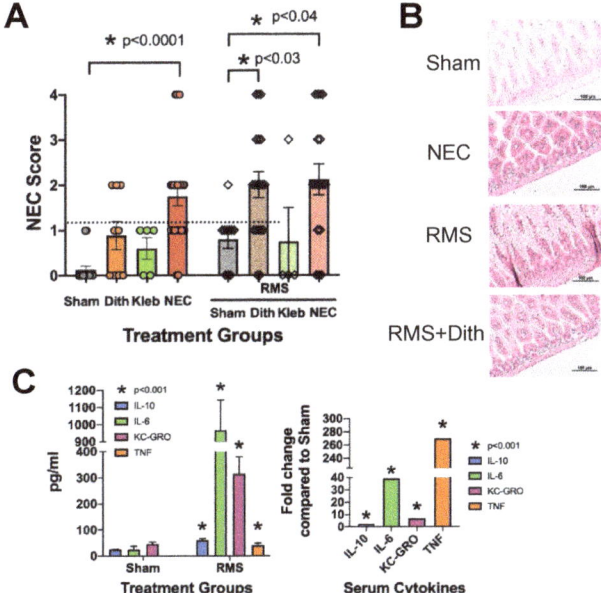

**Figure 1.** Formula feeding induces inflammation and removes the requirement for bacterial exposure to induce necrotizing enterocolitis (NEC)-like injury. C57Bl/6J mice (14–16 days old) were given an

intraperitoneal injection of dithizone (75 mg/kg), a gavage feeding of Klebsiella pneumonia, the combination of both, or sham controls ($n > 7$ for all groups). Only the group given both treatments had significantly elevated injury scores. A second group of mice was given the same treatments but was also fed four times with 250 µL/feed of prepared rodent milk substitute (RMS). In this group, both the dithizone alone and the dithizone plus Klebsiella groups had significant injury, showing that adding RMS feeds eliminated the requirement for bacterial exposure ($n > 7$ for all groups, p values as shown) (**A**). Representative histology is shown (**B**). Serum samples were obtained from sham and sham-RMS mice and quantified for IL-10, IL-6, KC/GRO, and TNF. Sham-RMS mice had significantly higher serum levels of all cytokines than non-RMS control groups ($p < 0.001$ for all cytokines, $n > 7$ for all groups) (**C**).

### 3.2. Paneth Cell Disruption/Formula-Induced NEC is not Dithizone-Dependent

We next sought to determine if the method of Paneth cell disruption in combination with RMS impacted the level of injury and inflammation. P14–P16 *PC-DTR* mice were intraperitoneally treated with 25 ng/g body weight diphtheria toxin to induce Paneth cell apoptosis in addition to four 250 µL RMS feeds given via gavage every three hours for a total of four feeds. Similar to the dithizone/RMS model, diphtheria toxin/RMS treatment induced significant increases in intestinal injury without needing the addition of *Klebsiella*-induced dysbiosis ($n > 5$ for all groups, $p < 0.0001$) (Figure 2A). Representative histology of all treatments can be seen in Figure 2B. We additionally quantified the inflammatory cytokines present in the serum of the *PC-DTR* mice and found significant increases in IL-6 and KC-GRO (Figure 2C).

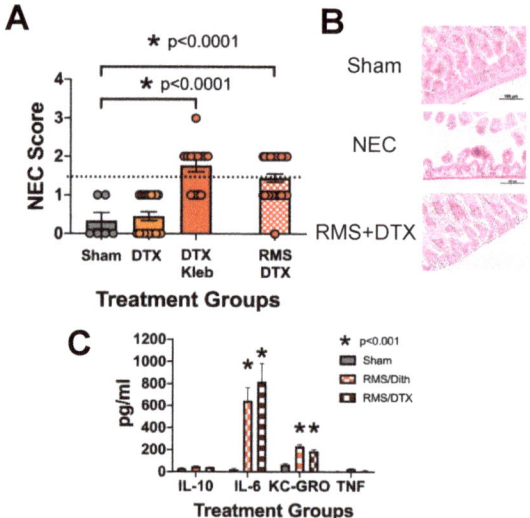

**Figure 2.** Formula feeding along with Paneth cell disruption resulting in NEC-like injury in the absence of bacterial dysbiosis is not dependent on the method of Paneth cell disruption. *PC-DTR* mice on a C57Bl/6J background (14–16 days old) were given an intraperitoneal injection of diphtheria toxin (40 ng/g), a gavage feeding of $1 \times 10^8$/g Klebsiella pneumonia, the combination of both, or RMS in place of K. pneumoniae ($n > 5$ for all groups). Mice fed formula along with diphtheria toxin-induced Paneth cell disruption experienced significant NEC-like injury in the absence of Klebsiella-induced dysbiosis (**A**). Representative histology is shown (**B**). Serum samples obtained from mice before tissue harvest depict significant increases in IL-6 and KC-GRO compared to controls in both dithizone/RMS and DTX/RMS ($n > 10$, $p < 0.001$) (**C**).

## 3.3. Immature Murine Generalized Intestinal Injury and Newborn Mortality Induced by Formula Feeding Is Osmolality-Dependent

RMS has an osmolality of 721 mOsm/kg $H_2O$, which is more than twice as high as either Pedialyte (250 mOsm/kg $H_2O$), saline (273 mOsm/kg $H_2O$), or most mammalian milk (300 mOsm/kg $H_2O$) [44,53]. To determine if isolated osmolality was responsible for the changes we observed in our NEC model, we fed mice every three hours for a total of four feeds with one of the following: saline (273 mOsm/kg $H_2O$), ad libitum dam feeding (300 mOsm/kg $H_2O$), RMS (721 mOsm/kg $H_2O$), 10% MAN in saline (873 mOsm/kg $H_2O$), or RMS + 10% MAN (RMS$^{MAN}$) (1491 mOsm/kg $H_2O$). Importantly, animals fed the highest osmolality formula (RMS$^{MAN}$) had a 50% mortality (most of them prior to the fourth feed) compared to 100% survival for all other feed types (Figure 3A). As mannitol can act as a significant diuretic, we also monitored weights of the animals at the beginning and end of experimentation (Figure 3B). While dam fed animals experienced a significant increase in weight (5.4% increase, $p = 0.009$), sham animals had negligible weight change. Animals fed RMS alone had a slight but non-significant weight increase (2.1%, $p = 0.27$). Animals fed MAN exhibited a significant loss of weight ($-13.6\%$, $p < 0.0001$), as did animals fed RMS$^{MAN}$ ($-7.8\%$, $p < 0.0001$). To quantify generalized intestinal injury, distal ileal sections were harvested at time of euthanasia and scored by two separate blinded investigators on a three-point scale of small intestinal injury described previously [55,58] that is distinct from the NEC injury scoring system (Figure 3C). Injury scores were significantly higher in the RMS, MAN, and RMS$^{MAN}$ groups compared to sham controls ($p = 0.0023$, $0.0009$, and $< 0.0001$ respectively) (Figure 3D).

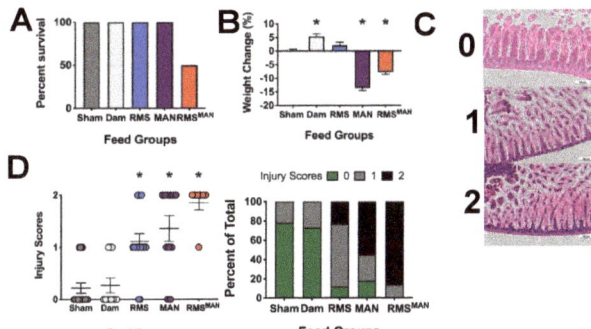

**Figure 3.** Exposure to increasing osmolality induces significant intestinal injury and mortality. C57BL/6J mice were given four 250 µL feeds with one of the following: sham Pedialyte (250 mOsm/kg $H_2O$), dam feeds (300 mOsm/kg $H_2O$), RMS (721 mOsm/kg $H_2O$), MAN in saline (873 mOsm/kg $H_2O$) or RMS + 10% mannitol (RMS$^{MAN}$) (1491 mOsm/kg $H_2O$). Mice fed RMS$^{MAN}$ had a 50% mortality compared to all other groups (**A**). Mouse weight significantly increased in dam fed animals (5.4% increase, $p = 0.009$) compared to controls. Animals fed MAN exhibited a significant loss of weight ($-13.6\%$, $p < 0.0001$), as did animals fed RMS$^{MAN}$ ($-7.8\%$, $p < 0.0001$) (**B**). Intestinal injury was determined on a three point injury scale as shown in (**C**). Intestinal injury scores were significantly higher in the RMS, MAN, and RMS$^{MAN}$ groups compared to sham controls ($p = 0.0023$, $0.0009$, and $< 0.0001$ respectively) (**D**).

Next, we wanted to assess the impact of these different osmolality feeds on serum inflammation (Figure 4A). Serum samples were obtained at the time of euthanasia and quantified for the presence of IL-6, IL-10, TNF, and KC-GRO. Sham and dam feeds showed similar levels of all four cytokines. RMS feeds significantly increased IL-6, TNF, and IL-10 levels compared to sham controls. Exposure to MAN feeds caused significant serum elevations of KC-GRO and IL-10, while feeding with the high osmolality RMS$^{MAN}$ induced significant elevations in all four cytokines ($n > 5$ in all groups and $p < 0.05$ with specific $p$ values shown). Lastly, we examined serum osmolality to ascertain if enteral feeds were impacting the animal systemically (Figure 4B). Serum was drawn from animals at time of euthanasia and measured for osmolality. Feeds with RMS, MAN, or RMS$^{MAN}$ all induced statistically significant elevations in serum osmolality, although the highest elevations were in feeds containing mannitol ($n > 5$, $p < 0.0001$ for all comparisons).

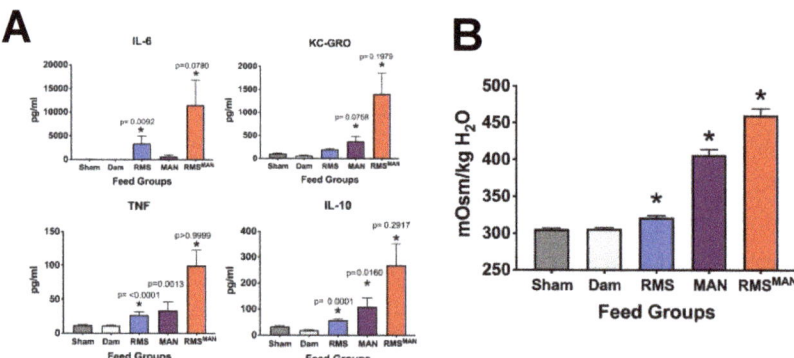

**Figure 4.** Exposure to increasing osmolality induces significant increases in serum inflammation. Serum samples were obtained at the time of euthanasia and quantified for the presence of IL-6, KC-GRO, TNF, and IL-10 (**A**). No significant differences were seen between sham and dam feeds. RMS feeds significantly induced IL-6, IL-10, and TNF levels. MAN feeds significantly increased serum levels of KC-GRO and IL-10, while RMS$^{MAN}$ feeds significantly increased serum levels of all cytokines evaluated ($n > 5$ for all groups, p values as shown) (**A**). Serum osmolality was also quantified to ascertain if enteral feeds were impacting the animal systemically. Feeds with MAN, RMS, or RMS$^{MAN}$ all significantly increased serum osmolality, although the highest elevations were in feeds containing mannitol ($n > 5$, $p < 0.0001$ for all comparisons) (**B**).

*3.4. Exposure to Mannitol-Increased Osmolality Induced Significant Alterations in the Composition of the Cecal Microbiome in the Immature Intestine*

One possible mechanism responsible for the osmolality-induced injury and inflammation was through alteration of the intestinal microbiome. To analyze this, cecal samples were collected following euthanasia and quantified for microbial composition. All mice receiving feeds experienced shifts in their cecal bacterial flora compared to those receiving only saline (Figure 5A). Mice fed RMS alone had a significant decrease in Firmicutes species similar to what was seen in dam fed mice. Interestingly, there were no differences in the microbiome between mice fed formula and mice that were dam fed. Mice fed either MAN or RMS$^{MAN}$ had significant increases in Proteobacteria with compensatory decreases in the relative number of Bacteroidetes and Firmicutes species. Principle coordinate analysis revealed that animals fed diets containing mannitol (MAN, RMS$^{MAN}$) had microbiome compositions that were discrete from those fed diets not containing mannitol (Sham, Dam, RMS) as depicted by the distinct clustering of the samples (Figure 5B). Within the Proteobacteria phylum, the families with the biggest increase in the MAN condition compared to sham or dam fed was Enterobacteriaceae and Pasteurellaceae (Figure 5C). Interestingly, in the RMS$^{MAN}$ condition trending increases were seen compared to sham or dam fed to approximately the same amount in Alcaligenaceae, Helicobacteraceae, Enterobacteriaceae, Pasteurellaceae, and Pseudomonadaceae (Figure 5C).

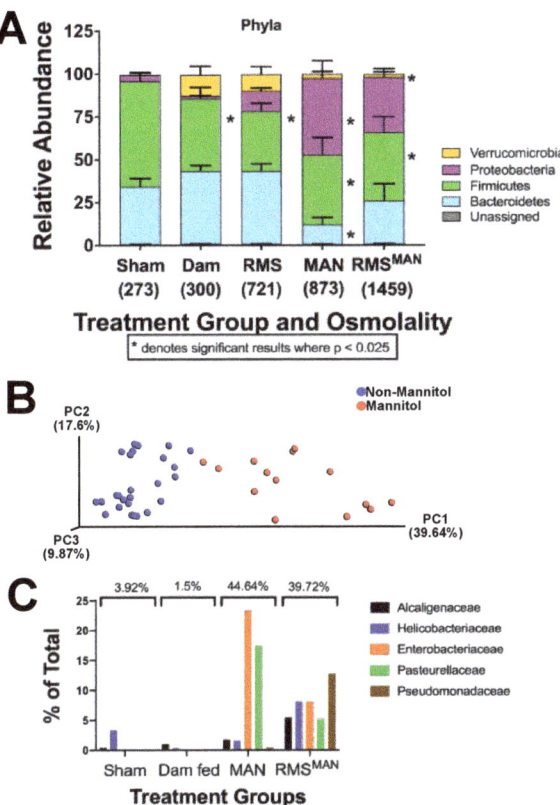

**Figure 5.** Exposure to increased osmolality induced significant alterations in the composition of the cecal microbiome in the immature intestine. Feed substance induced alterations in the microbial composition of the cecum. Dam fed and RMS fed mice had significantly less Firmicutes than sham controls, while mice fed MAN and RMS$^{MAN}$ had a shift in the microbiome resulting in a significant increase in Proteobacteria composition ($n$ = 9 animals per group, * represents a significant change from sham controls where $p$ < 0.025) (**A**). Principal coordinate analysis revealed that animals fed mannitol had distinct clustering of their flora compared to all other groups without mannitol in their feeds (**B**). Within the Proteobacteria phylum, the MAN condition resulted in increases in Enterobacteriaceae and Pasteurellaceae compared to controls (**C**). In the RMS$^{MAN}$ condition, increases were seen, compared to controls, to approximately the same amount in Alcaligenaceae, Helicobacteraceae, Enterobacteriaceae, Pasteurellaceae, and Pseudomonadaceae (**C**).

*3.5. Osmolality-Induced Effects Are Dependent on the Methodology Used to Increase the Solute Level*

To determine if increases in injury, inflammation, and bacterial dysbiosis were dependent on MAN or high osmolality, we created a formulation of RMS using three times the salt concentration in place of mannitol to induce a second method for obtaining a high osmolality (RMS$^{SALT}$) (982 mOsm/kg $H_2O$) feed. Experiments were performed as above using triple salt (SALT) in place of MAN.

As opposed to feeding with MAN, SALT feeds induced no mortality (data not shown as all animals survived), nor significant weight loss (Figure 6A). Further, no change in serum osmolality was seen from controls (Figure 6B). In looking at effects of SALT feeds on serum inflammation, feeding with SALT alone (equivalent salt concentration dissolved in saline) (581 mOsm/kg $H_2O$) had no significant effects on TNF, KC-GRO, IL-10, or IL-6 compared to controls, while feeding with RMS$^{SALT}$ (982 mOsm/kg

H$_2$O) significantly increased serum TNF, KC-GRO, and IL-6 levels (Figure 6C). Importantly, while RMS$^{SALT}$ feeds induced cytokine elevation, they were markedly less than what was seen from RMS$^{MAN}$ feeds (Figure 6C—data combined from 4A and 6C for ease of comparison). In quantifying intestinal injury, feeds with both SALT and RMS$^{SALT}$ had significantly increased injury scores compared to sham controls and were similar to those seen with RMS alone (Figure 7A). As was seen in our MAN experiments, the feeds with the highest osmolality (RMS$^{SALT}$) had the greatest percentage of maximal injury scores, however, as was seen in our cytokine levels, feeds with RMS$^{SALT}$ did not reach the same degree of injury as that seen in RMS$^{MAN}$. Interestingly, the microbiome showed no significant differences in any phyla when treatment groups were compared to the dam or to sham fed mice (Figure 7B). Although we did not see any shifts at the phylum level, when looking at changes in Proteobacteria families we did see trending increases in both Enterobacteriaceae and Pasteurellaceae in the SALT and RMS$^{SALT}$ conditions compared to sham- and dam fed mice (Figure 7C).

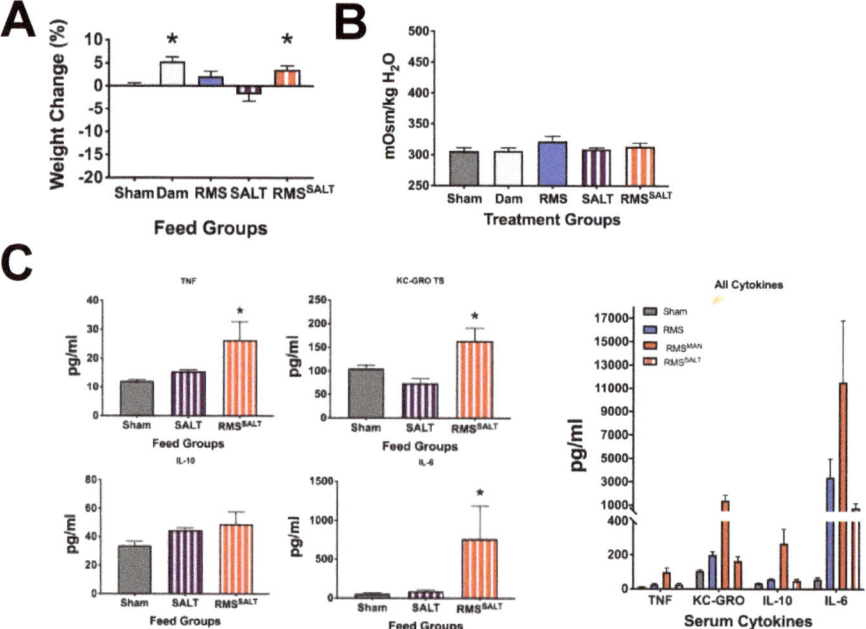

**Figure 6.** Osmolality-induced effects are methodology-dependent. To determine if our results were due to osmolality or to MAN, an additional high osmolality feed was generated by adding three times the salt concentration to standard RMS (RMS$^{SALT}$). Feeds with SALT and RMS$^{SALT}$ did not show the significant weight loss seen with MAN feeds (**A**), and no change in serum osmolality was observed in SALT or RMS$^{SALT}$ fed groups when compared to controls (**B**). SALT feeds had no significant impact on serum cytokine levels, while RMS$^{SALT}$ feeds induced significant increases in IL-6, KC-GRO, and TNF compared to sham controls ($n > 4$ for all experiments, $p = 0.0019, 0.0092$, and $0.0003$ respectively) (**C**). The far-right panel shows the combined MAN and SALT data for more direct comparison of the degree of inflammation generated by each feed type.

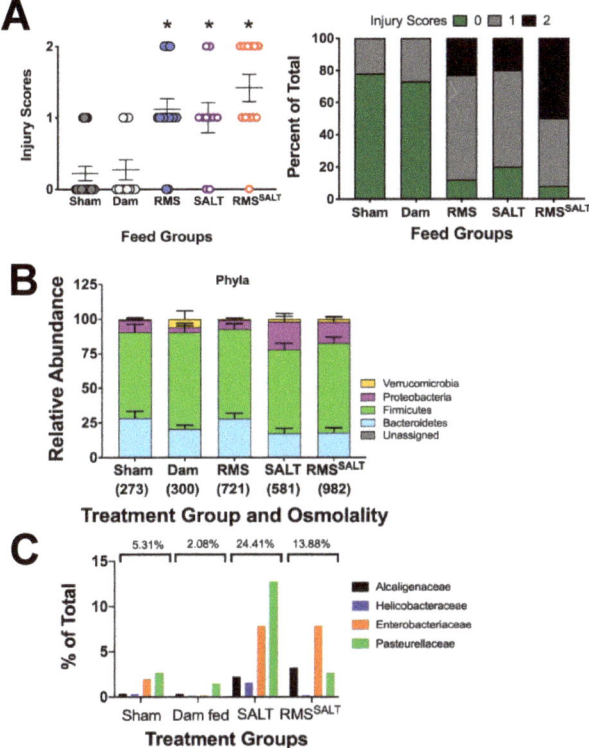

**Figure 7.** Alteration of the microbial composition is methodology-dependent, but intestinal injury is methodology-independent and is related instead to the height of osmolality achieved. Similar to our high osmolality MAN groups, feeding with either SALT alone (581 mOsm/kg H$_2$O) or RMS$^{SALT}$ (982 mOsm/kg H$_2$O) had significantly increased generalized injury scores compared to controls ($n = 7$, $p = 0.0196$ and $< 0.0001$ respectively) (**A**). However, no significant changes in microbial phylum composition were seen when comparing SALT and RMS$^{SALT}$ feeds to controls (**B**). When comparing changes in the Proteobacteria families similar to the comparison made in the mannitol conditions, trending increases were seen in both Enterobacteriaceae and Pasteurellaceae in the SALT and RMS$^{SALT}$ conditions compared to sham- and dam fed mice (**C**).

*3.6. High Osmolality RMS Deceased Survival When Included in Dithizone Paneth Cell Disruption and Formula Feeding NEC Model*

Our data shows that formula feeding along with Paneth cell disruption results in significant increases in inflammatory cytokines and in NEC-like injury. In addition, our data shows that exposure of the immature intestine to high osmolality formula (without Paneth cell disruption) significantly increases generalized intestinal injury and serum inflammation when compared to feeds with lower osmolality. Based on this data, we wanted to study the impact of high osmolality formula in one of our newly described RMS NEC models to determine the impact on survival. We disrupted Paneth cells using dithizone and gavage fed 250 μL of RMS with or without high salt to increase the osmolality (as seen in Figures 1 and 2). We found that in these conditions, mice that were fed high osmolality formula had higher mortality rates (93% mortality) compared to their regular RMS fed counterparts (75% mortality) (Figure 8).

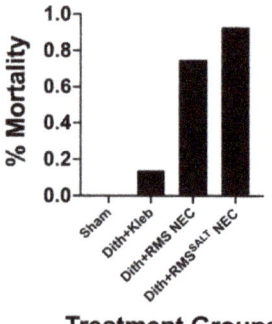

**Figure 8.** High osmolality formula combined with Paneth cell disruption results in increased mortality compared to regular formula. C57Bl/6J were injected with dithizone or an equivalent volume of LiCO$_3$ (controls animals) and exposed to feeds with Pedialyte, $1 \times 10^{11}$/kg *Klebsiella pneumonia*, regular RMS, or RMS$^{SALT}$ ($n$ = 11 Sham, 36 Dith+Kleb, 28 Dith+RMS, 28 Dith+RMS$^{SALT}$). Animals exposed to RMS$^{SALT}$ had increased mortality (93%) compared to those fed regular RMS (75%) or gavage of *K. pneumonia* (14%).

## 4. Discussion

The goal of this study was to determine the impact of formula feeding in combination with Paneth cell disruption and dysbiosis on rates and severity of injury to the immature intestine. Our secondary goals were to determine if high osmolality feeds would impact the immature intestine's susceptibility to injury, inflammation, or alterations in the microbiome composition, and to determine if high osmolality would exacerbate mortality in a formula NEC model. Our desire was to address gaps in knowledge regarding the mechanisms behind the increased rates of NEC in infants fed formula as well as questions regarding inconsistencies in data about the role of high osmolality and subsequent susceptibility to develop NEC. Our initial hypothesis was that formula feeding would exacerbate NEC-like injury in the Paneth cell-disruption NEC model. Interestingly, we found that formula feeding along with dithizone or diphtheria toxin to induce Paneth cell disruption caused NEC-like injury in our mice while eliminating the requirement of inducing a secondary bacterial dysbiosis. We further hypothesized that increased osmolality would lead to increased intestinal injury and inflammation through an alteration of the intestinal microbiome. Our novel data show that mice fed high osmolar feeds experience increased serum inflammation and increased levels of intestinal injury compared to sham controls. However, we found that these effects were independent from alterations in the microbiome. Finally, we hypothesized that high osmolar formula would exacerbate mortality seen in our formula NEC model and this was supported by our data. These data are critical to NEC biology and the field of neonatology as the imperative task of providing adequate nutrition to preterm infants requires the fortification of feeds to achieve the caloric requirements to maintain the fetal growth trajectory. Our data adds important insight into the role that formula feeds, and specifically high osmolar formula feeds, have on susceptibility to injury of the immature intestine.

The field of neonatology has advanced tremendously over the past few decades, yet despite these advances there has been slow progress on elucidating the pathophysiology behind NEC. While human breast milk is protective against NEC [17,35], it remains unknown why. The suggestion that hyperosmolality of prepared formulas could induce NEC was first postulated in the 1970s. In 1975, Santulli et al. published a case series reviewing 64 infants with NEC born from 1955 through June 1974. As part of the conclusion of this seminal work, Santulli suggested that hyperosmolar feeds may be causative of NEC as some of the infants who developed NEC had received hyperosmolar feedings (750 mOsm/L) [44,46]. That same year, Book et al. published a prospective study of 16 infants weighing less than 1200 g who were randomized to receive either elemental formula or cow milk formula [45].

Seven of eight (87.5%) infants fed the elemental formula (650 mOsm/L) and two of eight (25%) fed the standard cow milk formula (359 mOsm/L) developed necrotizing enterocolitis ($p < 0.02$). Based on these data, the authors concluded that the hypertonicity of the elemental diet may have contributed to the increased incidence of NEC in infants fed this formula. Following these two manuscripts, the American Academy of Pediatrics (AAP) in 1976 developed a recommendation that the osmolarity of infant formula should be less than 400 mOsm/L [47]. As osmolarity is defined as the number of solute particles in 1L of solvent and osmolality is the number of solute particles in 1kg of solvent, the AAP recommendations approximates to an osmolality of 450 mOsm/kg $H_2O$ [62]. This was a consensus view based on the observation that the milk of most mammalian species has an osmolarity of approximately 300 mOsm/L and that hyperosmolar formulas may be a causative factor in NEC. Despite (or perhaps because of) this consensus statement, little data has been generated to support the theory that osmolality is detrimental. Recent works by the Pierro lab have begun to address this gap in understanding. Their work utilizes five- to nine-day-old mice who were given systemic hypoxia over several days as well as hyperosmolar feeds laced with LPS three times a day. In their studies, the Pierro lab has shown that formula feeding induces changes in intestinal microcirculation and that the associated injury is not osmolality-dependent [48,49]. However, our data differs in that our mice were significantly older from a developmental pattern standpoint [20] and our studies used a much broader range of osmolalities as well as two different methods of altering feed osmolality. In this way, our data expands and adds to the important previous work of the Pierro group.

Although current neonatal practice is to use low osmolality feeds in the neonatal intensive care unit (NICU), these formulas are frequently fortified with supplemental protein, as well as other substances essential for growth such as vitamins or minerals to provide adequate nutrition. It is important to realize that use of the fortifiers and other supplements greatly increase osmolality. Our data show that feeding just four feeds of high osmolar formula to neonatal mice can provoke significant increases in serum inflammation and in epithelial damage in the immature small intestine. This appears to be dose-dependent, as feedings with higher osmolality had higher inflammation and injury scores. While breast milk, amniotic fluid, and Pedialyte all have osmolalities below 350 mOsm/kg $H_2O$, our formulas were significantly higher: SALT (581 mOsm/kg $H_2O$); RMS (721 mOsm/kg $H_2O$); MAN (873 mOsm/kg $H_2O$); $RMS^{SALT}$ (982 mOsm/kg $H_2O$); and $RMS^{MAN}$ (1491 mOsm/kg $H_2O$). Importantly, our injury scores for $RMS^{SALT}$ and MAN alone (982 and 873 mOsm/kg $H_2O$, respectively) were similar, as were the injury scores for RMS alone and SALT (721 and 581 mOsm/kg $H_2O$, respectively). The highest generalized injury scores were observed with the highest osmolality formula, $RMS^{MAN}$ (1491 mOsm/kg $H_2O$). While the osmolality of acceptable NICU feeds is below the levels that induced injury in our model, the formula and standard fortifiers commonly used do not take into consideration other substances that are often used with feeds in the NICU. A recent paper by Chandran et al. examined fourteen common medications utilized in the NICU [63]. Of these medications, nine had osmolalities too high to measure and the five additional medications were all above 450 mOsm/kg $H_2O$. This list included iron, multi-vitamins, NaCl, $NaPO_4$, and $KPO_4$, which are all common additives to feeds. To keep the osmolality below 450 mOsm/kg $H_2O$, the medications required significant dilutions of up to 1:40 when mixing the medication in preterm formulas and 1:250 when mixing with fortified expressed breast milk [63].

We observed a trend of increased injury being associated with higher osmolality feeds, but interestingly this trend was independent of the method for generating higher osmolality. While we were concerned that MAN would cause injury through dehydration, use of high salt formula did not impact weight while still inducing intestinal damage. This contrasts the work by Miyake et al. [48]. In this work, there were no differences seen in injury generation between formulas with an osmolality of 849 and 325 mOsm/kg $H_2O$. However, all animals also underwent exposure to LPS four mg/kg/day and hypoxia three times a day for 10-min time periods to induce NEC-like injury; thus, it is possible that the injury sustained in the hypoxia-formula model of NEC is severe enough that it would overwhelm any injury patterns seen in high osmolality alone. Although there is still conflicting data on the effect of formula osmolality and its relation to NEC likely due to conditional differences, our data highlights the danger of high osmolality not just in causing intestinal injury and inflammation, but also mortality as well when high osmolality formula is combined with Paneth cell disruption. Interestingly, our data suggested that the injury, inflammation, and mortality observed was related to the osmolality itself and could occur without changes in the microbiome, suggesting, at least for the microbiome, what is used to increase the osmolality is more indicative of community type than the osmolality itself. Additionally, it suggests that intestinal injury and inflammatory cytokine levels are likely independent of the microbiome in this particular model as intestinal injury and inflammation can be increased without shifts in the microbial community.

These findings were in direct contrast to our original hypothesis as we predicted increased osmolality would lead to increased intestinal injury and inflammation through an alteration of the intestinal microbiome. We were not surprised to find that different feed formulations had differential effects on the microbiome, but we were surprised to find that they were independent of injury scores. One finding was that feeds containing mannitol had significant expansions of the Proteobacteria phyla and more specifically Enterobacteriaceae. This is interesting as many studies have associated similar blooms with development of NEC [10,64]. Furthermore, many studies have linked formula feeding with NEC, and one connection made is that formula feeding tends to result in differential colonization of the infant gut compared to breast feeding. While breast fed infants tend to have a predominance of Firmicutes and Actinobacteria, formula-fed infants tend to have a predominance of Proteobacteria and more specifically Enterobacteriaceae, which can put them at higher risk for bacterial dysbiosis, which is another risk factor for NEC [65]. Another interesting finding was that in salt conditions we did not observe significant changes in the microbiome at the phylum level, but when looking at family level changes, we saw a trending increase in Enterobacteriaceae in the higher osmolality SALT and RMS$^{SALT}$ conditions. These conditions were associated with higher generalized injury scores; however, injury scores and inflammation were more consistent on overall osmolality than alterations in the cecal microbiome. One possibility for the increase in specific groups of organisms with mannitol feeds is that many Proteobacteria and Firmicutes species can utilize mannitol as an energy source allowing for a selective expansion of the bacteria that can utilize mannitol, which was supported by our data [66–68]. Additionally, Proteobacteria and Firmicutes species tend to be more tolerant to high salt conditions compared to other phyla of bacteria, which may explain why there were trending increases in some Proteobacteria families [69,70]. These data suggest that although changes in the microbiome were present in both the mannitol and salt related conditions, they likely occurred independent of the inflammation and injury we observed and were not causative in these experiments.

Although we did not observe microbiome alterations between dam fed and formula-fed mice, we did find significant increases in inflammation in formula-fed animals compared to dam fed animals. Formula feeding has been linked with increases in inflammation, which may explain why it can replace bacterial dysbiosis in our model and serve as a secondary hit in other NEC models [18]. Similar to other labs that have shown that formula feeding along with some other secondary form of insult such as hypoxia/hypothermia, LPS, or bacterial insult can induce NEC, we saw that when we induced Paneth cell disruption using either dithizone or diphtheria toxin and followed this with formula feeding of RMS we saw significant increases in NEC-like injury [13,15,18,48,59]. Unsurprisingly, the injury we observed was slightly different based on the type of Paneth cell disruption induced. Slightly higher NEC scores were found in the dithizone RMS NEC model and the damage in the intestine was mainly confined to the base and the core of the villi. While the scores were still significant in the diphtheria toxin RMS NEC mice, the scores trended to be slightly lower on average compared to the dithizone RMS NEC. Additionally, the damage pattern in the intestine included both the base of the villus as well as vacuolized cells at the top of the villus down compared to the damage pattern in the dithizone RMS NEC. This supports the findings of Lueschow et al. in 2018 showing that the NEC scores with diphtheria toxin and bacterial gavage, although still significant, trended slightly lower on average compared to the scores seen with dithizone and bacterial gavage [31]. Additionally, the difference in damage patterns of the intestine between dithizone and diphtheria toxin that we observed while formula feeding is complemented by the two different types of Paneth cell disruption described in Lueschow et al., 2018 where dithizone induces upregulation of autophagy pathways while diphtheria toxin induces apoptosis [31,71]. The findings that formula can replace induction of bacterial dysbiosis in a Paneth cell disruption NEC model highlights the potential dangers of formula feeding in premature infants at heightened risk for NEC.

Ultimately, the results of this paper demonstrate that formula feeding can induce NEC-like injury when combined with Paneth cell disruption without induction of bacterial dysbiosis, which is likely due to the inflammatory nature of the RMS formula without any additives. Additionally, high osmolality formula without Paneth cell disruption results in increased generalized intestinal injury and inflammation to a greater degree than formula feeding on its own in a microbiome independent manner. When high osmolality formula was combined with Paneth cell disruption, higher mortality rates were seen compared to when RMS alone was combined with Paneth cell disruption. Furthermore, the results show that changes in the microbiome can occur independent of injury and inflammation and were not causative in this case, as injury and inflammation were more closely connected with osmolality than changes in the microbiome. This is a critical point to consider as osmolality, microbiome composition, and intestinal injury can be interrelated or completely independent of each other depending on the conditions present. Therefore, as we consider optimized feeds that maximize nutrition for preterm infants, we must be vigilant of what we are giving to make sure we protect their immature intestinal tract.

**Author Contributions:** Conceptualization, S.L.K., J.L.S., S.J.C., S.J.M.; methodology, S.L.R., S.L.K., H.G., J.L.G., S.J.M., validation and formal analysis: S.R.L., S.L.K., H.G., J.L.G., S.J.M.; investigation: S.L.R., S.L.K., H.G., J.L.G., S.J.M.; resources, S.R.C., J.L.G., S.J.M.; data curation: S.R.L., S.L.K., H.G.; writing—original draft: S.L.K., J.L.S., S.J.M.; writing—editing: S.R.L., S.L.K., H.G., J.L.G., J.L.S., S.R.C., S.J.M.; supervision: S.J.M.; funding acquisition: J.L.G., S.J.M.; All authors have read and agreed to the published version of the manuscript.

**Funding:** This research received no external funding.

**Acknowledgments:** Support for this work was provided from the NIH, grants HL134850 and HL084207, The American Heart Association, grant 18EIA33890055, and the Stead Family Department of Pediatrics at the University of Iowa, and the Children's Miracle Network.

**Conflicts of Interest:** The authors declare no conflicts of interest.

## References

1. Fitzgibbons, S.C.; Ching, Y.; Yu, D.; Carpenter, J.; Kenny, M.; Weldon, C.; Lillehei, C.; Valim, C.; Horbar, J.D.; Jaksic, T. Mortality of necrotizing enterocolitis expressed by birth weight categories. *J. Pediatr. Surg.* **2009**, *44*, 1072–1075. [CrossRef] [PubMed]
2. Patel, R.M.; Kandefer, S.; Walsh, M.C.; Bell, E.F.; Carlo, W.A.; Laptook, A.R.; Sanchez, P.J.; Shankaran, S.; Van Meurs, K.P.; Ball, M.B.; et al. Causes and timing of death in extremely premature infants from 2000 through 2011. *N. Engl. J. Med.* **2015**, *372*, 331–340. [CrossRef] [PubMed]
3. Lin, P.W.; Nasr, T.R.; Stoll, B.J. Necrotizing enterocolitis: Recent scientific advances in pathophysiology and prevention. *Semin. Perinatol.* **2008**, *32*, 70–82. [CrossRef] [PubMed]
4. Chen, A.C.; Chung, M.Y.; Chang, J.H.; Lin, H.C. Pathogenesis implication for necrotizing enterocolitis prevention in preterm very-low-birth-weight infants. *J. Pediatr. Gastroenterol. Nutr.* **2014**, *58*, 7–11. [CrossRef] [PubMed]
5. Cho, I.; Blaser, M.J. The human microbiome: At the interface of health and disease. *Nat. Rev. Genet* **2012**, *13*, 260–270. [CrossRef]
6. Elgin, T.G.; Kern, S.L.; McElroy, S.J. Development of the neonatal intestinal microbiome and its association with necrotizing enterocolitis. *Clin. Ther.* **2016**, *38*, 706–715. [CrossRef]
7. Morrow, A.L.; Lagomarcino, A.J.; Schibler, K.R.; Taft, D.H.; Yu, Z.; Wang, B.; Altaye, M.; Wagner, M.; Gevers, D.; Ward, D.V.; et al. Early microbial and metabolomic signatures predict later onset of necrotizing enterocolitis in preterm infants. *Microbiome* **2013**, *1*, 13. [CrossRef]

8. Niemarkt, H.J.; de Meij, T.G.; van de Velde, M.E.; van der Schee, M.P.; van Goudoever, J.B.; Kramer, B.W.; Andriessen, P.; de Boer, N.K. Necrotizing enterocolitis: A clinical review on diagnostic biomarkers and the role of the intestinal microbiota. *Inflamm. Bowel Dis.* **2015**, *21*, 436–444. [CrossRef]
9. Lu, C.Y.; Ni, Y.H. Gut microbiota and the development of pediatric diseases. *J. Gastroenterol.* **2015**, *50*, 720–726. [CrossRef]
10. Claud, E.C.; Keegan, K.P.; Brulc, J.M.; Lu, L.; Bartels, D.; Glass, E.; Chang, E.B.; Meyer, F.; Antonopoulos, D.A. Bacterial community structure and functional contributions to emergence of health or necrotizing enterocolitis in preterm infants. *Microbiome* **2013**, *1*, 20. [CrossRef]
11. Pammi, M.; Cope, J.; Tarr, P.I.; Warner, B.B.; Morrow, A.L.; Mai, V.; Gregory, K.E.; Kroll, J.S.; McMurtry, V.; Ferris, M.J.; et al. Intestinal dysbiosis in preterm infants preceding necrotizing enterocolitis: A systematic review and meta-analysis. *Microbiome* **2017**, *5*, 31. [CrossRef] [PubMed]
12. Good, M.; Siggers, R.H.; Sodhi, C.P.; Afrazi, A.; Alkhudari, F.; Egan, C.E.; Neal, M.D.; Yazji, I.; Jia, H.; Lin, J.; et al. Amniotic fluid inhibits Toll-like receptor 4 signaling in the fetal and neonatal intestinal epithelium. *Proc. Natl. Acad. Sci. USA* **2012**, *109*, 11330–11335. [CrossRef] [PubMed]
13. Good, M.; Sodhi, C.P.; Egan, C.E.; Afrazi, A.; Jia, H.; Yamaguchi, Y.; Lu, P.; Branca, M.F.; Ma, C.; Prindle, T., Jr.; et al. Breast milk protects against the development of necrotizing enterocolitis through inhibition of Toll-like receptor 4 in the intestinal epithelium via activation of the epidermal growth factor receptor. *Mucosal Immunol.* **2015**, *8*, 1166–1179. [CrossRef] [PubMed]
14. Neal, M.D.; Sodhi, C.P.; Dyer, M.; Craig, B.T.; Good, M.; Jia, H.; Yazji, I.; Afrazi, A.; Richardson, W.M.; Beer-Stolz, D.; et al. A critical role for TLR4 induction of autophagy in the regulation of enterocyte migration and the pathogenesis of necrotizing enterocolitis. *J. Immunol.* **2013**, *190*, 3541–3551. [CrossRef] [PubMed]
15. Hunter, C.J.; Singamsetty, V.K.; Chokshi, N.K.; Boyle, P.; Camerini, V.; Grishin, A.V.; Upperman, J.S.; Ford, H.R.; Prasadarao, N.V. Enterobacter sakazakii enhances epithelial cell injury by inducing apoptosis in a rat model of necrotizing enterocolitis. *J. Infect. Dis.* **2008**, *198*, 586–593. [CrossRef] [PubMed]
16. Managlia, E.; Liu, S.X.L.; Yan, X.; Tan, X.D.; Chou, P.M.; Barrett, T.A.; De Plaen, I.G. Blocking NF-kappaB Activation in Ly6c(+) Monocytes Attenuates Necrotizing Enterocolitis. *Am. J. Pathol.* **2019**, *189*, 604–618. [CrossRef]
17. Lucas, A.; Cole, T.J. Breast milk and neonatal necrotising enterocolitis. *Lancet* **1990**, *336*, 1519–1523. [CrossRef]
18. Liu, Y.; Fatheree, N.Y.; Mangalat, N.; Rhoads, J.M. Lactobacillus reuteri strains reduce incidence and severity of experimental necrotizing enterocolitis via modulation of TLR4 and NFkappaB signaling in the intestine. *Am. J. Physiol. Gastrointest. Liver Physiol.* **2011**. [CrossRef]
19. McElroy, S.J.; Weitkamp, J.H. Innate immunity in the small intestine of the preterm infant. *NeoReviews* **2011**, *12*, e517–e526. [CrossRef]
20. Stanford, A.H.; Gong, H.; Noonan, M.; Lewis, A.N.; Gong, Q.; Lanik, W.E.; Hsieh, J.J.; Lueschow, S.R.; Frey, M.R.; Good, M.; et al. A direct comparison of mouse and human intestinal development using epithelial gene expression patterns. *Pediatr. Res.* **2019**. [CrossRef]
21. Fung, C.M.; White, J.R.; Brown, A.S.; Gong, H.; Weitkamp, J.H.; Frey, M.R.; McElroy, S.J. Intrauterine growth restriction alters mouse intestinal architecture during development. *PLoS ONE* **2016**, *11*, e0146542. [CrossRef] [PubMed]
22. McElroy, S.J.; Castle, S.L.; Bernard, J.K.; Almohazey, D.; Hunter, C.J.; Bell, B.A.; Al Alam, D.; Wang, L.; Ford, H.R.; Frey, M.R. The ErbB4 ligand neuregulin-4 protects against experimental necrotizing enterocolitis. *Am. J. Pathol.* **2014**, *184*, 2768–2778. [CrossRef] [PubMed]
23. Zhang, C.; Sherman, M.P.; Prince, L.S.; Bader, D.; Weitkamp, J.H.; Slaughter, J.C.; McElroy, S.J. Paneth cell ablation in the presence of Klebsiella pneumoniae induces necrotizing enterocolitis (NEC)-like injury in the small intestine of immature mice. *Dis. Models Mech.* **2012**, *5*, 522–532. [CrossRef] [PubMed]
24. White, J.R.; Gong, H.; Pope, B.; Schlievert, P.; McElroy, S.J. Paneth-cell-disruption-induced necrotizing enterocolitis in mice requires live bacteria and occurs independently of TLR4 signaling. *Dis. Models Mech.* **2017**, *10*, 727–736. [CrossRef]
25. McElroy, S.J.; Prince, L.S.; Weitkamp, J.H.; Reese, J.; Slaughter, J.C.; Polk, D.B. Tumor necrosis factor receptor 1-dependent depletion of mucus in immature small intestine: A potential role in neonatal necrotizing enterocolitis. *Am. J. Physiol. Gastrointest. Liver Physiol.* **2011**, *301*, G656–G666. [CrossRef]
26. McElroy, S.J.; Underwood, M.A.; Sherman, M.P. Paneth cells and necrotizing enterocolitis: A novel hypothesis for disease pathogenesis. *Neonatology* **2013**, *103*, 10–20. [CrossRef]

27. Coutinho, H.B.; da Mota, H.C.; Coutinho, V.B.; Robalinho, T.I.; Furtado, A.F.; Walker, E.; King, G.; Mahida, Y.R.; Sewell, H.F.; Wakelin, D. Absence of lysozyme (muramidase) in the intestinal Paneth cells of newborn infants with necrotising enterocolitis. *J. Clin. Pathol.* **1998**, *51*, 512–514. [CrossRef]
28. Markasz, L.; Wanders, A.; Szekely, L.; Lilja, H.E. Diminished DEFA6 expression in paneth cells is associated with necrotizing enterocolitis. *Gastroenterol. Res. Pract.* **2018**, *2018*, 7345426. [CrossRef]
29. Franklin, A.L.; Said, M.; Cappiello, C.D.; Gordish-Dressman, H.; Tatari-Calderone, Z.; Vukmanovic, S.; Rais-Bahrami, K.; Luban, N.L.; Devaney, J.M.; Sandler, A.D. Are immune modulating single nucleotide polymorphisms associated with necrotizing enterocolitis? *Sci. Rep.* **2015**, *5*, 18369. [CrossRef]
30. Berger, J.N.; Gong, H.; Good, M.; McElroy, S.J. Dithizone-induced Paneth cell disruption significantly decreases intestinal perfusion in the murine small intestine. *J. Pediatr. Surg.* **2019**, *54*, 2402–2407. [CrossRef]
31. Lueschow, S.R.; Stumphy, J.; Gong, H.; Kern, S.L.; Elgin, T.G.; Underwood, M.A.; Kalanetra, K.M.; Mills, D.A.; Wong, M.H.; Meyerholz, D.K.; et al. Loss of murine Paneth cell function alters the immature intestinal microbiome and mimics changes seen in neonatal necrotizing enterocolitis. *PLoS ONE* **2018**, *13*, e0204967. [CrossRef]
32. Garabedian, E.M.; Roberts, L.J.; McNevin, M.S.; Gordon, J.I. Examining the role of Paneth cells in the small intestine by lineage ablation in transgenic mice. *J. Biol. Chem.* **1997**, *272*, 23729–23740. [CrossRef]
33. O'Connor, D.L.; Gibbins, S.; Kiss, A.; Bando, N.; Brennan-Donnan, J.; Ng, E.; Campbell, D.M.; Vaz, S.; Fusch, C.; Asztalos, E.; et al. Effect of supplemental donor human milk compared with preterm formula on neurodevelopment of very low-birth-weight infants at 18 months: A randomized clinical trial. *JAMA* **2016**, *316*, 1897–1905. [CrossRef]
34. Sullivan, S.; Schanler, R.J.; Kim, J.H.; Patel, A.L.; Trawoger, R.; Kiechl-Kohlendorfer, U.; Chan, G.M.; Blanco, C.L.; Abrams, S.; Cotten, C.M.; et al. An exclusively human milk-based diet is associated with a lower rate of necrotizing enterocolitis than a diet of human milk and bovine milk-based products. *J. Pediatr.* **2010**, *156*, 562–567. [CrossRef]
35. Miller, J.; Tonkin, E.; Damarell, R.A.; McPhee, A.J.; Suganuma, M.; Suganuma, H.; Middleton, P.F.; Makrides, M.; Collins, C.T. A systematic review and meta-analysis of human milk feeding and morbidity in very low birth weight infants. *Nutrients* **2018**, *10*, 707. [CrossRef]
36. Underwood, M.A. Human milk for the premature infant. *Pediatr. Clin. N. Am.* **2013**, *60*, 189–207. [CrossRef]
37. Breastfeeding, S.O. Breastfeeding and the use of human milk. *Pediatrics* **2012**, *129*, e827–e841. [CrossRef]
38. Wojcik, K.Y.; Rechtman, D.J.; Lee, M.L.; Montoya, A.; Medo, E.T. Macronutrient analysis of a nationwide sample of donor breast milk. *J. Am. Diet. Assoc.* **2009**, *109*, 137–140. [CrossRef]
39. Vieira, A.A.; Soares, F.V.; Pimenta, H.P.; Abranches, A.D.; Moreira, M.E. Analysis of the influence of pasteurization, freezing/thawing, and offer processes on human milk's macronutrient concentrations. *Early Hum. Dev.* **2011**, *87*, 577–580. [CrossRef]
40. Wood, N.S.; Costeloe, K.; Gibson, A.T.; Hennessy, E.M.; Marlow, N.; Wilkinson, A.R.; Group, E.P.S. The EPICure study: Growth and associated problems in children born at 25 weeks of gestational age or less. *Arch. Dis. Child. Fetal Neonatal Ed.* **2003**, *88*, F492–F500. [CrossRef]
41. Ehrenkranz, R.A.; Dusick, A.M.; Vohr, B.R.; Wright, L.L.; Wrage, L.A.; Poole, W.K. Growth in the neonatal intensive care unit influences neurodevelopmental and growth outcomes of extremely low birth weight infants. *Pediatrics* **2006**, *117*, 1253–1261. [CrossRef] [PubMed]
42. Farooqi, A.; Hagglof, B.; Sedin, G.; Gothefors, L.; Serenius, F. Growth in 10- to 12-year-old children born at 23 to 25 weeks' gestation in the 1990s: A Swedish national prospective follow-up study. *Pediatrics* **2006**, *118*, e1452–e1465. [CrossRef] [PubMed]
43. Srinivasan, L.; Bokiniec, R.; King, C.; Weaver, G.; Edwards, A.D. Increased osmolality of breast milk with therapeutic additives. *Arch. Dis. Child. Fetal Neonatal Ed.* **2004**, *89*, F514–F517. [CrossRef] [PubMed]
44. Pearson, F.; Johnson, M.J.; Leaf, A.A. Milk osmolality: Does it matter? *Arch. Dis. Child. Fetal Neonatal Ed.* **2013**, *98*, F166–F169. [CrossRef] [PubMed]
45. Book, L.S.; Herbst, J.J.; Atherton, S.O.; Jung, A.L. Necrotizing enterocolitis in low-birth-weight infants fed an elemental formula. *J. Pediatr.* **1975**, *87*, 602–605. [CrossRef]
46. Santulli, T.V.; Schullinger, J.N.; Heird, W.C.; Gongaware, R.D.; Wigger, J.; Barlow, B.; Blanc, W.A.; Berdon, W.E. Acute necrotizing enterocolitis in infancy: A review of 64 cases. *Pediatrics* **1975**, *55*, 376–387.
47. Commentary on breast-feeding and infant formulas, including proposed standards for formulas. *Pediatrics* **1976**, *57*, 278–285.

48. Miyake, H.; Chen, Y.; Koike, Y.; Hock, A.; Li, B.; Lee, C.; Zani, A.; Pierro, A. Osmolality of enteral formula and severity of experimental necrotizing enterocolitis. *Pediatr. Surg. Int.* **2016**, *32*, 1153–1156. [CrossRef]
49. Chen, Y.; Koike, Y.; Chi, L.; Ahmed, A.; Miyake, H.; Li, B.; Lee, C.; Delgado-Olguin, P.; Pierro, A. Formula feeding and immature gut microcirculation promote intestinal hypoxia, leading to necrotizing enterocolitis. *Dis. Models Mech.* **2019**, *12*. [CrossRef]
50. Bry, L.; Falk, P.; Huttner, K.; Ouellette, A.; Midtvedt, T.; Gordon, J.I. Paneth cell differentiation in the developing intestine of normal and transgenic mice. *Proc. Natl. Acad. Sci. USA* **1994**, *91*, 10335–10339. [CrossRef]
51. Heida, F.H.; Beyduz, G.; Bulthuis, M.L.; Kooi, E.M.; Bos, A.F.; Timmer, A.; Hulscher, J.B. Paneth cells in the developing gut: When do they arise and when are they immune competent? *Pediatr. Res.* **2016**, *80*, 306–310. [CrossRef] [PubMed]
52. Yee, W.H.; Soraisham, A.S.; Shah, V.S.; Aziz, K.; Yoon, W.; Lee, S.K. Incidence and timing of presentation of necrotizing enterocolitis in preterm infants. *Pediatrics* **2012**, *129*, e298–e304. [CrossRef] [PubMed]
53. Dvorak, B.; McWilliam, D.L.; Williams, C.S.; Dominguez, J.A.; Machen, N.W.; McCuskey, R.S.; Philipps, A.F. Artificial formula induces precocious maturation of the small intestine of artificially reared suckling rats. *J. Pediatr. Gastroenterol. Nutr.* **2000**, *31*, 162–169. [CrossRef]
54. White, J.R.; Gong, H.; Colaizy, T.T.; Moreland, J.G.; Flaherty, H.; McElroy, S.J. Evaluation of hematologic composition in newborn C57/BL6 mice up to day 35. *Vet. Clin. Pathol.* **2015**. [CrossRef]
55. Fricke, E.M.; Elgin, T.G.; Gong, H.; Reese, J.; Gibson-Corley, K.N.; Weiss, R.M.; Zimmerman, K.; Bowdler, N.C.; Kalantera, K.M.; Mills, D.A.; et al. Lipopolysaccharide-induced maternal inflammation induces direct placental injury without alteration in placental blood flow and induces a secondary fetal intestinal injury that persists into adulthood. *Am. J. Reprod. Immunol.* **2018**, *79*, e12816. [CrossRef]
56. Underwood, M.A.; German, J.B.; Lebrilla, C.B.; Mills, D.A. Bifidobacterium longum subspecies infantis: Champion colonizer of the infant gut. *Pediatr. Res.* **2015**, *77*, 229–235. [CrossRef]
57. Caporaso, J.G.; Kuczynski, J.; Stombaugh, J.; Bittinger, K.; Bushman, F.D.; Costello, E.K.; Fierer, N.; Pena, A.G.; Goodrich, J.K.; Gordon, J.I.; et al. QIIME allows analysis of high-throughput community sequencing data. *Nat. Methods* **2010**, *7*, 335–336. [CrossRef]
58. Wynn, J.L.; Wilson, C.S.; Hawiger, J.; Scumpia, P.O.; Marshall, A.F.; Liu, J.H.; Zharkikh, I.; Wong, H.R.; Lahni, P.; Benjamin, J.T.; et al. Targeting IL-17A attenuates neonatal sepsis mortality induced by IL-18. *Proc. Natl. Acad. Sci. USA* **2016**, *113*, E2627–E2635. [CrossRef]
59. Jilling, T.; Simon, D.; Lu, J.; Meng, F.J.; Li, D.; Schy, R.; Thomson, R.B.; Soliman, A.; Arditi, M.; Caplan, M.S. The roles of bacteria and TLR4 in rat and murine models of necrotizing enterocolitis. *J. Immunol.* **2006**, *177*, 3273–3282. [CrossRef]
60. Sangild, P.T.; Siggers, R.H.; Schmidt, M.; Elnif, J.; Bjornvad, C.R.; Thymann, T.; Grondahl, M.L.; Hansen, A.K.; Jensen, S.K.; Boye, M.; et al. Diet- and colonization-dependent intestinal dysfunction predisposes to necrotizing enterocolitis in preterm pigs. *Gastroenterology* **2006**, *130*, 1776–1792. [CrossRef]
61. Maheshwari, A.; Schelonka, R.L.; Dimmitt, R.A.; Carlo, W.A.; Munoz-Hernandez, B.; Das, A.; McDonald, S.A.; Thorsen, P.; Skogstrand, K.; Hougaard, D.M.; et al. Cytokines associated with necrotizing enterocolitis in extremely-low-birth-weight infants. *Pediatr. Res.* **2014**, *76*, 100–108. [CrossRef] [PubMed]
62. Koeppen, B.M.; Stanton, B.A. *Renal Physiology*, 5th ed.; Elsevier Mosby: Philadelphia, PA, USA, 2013; 240p.
63. Chandran, S.; Chua, M.C.; Lin, W.; Min Wong, J.; Saffari, S.E.; Rajadurai, V.S. Medications that increase osmolality and compromise the safety of enteral feeding in preterm infants. *Neonatology* **2017**, *111*, 309–316. [CrossRef] [PubMed]
64. Warner, B.B.; Deych, E.; Zhou, Y.; Hall-Moore, C.; Weinstock, G.M.; Sodergren, E.; Shaikh, N.; Hoffmann, J.A.; Linneman, L.A.; Hamvas, A.; et al. Gut bacteria dysbiosis and necrotising enterocolitis in very low birthweight infants: A prospective case-control study. *Lancet* **2016**, *387*, 1928–1936. [CrossRef]
65. Torrazza, R.M.; Neu, J. The altered gut microbiome and necrotizing enterocolitis. *Clin. Perinatol.* **2013**, *40*, 93–108. [CrossRef] [PubMed]
66. La Scola, B.; Barrassi, L.; Raoult, D. Isolation of new fastidious alpha Proteobacteria and Afipia felis from hospital water supplies by direct plating and amoebal co-culture procedures. *FEMS Microbiol. Ecol.* **2000**, *34*, 129–137. [PubMed]

67. Haahtela, K.; Kari, K.; Sundman, V. Nitrogenase activity (acetylene reduction) of root-associated, cold-climate azospirillum, enterobacter, Klebsiella, and pseudomonas species during growth on various carbon sources and at various partial pressures of oxygen. *Appl. Environ. Microbiol.* **1983**, *45*, 563–570. [CrossRef]
68. Gupta, P.K.; Mital, B.K.; Garg, S.K. Characterization of Lactobacillus acidophilus strains for use as dietary adjunct. *Int. J. Food Microbiol.* **1996**, *29*, 105–109. [CrossRef]
69. Genderjahn, S.; Alawi, M.; Mangelsdorf, K.; Horn, F.; Wagner, D. Desiccation- and saline-tolerant bacteria and archaea in kalahari pan sediments. *Front. Microbiol.* **2018**, *9*, 2082. [CrossRef]
70. Oren, A. Microbial life at high salt concentrations: Phylogenetic and metabolic diversity. *Saline Syst.* **2008**, *4*, 2. [CrossRef]
71. Alouf, J.E.; Popoff, M.R. *The Comprehensive Sourcebook of Bacterial Protein Toxins*, 3rd ed.; Elsevier: Amsterdam, The Netherlands, 2006; 1047p.

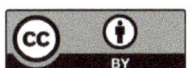

© 2020 by the authors. Licensee MDPI, Basel, Switzerland. This article is an open access article distributed under the terms and conditions of the Creative Commons Attribution (CC BY) license (http://creativecommons.org/licenses/by/4.0/).

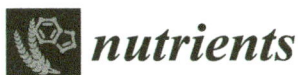 

*Review*

# Nutrition in Necrotizing Enterocolitis and Following Intestinal Resection

**Jocelyn Ou** [1,†], **Cathleen M. Courtney** [2,†], **Allie E. Steinberger** [2], **Maria E. Tecos** [2] **and Brad W. Warner** [2,*]

1. Department of Pediatrics, Division of Newborn Medicine, Washington University School of Medicine, St. Louis, MO 63110, USA; jocelyn.ou@wustl.edu
2. Department of Surgery, Division of Pediatric Surgery, Washington University School of Medicine, St. Louis, MO 63110, USA; c.courtney@wustl.edu (C.M.C.); allie.steinberger@wustl.edu (A.E.S.); metecos@wustl.edu (M.E.T.)
* Correspondence: brad.warner@wustl.edu; Tel.: 314-454-6022
† These authors contributed equally to this work.

Received: 16 January 2020; Accepted: 14 February 2020; Published: 18 February 2020

**Abstract:** This review aims to discuss the role of nutrition and feeding practices in necrotizing enterocolitis (NEC), NEC prevention, and its complications, including surgical treatment. A thorough PubMed search was performed with a focus on meta-analyses and randomized controlled trials when available. There are several variables in nutrition and the feeding of preterm infants with the intention of preventing necrotizing enterocolitis (NEC). Starting feeds later rather than earlier, advancing feeds slowly and continuous feeds have not been shown to prevent NEC and breast milk remains the only effective prevention strategy. The lack of medical treatment options for NEC often leads to disease progression requiring surgical resection. Following resection, intestinal adaptation occurs, during which villi lengthen and crypts deepen to increase the functional capacity of remaining bowel. The effect of macronutrients on intestinal adaptation has been extensively studied in animal models. Clinically, the length and portion of intestine that is resected may lead to patients requiring parenteral nutrition, which is also reviewed here. There remain significant gaps in knowledge surrounding many of the nutritional aspects of NEC and more research is needed to determine optimal feeding approaches to prevent NEC, particularly in infants younger than 28 weeks and <1000 grams. Additional research is also needed to identify biomarkers reflecting intestinal recovery following NEC diagnosis individualize when feedings should be safely resumed for each patient.

**Keywords:** necrotizing enterocolitis; prematurity; intestinal resection; short bowel syndrome; intestinal adaptation; microbiome; parenteral nutrition; hormones; breast milk

## 1. Introduction

Necrotizing enterocolitis (NEC) remains one of the most devastating diagnoses in premature neonates. Although its incidence varies amongst different neonatal intensive care units, the mean prevalence of NEC is 7% in infants between 500–1500 grams and the disease has a high morbidity and mortality [1]. The exact pathophysiology of NEC is unknown, but the immature intestinal barrier and intestinal dysbiosis are two important factors that likely contribute to intestinal inflammation and injury seen in the disease [1,2]. Because of its nonspecific symptoms, NEC is difficult to diagnose. Currently, Bell's staging, first introduced in 1978 by Bell et al. and modified by Kligeman and Walsh in 1986, is widely used to stratify disease severity and guide treatment (Figure 1). For Bell's stage 1 (suspected, but not confirmed NEC) and Bell's stage 2 (confirmed pneumatosis intestinalis with or without portal venous gas) [2], parenteral nutrition (PN) and broad-spectrum antibiotics are initiated, and enteral feeds are held for 7–14 days. Because the management of disease in these stages is non-operative,

Bell's stage 1 and Bell's stage 2 are also known as "medical NEC." If disease progresses despite holding feeds and starting antibiotics, surgery is required in Bell's stage 3, which is characterized by hemodynamic instability in addition to severe thrombocytopenia, disseminated intravascular coagulopathy, and peritonitis (IIA) or pneumoperitoneum (IIB) [2,3]. Surgical NEC increases disease mortality from 3% to 30% [4]. Not infrequently, the length of bowel needed to be removed can be significant, resulting in short bowel syndrome.

On a cellular level, intestinal adaptation occurs after massive bowel resection as a compensatory response by the remnant bowel wherein villi elongate, crypts deepen, and enterocyte proliferation is enhanced. Together, these changes function to increase the functional absorptive capacity per unit length of the remnant bowel [5]. This review aims to summarize the role of nutrition in NEC, including its prevention, complications, and sequelae of surgical treatment. A thorough PubMed search was performed using search terms that included "preterm enteral feeding", "early enteral feeding", "feeding necrotizing enterocolitis", "intestinal adaptation", "intestinal adaptation macronutrients" and "parenteral nutrition necrotizing enterocolitis." Meta-analyses and randomized controlled trials were reviewed on these topics when available; otherwise, pre-clinical animal trials were reviewed. We included studies pertaining to nutrition in NEC, specifically those examining feeding comparisons in which NEC was a primary or secondary outcome. Reports not focused on NEC as a primary or secondary outcome or those discussing NEC without a clear definition were excluded.

## 2. NEC Prevention

### 2.1. Delivery of Feeds

#### 2.1.1. Initiation of Feeds

Historically, it was thought that delaying enteral feeds would decrease the incidence of NEC. However, a 2013 Cochrane review found that there was no increased incidence of NEC when beginning trophic feeds early (within 96 hours of birth) and continuing them for a week compared to fasting and starting feeds at 7 or more days of life in very preterm (<32 weeks) or very low birthweight (<1500 grams) infants [6]. Starting enteral nutrition early also was not protective against NEC in this population. Initiating enteral feeds early appears to be safe for preterm and very low birthweight infants and beginning feeds at a higher volume may also be beneficial. A 2019 meta-analysis conducted by Alshaikh, et al. compared the safety of starting total enteral feeds at 80 ml/kg/d to starting enteral feeds at the conventional volume of 20 ml/kg/d. There was no difference in the incidence of NEC or feeding intolerance when starting early total enteral feeds, with the added benefit of decreased late-onset sepsis and decreased length of hospital stay by 1.3 days [7]. However, the conclusions that can be drawn from this meta-analysis for infants <1000 g and <28 weeks are limited, as the studies included in the analysis included infants between 28–36 weeks' gestational age and between 1000–1500 g. In a 2019 randomized controlled trial, Nangia, et al. compared starting very low birthweight infants between 28–34 weeks' gestational age on total enteral feeds (80 ml/kg/day) on the first day of life to starting infants at the conventional enteral feeding volume (20 ml/kg/day) supplemented with intravenous fluids. The study found no difference in the incidence of NEC between the two groups, with 1.1% in the early total enteral feeding group compared to 5.8% in the conventional enteral feeding group ($p = 0.12$). However, infants in the early total enteral feeding group reached goal feeds on average of 3.6 days sooner. This group also had fewer complications such as sepsis or feeding intolerance, and ultimately had shorter lengths of stay [8].

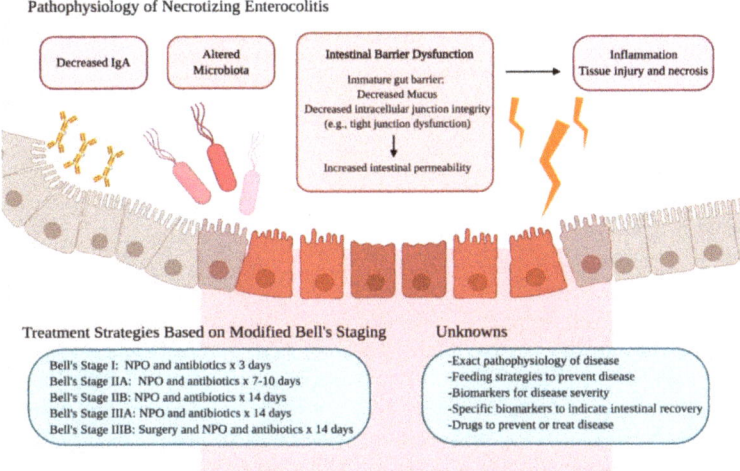

**Figure 1.** Summary of the Pathophysiology, Treatment Strategies, and Unknowns of Necrotizing Enterocolitis. The pathophysiology of NEC is multi-faceted, involving intestinal barrier dysfunction, decreased IgA, and altered microbiota. Current treatment strategies include stopping feeds and starting antibiotics based on disease severity, as classified by Bell's staging. Much remains unknown about disease prevention, diagnosis, and treatment. Figure created with Biorender.com. Abbreviations: Immunoglobulin A (IgA), NEC (Necrotizing enterocolitis), NPO (*nil per os*).

2.1.2. Feeding Advancement

Once feeds are successfully initiated and tolerated, the next consideration is the rate of feed advancement. Although there is significant variation in advancement protocols amongst different neonatal intensive care units, feeds are typically increased by 15–35 ml/kg each day, depending on infant size. Dorling, et al. conducted a randomized controlled trial comparing slow (18 ml/kg/day) and rapid (30 ml/kg/day) feed advancement that showed no significant difference in survival without moderate or severe neurologic deficits at 24 months in very preterm (<32 weeks) and very low birth weight infants [9]. Rapid advancement of feeds also did not increase the incidence of NEC when compared to slow advancement. Advancing feeds more rapidly and thus allowing infants to reach full feeds sooner may lead to increased caloric intake and better growth, as well as decreased duration of parenteral nutrition.

2.1.3. Bolus and Continuous Feeding

Bolus feeding has the advantage of gut stimulation, which promotes normal functioning and tissue maturation. Conversely, continuous feeding provides an opportunity for slow and steady nutrient introduction, which may allow for better tolerance and absorption in the setting of less distension and diarrhea [10,11]. In a recent meta-analysis, Wang, et al. found that although there was no difference in growth parameters or length of hospitalization, bolus-fed preterm (<37 weeks' gestational age), low birthweight (<2500 grams) infants reached feeds sooner (mean difference 0.98 days) with a similar incidence of NEC compared to infants receiving continuous feeds [12]. This meta-analysis includes infants up to 2500 grams, but found no differences in subgroup analysis of infants with birthweight <1000 grams and >1000 grams.

Randomized controlled trials have disproven previous observational data that delaying the initiation of feeds, starting at a smaller volume, and advancing feeds slowly may decrease the incidence of NEC. Evidence remains limited in extremely preterm and extremely low birthweight infants;

a feasible approach to feeding preterm infants may be initiating feeds as soon as an infant is clinically stable and advancing by 30 ml/kg/day as tolerated. For very low birthweight infants, starting feeds within 96 hours of birth and advancing at 30 ml/kg/day have both been shown to be safe and allow infants to reach full feeds sooner. However, despite decreasing the number of days infants require parenteral nutrition, advancing feeds faster does not decrease the incidence of late-onset sepsis and in general, the benefit of reaching full feeds faster may be limited. The most beneficial approach may be for each neonatal intensive care unit to standardize their feeding protocols and ensure that are consistently followed.

*2.2. Composition of Feeds*

2.2.1. Osmolality

Human breast milk has an osmolality of around 300 mOsm/l, whereas commercially available enteral formulas have osmolalities of less than 450 mOsm/l [13]. In order to meet a preterm infant's nutritional and growth requirements, both breast milk and infant formulas require caloric fortification and supplements, thereby increasing osmolarity. Multi-nutrient fortification adds protein, vitamins, and other minerals and increases the osmolality of breast milk to 400 mOsm/l [13]. Historically, administration of hyperosmolar formula was thought to be associated with an increased risk for the development of necrotizing enterocolitis (NEC). This was based on a handful of small-scale studies in the 1970s, all of which failed to provide a durable mechanism of mucosal injury [14,15]. More recently, Miyake, et al. looked at hyperosmolar enteral formula compared to diluted formula in a mouse model of NEC. They found that the inflammatory response, mucosal injury, and incidence of NEC was the same in both experimental groups [16]. In other animal studies, the only reported adverse outcome associated with hyperosmolar feeds was delayed gastric emptying [13]. Lastly, in humans, a 2016 Cochrane review concluded that there is weak evidence showing that nutrient fortification does not increase the incidence of NEC in preterm infants. It does increase in-hospital growth rate (weight 1.81 g/kg/day, length 0.12 cm/week, head circumference 0.08 cm/week), but does not seem to improve long-term growth and development [17]. Because in-hospital growth rates are improved and the incidence of NEC is not increased with hyperosmolar feeds, the benefit of additional nutrients and other supplements warrants fortification of human breast milk. The data on the effect of fortification on neurodevelopment and growth beyond infancy is very limited and needs to be studied further.

2.2.2. Breast Milk

Human milk is the only modifiable risk factor that has been consistently shown to protect against the development of NEC [18,19]. Since the 1990s, the incidence of NEC has been described as 6–10 times higher in exclusively formula-fed infants compared to exclusively breastfed infants [20]. The specific mechanisms by which breast milk is protective continue to be studied. However, several non-nutrient components have been found to contribute to the immune functions of the gastrointestinal tract and augment mucosal integrity [21,22]. These include secretory IgA, growth hormones (epidermal growth factor, insulin, and insulin-like growth factor), polyunsaturated fatty acids, and oligosaccharides. A 2019 study found that not only is an infant's IgA largely derived from maternal milk in the first month of life, but also that infants with NEC have larger proportions of IgA-unbound bacteria compared to age-matched controls. In the same study, Gopalakrishna, et al. used a murine model and concluded that pups reared by IgA-deficient mothers were not protected from NEC [23]. It has also been hypothesized that the beneficial effects of human milk relate to how diet affects gut microbiota and the developing immune system. Human breast milk contains oligosaccharides known to stimulate "healthy" bacteria and in a murine model, has been shown to downregulate bacterial related inflammatory signaling pathways [24].

2.2.3. Donor Breast Milk

Although mother's own milk is preferred for preterm and low birth weight infants, infants often need to be supplemented with donor breast milk or formula when maternal supply is inadequate. Donor milk has also been shown to have a protective effect on NEC incidence when compared to cow's milk and other formulas, with a 79% reduced risk [25–28]. A 2019 Cochrane Database review of 12 trials found that although formula-fed or supplemented preterm and low birth weight infants did have increased growth compared to those fed with donor breast milk, they also exhibited a higher risk of NEC (typical risk ratio 1.87) [29].

2.2.4. Cow's Milk Formula

Prior literature has established a higher incidence of NEC when cow's milk formula is used instead of mother's own milk [25,30]. In addition to the protective factors that breast milk contains, it's been hypothesized that the intestinal reaction to cow's milk proteins could also contribute to disease pathogenesis. In small cohorts of infants with NEC, a group has found an increase in cytokine response (interferon-$\gamma$, IL-4, and IL-5) to cow's milk proteins beta-lactoglobulin and casein [31]. Interestingly, bovine milk-derived exosomes have been shown to combat experimentally induced NEC by stimulating goblet cells and mitigating decreases in mucin 2 (MUC2) and glucose regulated protein 94 (GRP94). Isolation and administration of such exosomes could be useful for infants at high risk for NEC for whom breast milk cannot be obtained [32].

## 3. Medical NEC

Symptoms seen in the early stages of NEC may mimic feeding intolerance or other abdominal pathologies. The modified Bell's staging criteria include neutropenia, thrombocytopenia, coagulation factors, and metabolic acidosis as laboratory markers that can aid clinicians in diagnosing more advanced NEC [3]. However, these laboratory values are non-specific and are less likely to be reliable markers for disease in early stages or to predict intestinal recovery and safety to restart feeds. In addition to antibiotics, current nutritional management for NEC includes stopping feeds and starting parenteral nutrition.

*3.1. NPO Duration*

Patients' *nil per os* (NPO) status is largely driven by clinical assessment. Decreased apneic and bradycardic events in conjunction with laboratory values including blood gas, white count, and thrombocytopenia, as well as abdominal imaging without the appearance of portal venous gas or pneumatosis intestinalis are indications of improving clinical status [33]. Despite apparent improvement in clinical status, clinicians may hesitate to restart feeds after an NPO period, as objective evidence reflecting the optimal time to begin feeding is lacking. A meta-analysis conducted by Hock, et al. found no significant difference in adverse outcomes in patients given early (within 5 days of NEC diagnosis) and late (>5 days after NEC diagnosis) feeds [34]. Bonhorst, et al. utilized ultrasonography and compared outcomes following restarting feeding after 3 consecutive days without portal venous gas to restarting feeding after 10 days without portal venous gas. Earlier feeds were associated with fewer complications, shorter antibiotic courses, quicker progression to goal feeds, and shorter length of stay [35].

In addition to using imaging as an objective measure for readiness and safety to restart feeds, specific laboratory values and biomarkers would be useful. In a 2019 prospective observational cohort study, Kuik, et al. measured the regional intestinal oxygen saturation ($r_{int}SO_2$) by near-infrared spectroscopy (NIRS) and intestinal fatty acid binding protein (I-FABP$_u$) in the urine of 27 preterm infants. The study found that when measured after the first re-feed, these markers were predictive of post-NEC stricture, though not of recurrent NEC [36]. Additionally, a recent study on infants between 24–40 weeks postmenstrual age found high intestinal alkaline phosphatase (IAP) in stool and low

IAP enzyme activity in patients with NEC compared to those without disease; IAP also was a useful biomarker for disease severity [37]. Clinicians should attempt to minimize NPO time and begin refeeding patients as soon as clinical improvement is determined by vital sign stability and abdominal examination, as well as resolving thrombocytopenia and abdominal radiography or ultrasonography. Identifying biomarkers such as IAP that reflect a patient's disease severity and intestinal recovery could be useful in individualizing NPO duration to minimize complications associated with prolonged NPO status.

*3.2. Parenteral Nutrition*

PN is initiated in patients who are made NPO following NEC diagnosis. It is comprised of carbohydrates, amino acids, lipids, electrolytes, minerals, and vitamins administered intravenously to allow for bowel rest. PN should be started early with adequate protein (3.5–4 g/kg/day) to maintain a positive nitrogen balance, improve weight gain, and to allow repair of injured tissue [1,38–40]. However, it has been shown that supplemental PN at NEC onset does not appear to significantly improve outcomes, with no decrease in the rate of surgical intervention or in-hospital mortality [41]. PN is discontinued once enteral feedings approach goal volumes [42].

**4. Surgical NEC**

In cases of NEC refractory to medical management or NEC leading to intestinal perforation, surgery is indicated (i.e., "surgical NEC"). A complication of NEC following extensive intestinal resection is short bowel syndrome (SBS) and subsequent intestinal failure (IF) wherein the small bowel is unable to adequately absorb fluids, electrolytes, and nutrients required to support growth and development [43]. Nutrition therefore must be provided through parenteral nutrition. The key compensatory process involved in reaching enteral autonomy is intestinal adaptation. Adaptation is characterized by structural and functional changes that compensate for the loss of intestinal mucosal surface area [44] and involves an increase in villus height and crypt depth, myocyte and enterocyte proliferation, a decrease in enterocyte apoptosis, and elongation and dilatation of the remnant small bowel [45]. Therefore, post-operative nutrition strategies focused on enhancing the intestinal adaptive response remain a cornerstone of treatment. Factors known to play important roles in adaptation and enteral autonomy include length of remnant bowel, specific macronutrients, and the composition of PN.

*4.1. Enteral Feeding*

While the optimal enteral formulation for pediatric SBS is still unknown, the data consistently supports the benefit of breast milk in intestinal adaptation [46]. In addition to growth factors and immunoglobulins, breast milk contains key oligosaccharides that act in a prebiotic manner to stimulate enterocyte proliferation and positively regulate the intestinal microbiome [47]. The most abundant of these is 2'-fucosyllactose (2'-FL). A few preclinical studies have investigated the effects of 2'-FL enteral supplementation on various intestinal inflammatory diseases. Mezoff, et al. demonstrated that 2'-FL augments intestinal adaptation after ileocecal resection by optimizing energy processing by the gut microbiome [48]. Another group showed that 2'-FL significantly decreased the severity of colitis in interleukin-10 null mice through enhanced epithelial integrity and expansion of a positive gut microbial environment [47].

*4.2. Anatomical Considerations*

4.2.1. Intestinal Length

Following surgical NEC, remnant length and anatomy become major determinants of disease severity [49]. It is well demonstrated that residual intestinal length is inversely proportional both to duration of PN and mortality [50–52]. While there is no definitive threshold, data suggests that greater than 40 cm of remnant small bowel length (SBL) in the presence or absence of an ileocecal valve (ICV) is associated with improved outcomes [50]. The effect of an intact ICV is somewhat controversial and likely a surrogate for the presence of colonic mucosa. This may be more important in patients with less than 15 cm [53]. Quiros-Tejeira, et al. showed that both survival and enteral adaptation were increased when more than 38 cm of small bowel length remained [50]. Lastly, Goulet, et al. analyzed 87 SBS children based on PN weaning and reported that all patients in the PN-dependent group had less than 40 cm of SBL and/or absent ICV. Conversely, patients with persistent enteral independence had SBL of 57 +/− 19 cm [51]. Given the rapid intestinal elongation that normally occurs in late gestation, studies have recommended using the percentage of expected length as opposed to absolute remnant length in neonates. By this metric, Spencer, et al. found that greater than 10% age-adjusted remnant bowel length was highly predictive of both survival and enteral autonomy [52].

4.2.2. Segment Functionality

Given the segmental functionality of the gastrointestinal tract, the site of bowel resection has a substantial impact on the need for long-term nutritional support [54]. The three most common resection patterns in SBS are jejunoileal anastomosis, jejunocolic anastomosis, and jejunostomy. These anatomical permutations are associated with a predictable range of outcomes based on digestive and absorptive capacity.

Patients with jejunoileal anastomoses (mostly jejunum removed) have the highest likelihood of achieving enteral autonomy. This proximal resection spares the ileum, which has the greatest capacity for structural and functional adaptation [55]. In addition, the presence of the ileocecal valve and colonic continuity may mitigate intestinal transit time and excessive fluid losses [54]. Despite the intestinal adaptive capacity of patients with jejunoileal anastamoses, this population still experiences gastric hypersecretion secondary to loss of regulatory humoral action (cholecystokinin, secretin, vasoactive intestinal peptide, and serotonin) in the jejunum. This can transiently affect intestinal motility and increase gastric emptying and acid output. Administration of $H_2$ antagonists and proton pump inhibitors may be helpful [56].

Patients with jejunocolic anastomoses (mostly ileum removed) are often more difficult to manage, as the jejunum lacks the robust adaptive capacity of the distal small bowel [56]. Decreased water absorption along the proximal remnant length overwhelms the compensatory abilities of the colon, leading to fluid and electrolyte losses through diarrhea [54]. Furthermore, the ileum is the primary site of vitamin B12 and bile salt absorption. Consequent disruptions of the enterohepatic circulation result in fat malabsorption, steatorrhea, marked vitamin deficiencies, and renal oxalate stones [56]. Lastly, ileal resection can impact local hormonal control of gut motility through dysregulation of enteroglucagon and peptide YY [54]. As discussed above, loss of the ICV may be a negative predictor of long-term enteral autonomy. The ICV may play a role in the prevention of colonic bacterial migration into a small bowel environment that is vulnerable to bacterial overgrowth [57]. Ileocolic resections will result in variable PN dependence, which is higher when less than 60 cm of proximal SBL remains [54].

End jejunostomy patients have the most severe malabsorptive phenotype and the highest likelihood of requiring long-term parenteral support [55]. In addition to the specific issues encountered with ileal resections, this population also lacks any of the absorptive, digestive and energy-salvaging compensation afforded by colonic continuity [54]. Accelerated rates of gastric emptying and intestinal transit due to changes in the intestinal hormonal milieu further minimize nutrient interaction with jejunal luminal mucosa. Net losses of fluid and electrolytes from high enterostomy output often exceed patient intake, necessitating supplementation with PN and intravenous fluid administration [56]. These patients must be carefully monitored for dehydration, metabolic disturbances and nutrient deficiencies.

4.3. Ostomy Replacement

Fluid and electrolyte losses are significant problems in the pediatric SBS population and require diligent monitoring and repletion. This is especially true for children with small bowel ostomies.

The degree of malabsorption, dehydration and metabolic disturbances are commensurate to the length of small intestine remaining and the site of resection [58]. While an adaptive compensatory response is seen in patients with ileostomies, there is little evidence of structural or functional adaptation in those with jejunostomies. Despite optimized nutritional management and fluid balance, these patients are likely to require prolonged PN [58]. Furthermore, if less than 75 cm of small bowel remains in the presence of a jejunostomy, the ability to wean from parenteral nutritional or saline support is significantly impaired [58]. Patients with SBS and enterostomies tend to lose considerable amounts of sodium in stool causing secondary hyperaldosteronemia and significant potassium losses in the urine [59]. This often requires separate parenteral saline repletion in addition to the sodium provided from PN in amounts up to 8–10 mEq/kg/day [59]. Ostomy output and electrolytes should be closely observed to maintain hydration with urine output of at least 1–2 ml/kg/day and urine sodium >30 mEq/L [59].

High ostomy output is generally defined as greater than 40 ml/kg per 24 hours, with the severity of losses highly dependent on the length and site of remaining bowel. Provision of adequate fluids to prevent and treat dehydration is tantamount in this population, as the risk of hypotension and pre-renal failure are high [58]. Fluid needs are typically delivered through a combination of PN and EN, but may require supplemental intravenous fluids in cases of excessive loss [49].

*4.4. Macronutrients*

4.4.1. Fat

Several preclinical studies have shown that lipids in particular are associated with an enhanced adaptation response. Rats fed high fat diets (HFD) had significantly increased bowel weight and villus height post-resection when compared to those fed standard chow [60]. Choi, et al. randomized mice to low (12% kcal fat), medium (44% kcal fat) and high (71% kcal fat) fat diets after 50% proximal small bowel resection (SBR) and demonstrated that increased enteral fat concentration (HFD) optimally prevented postoperative catabolic responses and increased lean mass after SBR [61]. Conversely, in another rat model, low fat diets, despite comparable caloric intake, negatively impacted adaptation as evidenced by decreased body weight, reduced expression of fat transporters and attenuated villus height and enterocyte proliferation [62].

Moreover, the specific kind of enteral fat appears to play an important role in intestinal adaptation. In rats, long-chain fatty acids (LCFA) are superior to medium-chain fatty acids (MCFA) in augmenting both the structural and functional intestinal response following SBR [63]. While most studies have focused on polyunsaturated LCFA (LCPUFAs) such as menhaden oil, the relative benefit compared to saturated FAs is still debated. Menhaden oil is an excellent source of the omega-3 fatty acids eicosapentaenoic acid (EPA) and docosahexanoic acid (DHA) [64]. EPA and DHA are not only precursors of anti-inflammatory prostaglandins and associated with improved cardiovascular profiles, but they have also been shown to enhance intestinal adaptation after massive small bowel resection. Kollman, et al. demonstrated that resected rats fed LCPUFA-enhanced diets demonstrated significantly increased intestinal mucosal mass in a dose-dependent manner [65]. Another study found that in a mouse model, menhaden oil (versus saturated and monounsaturated fats) resulted in the highest percent of lean mass and greatest weight retention after SBR, though adaptation was indistinguishable across diets [66]. The benefit of LCFAs is attributed to its anti-inflammatory metabolite (prostaglandins), as inhibition with aspirin, a cyclo-oxygenase inhibitor, reduces the predicted intestinal adaptive response [67]. Although LCFAs have the greatest trophic yield, their absorption can be suboptimal in patients with extensive distal resections due to compromised enterohepatic circulation. While MCFAs are more water soluble, they have not been shown to have a robust effect on adaptation in mice and have significant osmotic sequelae which can exacerbate diarrhea and fluid losses [68]. Most of what is known about the effect of fats on adaptation is from preclinical animal models, but a high fat diet, specifically with LCFA, have been shown to support adaptation in these models and could potentially increase intestinal adaptation in patients following resection as well.

4.4.2. Protein

Most of the literature surrounding the protein composition of enteral nutrition is focused on absorption rather than adaptation. Elemental (fully digested) or semi-elemental (partially digested) enteral formulas have historically been preferred in infants with SBS in an effort to maximize absorption in the remnant bowel. For a subset of patients, losses can occur both in the bowel effluent and through loss of protein exudate. This double hit is akin to a protein-losing enteropathy, necessitating increased protein requirements for adequate growth. The extent to which children with persistent malabsorption and intolerance may benefit from a hydrolyzed formula is not known. A small study of four children with SBS found that after initiating a hydrolyzed formula, subjects that previously had persistent feeding intolerance were able to be weaned off parenteral nutrition within 15 months [69]. A possible explanation for improved tolerance on hydrolyzed formula could be non-IgE mediated cow's milk protein sensitization seen in infants with NEC [31]. However, it is difficult to draw conclusions from the small population that was observed. Additionally, it has been shown that 70–90% of protein absorption ability is retained after massive intestinal resection in human neonates [70]. It was previously theorized that the lack of MCTs and lactose in extensively hydrolyzed formulas may lead to easier digestion in patients with SBS. However, in a randomized crossover trial comparing protein hydrosylate formula to standard formulas in children with SBS, Ksiazyk et al. found no differences in intestinal permeability, energy expenditure, or nitrogen balance [46].

Providing adequate amino acids after intestinal resection is important. Glutamine serves as the primary fuel substrate for intestinal cells, promoting enterocyte proliferation and protein synthesis [71]. In preclinical rat models, there is a marked increase in glutamine and total amino acid uptake in the early adaptive phases following SBR. Unfortunately, supplementing enteral nutrition with glutamine or arginine after massive intestinal loss in humans has failed to improve adaptive responses and thus remains controversial [71,72]. Additionally, recent data suggests that complex nutrients promote greater intestinal adaptation. In this "functional workload" hypothesis, the remnant bowel meets the digestive demand of the nutrients encountered and there is thus a more robust compensatory response when infants are fed a non-hydrolyzed formula [57].

Ultimately, optimal protein intake from enteral nutrition should take into consideration remnant bowel length, absorptive capacity, and feeding tolerance. The goal is to achieve a positive nitrogen balance through improved nitrogen absorption. The data on the impact of formula protein content and composition on intestinal adaptation is sparse and the variation amongst formulas makes comparison of studies difficult. Although there is no robust evidence that elemental formula is superior to non-hydrolyzed formula, there is data showing that patients with SBS may tolerate it better and it is commonly used in the pediatric SBS population.

4.4.3. Oligosaccharides

After intestinal resection, the bowel undergoes significant functional adaptation as evidenced in a rat model by increased densities of both key digestive enzymes and glucose transporters [64]. Excessive administration of simple carbohydrates should be avoided given their considerable osmotic effects.

Energy can be derived from complex carbohydrates and soluble fibers processed in the colon. These undigested macromolecules are metabolized by colonic bacteria to produce short chain fatty acids (SCFAs) such as butyrate [67]. Butyrate is the primary fuel substrate for colonocytes and has been shown to play an important role in intestinal adaptation in both rats [73] and piglets [48]. In neonatal piglets that underwent 80% distal SBR, butyrate supplementation markedly increased the structural and functional indices of intestinal adaptation in both the acute and chronic phases [48]. Similar findings were recapitulated using a rodent SBS model. DNA, RNA and protein content per unit mucosal weight all increased post-resection in fiber- and butyrate-supplemented diet compared to controls [73]. In humans, these benefits are mitigated by the length of residual colon and colonic continuity. Furthermore, simple carbohydrates in excess also have significant osmotic influence that may exacerbate diarrhea and extraneous losses [57]. Preferably, carbohydrates should comprise no more than 40% of the total caloric provision [57].

*4.5. Parenteral Nutrition*

Surgical NEC typically delays the time until enteral autonomy and prolonged PN use (>21 days) may be required. Allin, et al. demonstrated that the need for PN support at 28 days post-decision to intervene surgically is associated with increased one-year mortality [74]. In clinical practice, intestinal insufficiency may be indirectly measured by the level of PN required for normal or catch up growth [75]. Patients with less remaining bowel require more PN and a residual length of 15–40 cm is associated with PN weaning [50,51,76–78]. The primary metabolic complication associated with PN is intestinal failure associated liver disease (IFALD), which is characterized by direct hyperbilirubinemia, elevated transaminases, and liver synthetic dysfunction [53]. Some modifications to PN can be made to reduce the risk for liver injury, such as not overfeeding and cycling infusions [42]. Improvement of cholestasis also depends on maintaining an appropriate protein-to-energy ratio in PN [79]. However, the most heavily studied factor implicated in PN-associated liver disease is intravenous lipid emulsions (ILE).

PN Lipid Source

ILEs are a crucial component of PN, as they are a source of essential fatty acids and non-protein calories. Several factors should be taken into consideration when choosing an ILE for parenteral use: the content of essential fatty acids (FAs), the ratio of polyunsaturated fatty acids omega-6 to omega-3, the quantity of α-tocopherol, and phytosterols. Monitoring FA profiles of children with IF is critical to their nutrition management.

Soybean-based (SO) lipid emulsions were previously considered the standard of care for providing fatty acids to children with intestinal failure. However, SO contains a 7:1 ratio of omega-6: omega-3, whereas the optimal ratio is 4:1 to minimize the production of inflammatory mediators [80,81]. It also has a high concentration of phytosterols, which have been associated with hepatic inflammation and cholestasis [82,83]. The SO factor, stigmasterol, has also been shown in a murine model to promote cholestasis, liver injury, and liver macrophage activation [84]. In 2012, Teitelbaum and colleagues described a significant reduction in cholestasis in a cohort of pediatric IF whose SO lipid dose was restricted to 1 g/kg/day compared to the historical dose of 3 g/kg/day [85]. Subsequent studies demonstrated that this lipid reduction strategy does not decrease the incidence of IFALD, but may slow its progression [86].

In 2018, the United States Food and Drug Administration approved a fish-oil (FO)-based lipid emulsion (Omegaven®) for the treatment of pediatric intestinal failure associated liver disease (IFALD). Unlike SO-based lipid emulsion, FO is composed primarily of anti-inflammatory omega-3 FA (docosahexaenoic and eicosapentaenoic acids) and contains a small amount of the essential FA (linoleic and alpha-linolenic acids) [87]. FO-based lipids are rich in α-tocopherol, which scavenges free radicals from peroxidized lipids to prevent propagation of oxidative lipid damage [88]. IV FO treatment results in a biochemical reversal of cholestasis and is associated with reduction in plasma phytosterols, cytokines, and bile acids. However, despite biochemical and histologic improvement in cholestasis, there is persistent significant liver fibrosis on histology [89,90]. There is also concern that because FO provides fewer essential omega-6 FAs than that recommended in children, it could cause essential fatty acid deficiency (EFAD). However, Calkins, et al. found in a cohort of PN-dependent children, switching from SO to FO for six months led to a decrease in essential FA concentrations, but no evidence of EFAD [91]. These findings were supported in a long term study conducted over three years by Puder, et al. [92]. Newer preparations such as Smoflipid® (Fresenius-Kabi, Uppsala, Sweden) combine soybean oil (30%), coconut oil (30%), olive oil (25%) and fish oil (15%) and have proven to be of benefit in patients with IFALD. Randomized controlled trials in preterm infants have shown that Smoflipid® emulsion increases the content of eicosapentaenoic acid (EPA) and docosahexaenoic acids [93]. Muhammed, et al. reported rapid and marked improvement in biochemical liver function tests in children with cholestatic jaundice after switching from a SO-based ILE to Smoflipid® [94]. Smoflipid® has a positive impact on liver enzymes due low phytosterol and high vitamin E content; in addition, its use leads to a decrease in lipid peroxidation and an improvement on the $\omega$-3:$\omega$-6 PUFA ratio, producing a less proinflammatory profile [95].

## 5. Conclusions

Providing infants breast milk has been the mainstay of nutritional therapy in NEC prevention and is also beneficial for infants following surgery in stage III NEC [19,20,46]. Unfortunately, there have been no feeding strategies proven to prevent NEC, such as initiating feeds later, advancing feeds more slowly, or bolus versus continuous feeds; however, it is safe to start feeds within 96 hours of birth, advance more rapidly, and bolus feed [7,9,12]. Because there is great variability in individual feeding practices, it is important that each NICU has a standardized protocol to approaching feeds in order to ensure appropriate nutrition and minimize complications. Additional studies focusing on more premature and smaller infants should be conducted, as most studies that are currently available are limited to infants >1000 g and between 28–32 weeks. Younger and smaller infants may respond differently than older infants to alternate feeding approaches. Additionally, identifying more specific biomarkers for NEC severity and intestinal recovery is necessary to provide appropriate treatment and assist clinicians in determining intestinal recovery after disease.

Finally, more diet studies on the effect of macronutrients on recovery after surgical NEC are required. The majority of current data on intestinal adaptation shows the benefit of a high fat diet but is limited to animal studies [61]. Using hydrolyzed formula in patients with SBS is common but has only been studied in a small population and lacks robust evidence [69]. Since parenteral nutrition is often required following resection, it is important to understand its complications. Omegaven® and Smoflipid® both are less likely to lead to cholestasis and IFALD without causing essential fatty acid deficiency and may be more beneficial as a fat source than the traditionally used intralipids [92,95].

**Author Contributions:** J.O., C.M.C., A.E.S., and M.E.T. contributed to the writing—original draft preparation, review, and editing of the initial version manuscript. J.O., C.M.C., and B.W.W. edited and revised the manuscript. All authors have read and agreed to the published version of the manuscript.

**Funding:** B.W. is funded by NIHR01DK104698, R01DK112378, and the Children's Surgical Sciences Research Institute of St. Louis Children's Hospital Foundation CMC is supported by the Marion and van Black Research Fellowship. AES is funded by T32DK077653-28. MET is funded by T32DK007120.

**Conflicts of Interest:** The authors declare no conflict of interest.

## References

1. Neu, J.; Walker, W.A. Necrotizing enterocolitis. *N. Engl. J. Med.* **2011**, *364*, 255–264. [CrossRef]
2. Bell, M.J.; Ternberg, J.L.; Feigin, R.D.; Keating, J.P.; Marshall, R.; Barton, L.; Brotherton, T. Neonatal necrotizing enterocolitis. Therapeutic decisions based upon clinical staging. *Ann. Surg.* **1978**, *187*, 1–7. [CrossRef]
3. Walsh, M.C.; Kliegman, R.M. Necrotizing Enterocolitis: Treatment Based on Staging Criteria. *Pediatr. Clin. North Am.* **1986**, *33*, 179–201. [CrossRef]
4. Schnabl, K.L.; E Van Aerde, J.; Thomson, A.B.; Clandinin, M.T. Necrotizing enterocolitis: A multifactorial disease with no cure. *World J. Gastroenterol.* **2008**, *14*, 2142–2161. [CrossRef]
5. Warner, B.W. The Pathogenesis of Resection-Associated Intestinal Adaptation. *Cell. Mol. Gastroenterol. Hepatol.* **2016**, *2*, 429–438. [CrossRef]
6. Morgan, J.; Bombell, S.; McGuire, W. Early trophic feeding versus enteral fasting for very preterm or very low birth weight infants. *Cochrane Database Syst. Rev.* **2013**, *2013*, CD000504. [CrossRef]
7. AlShaikh, B.; Dharel, D.; Yusuf, K.; Singhal, N. Early total enteral feeding in stable preterm infants: a systematic review and meta-analysis. *J. Matern. Neonatal Med.* **2019**, 1–8. [CrossRef]
8. Nangia, S.; Vadivel, V.; Thukral, A.; Saili, A. Early Total Enteral Feeding versus Conventional Enteral Feeding in Stable Very-Low-Birth-Weight Infants: A Randomised Controlled Trial. *Neonatol.* **2019**, *115*, 256–262. [CrossRef]

9. Dorling, J.; Abbott, J.; Berrington, J.; Bosiak, B.; Bowler, U.; Boyle, E.; Embleton, N.; Hewer, O.; Johnson, S.; Juszczak, E.; et al. Controlled Trial of Two Incremental Milk-Feeding Rates in Preterm Infants. *New Engl. J. Med.* **2019**, *381*, 1434–1443. [CrossRef]
10. Olieman, J.F.; Penning, C.; Ijsselstijn, H.; Escher, J.C.; Joosten, K.F.; Hulst, J.M.; Tibboel, D. Enteral Nutrition in Children with Short-Bowel Syndrome: Current Evidence and Recommendations for the Clinician. *J. Am. Diet. Assoc.* **2010**, *110*, 420–426. [CrossRef]
11. Davis, T.A.; Fiorotto, M.L.; Suryawan, A. Bolus vs. continuous feeding to optimize anabolism in neonates. *Curr. Opin. Clin. Nutr. Metab. Care* **2015**, *18*, 102–108. [CrossRef]
12. Wang, Y.; Zhu, W.; Luo, B.-R. Continuous feeding versus intermittent bolus feeding for premature infants with low birth weight: a meta-analysis of randomized controlled trials. *Eur. J. Clin. Nutr.* **2019**, 1–9. [CrossRef]
13. Pearson, F.; Johnson, M.J.; Leaf, A.A. Leaf, Milk osmolality: does it matter? *Arch. Dis. Child. Fetal Neonatal. Ed.* **2013**, *98*, F166–F169. [CrossRef]
14. Willis, D.M.; Chabot, J.; Radde, I.C.; Chance, G.W. Unsuspected hyperosmolality of oral solutions contributing to necrotizing enterocolitis in very-low-birth-weight infants. *Pediatrics* **1977**, *60*, 535–538.
15. Sántulli, T.V.; Schullinger, J.N.; Heird, W.C.; Gongaware, R.D.; Wigger, J.; Barlow, B.; Blanc, W.A.; Berdon, W.E. Acute necrotizing enterocolitis in infancy: A review of 64 cases. *Pediatrics* **1975**, *55*, 376–387.
16. Miyake, H.; Chen, Y.; Koike, Y.; Hock, A.; Lee, C.; Zani, A.; Pierro, A.; Li, B. Osmolality of enteral formula and severity of experimental necrotizing enterocolitis. *Pediatr. Surg. Int.* **2016**, *32*, 1153–1156. [CrossRef]
17. Brown, J.V.E.; Embleton, N.; Harding, J.E.; McGuire, W. Multi-nutrient fortification of human milk for preterm infants. *Cochrane Database Syst. Rev.* **2016**, *2016*, CD000343. [CrossRef]
18. Meinzen-Derr, J.; Poindexter, B.; Wrage, L.; Morrow, A.L.; Stoll, B.; Donovan, E.F. Role of human milk in extremely low birth weight infants' risk of necrotizing enterocolitis or death. *J. Perinatol.* **2009**, *29*, 57–62. [CrossRef]
19. Sisk, P.M.; A Lovelady, C.; Dillard, R.G.; Gruber, K.; O'Shea, T.M. Early human milk feeding is associated with a lower risk of necrotizing enterocolitis in very low birth weight infants. *J. Perinatol.* **2007**, *27*, 428–433. [CrossRef]
20. Lucas, A.; Cole, T. Breast milk and neonatal necrotising enterocolitis. *Lancet* **1990**, *336*, 1519–1523. [CrossRef]
21. Hanson, L.Å.; Strömbäck, L.; Erling, V.; Zaman, S.; Olcén, P.; Telemo, E. The immunological role of breast feeding. *Pediatr. Allergy Immunol.* **2001**, *12*, 15–19. [CrossRef]
22. Walsh, V.; McGuire, W. Immunonutrition for Preterm Infants. *Neonatol.* **2019**, *115*, 398–405. [CrossRef]
23. Gopalakrishna, K.P.; Macadangdang, B.R.; Rogers, M.B.; Tometich, J.T.; Firek, B.A.; Baker, R.; Ji, J.; Burr, A.H.P.; Ma, C.; Good, M.; et al. Maternal IgA protects against the development of necrotizing enterocolitis in preterm infants. *Nat. Med.* **2019**, *25*, 1110–1115. [CrossRef]
24. Good, M.; Sodhi, C.P.; Egan, C.E.; Afrazi, A.; Jia, H.; Yamaguchi, Y.; Lu, P.; Branca, M.F.; Ma, C.; Prindle, T.; et al. Breast milk protects against the development of necrotizing enterocolitis through inhibition of Toll-like receptor 4 in the intestinal epithelium via activation of the epidermal growth factor receptor. *Mucosal Immunol.* **2015**, *8*, 1166–1179. [CrossRef]
25. Sullivan, S.; Schanler, R.J.; Kim, J.H.; Patel, A.; Trawöger, R.; Kiechl-Kohlendorfer, U.; Chan, G.M.; Blanco, C.L.; Abrams, S.A.; Cotten, C.M.; et al. An Exclusively Human Milk-Based Diet Is Associated with a Lower Rate of Necrotizing Enterocolitis than a Diet of Human Milk and Bovine Milk-Based Products. *J. Pediatr.* **2010**, *156*, 562–567. [CrossRef]
26. Schanler, R.J.; Lau, C.; Hurst, N.M.; Smith, E.O. Randomized Trial of Donor Human Milk Versus Preterm Formula as Substitutes for Mothers' Own Milk in the Feeding of Extremely Premature Infants. *Pediatrics* **2005**, *116*, 400–406. [CrossRef]
27. Cristofalo, E.A.; Schanler, R.J.; Blanco, C.L.; Sullivan, S.; Trawoeger, R.; Kiechl-Kohlendorfer, U.; Dudell, G.; Rechtman, D.J.; Lee, M.L.; Lucas, A.; et al. Randomized Trial of Exclusive Human Milk versus Preterm Formula Diets in Extremely Premature Infants. *J. Pediatr.* **2013**, *163*, 1592–1595. [CrossRef]
28. Boyd, C.A.; Quigley, M.A.; Brocklehurst, P. Donor breast milk versus infant formula for preterm infants: systematic review and meta-analysis. *Arch. Dis. Child. Fetal Neonatal Ed.* **2007**, *92*, F169–F175. [CrossRef]
29. Quigley, M.; Embleton, N.D.; McGuire, W. Formula versus donor breast milk for feeding preterm or low birth weight infants. *Cochrane Database Syst. Rev.* **2019**, *7*, CD002971. [CrossRef]

30. Chowning, R.; Radmacher, P.; Lewis, S.; Serke, L.; Pettit, N.; Adamkin, D.H. A retrospective analysis of the effect of human milk on prevention of necrotizing enterocolitis and postnatal growth. *J. Perinatol.* **2016**, *36*, 221–224. [CrossRef]
31. Chuang, S.-L.; Hayes, P.J.; Ogundipe, E.; Haddad, M.; Macdonald, T.T.; Fell, J.M. Cow's milk protein-specific T-helper type I/II cytokine responses in infants with necrotizing enterocolitis. *Pediatr. Allergy Immunol.* **2009**, *20*, 45–52. [CrossRef] [PubMed]
32. Li, B.; Hock, A.; Wu, R.Y.; Minich, A.; Botts, S.; Lee, C.; Antounians, L.; Miyake, H.; Koike, Y.; Chen, Y.; et al. Bovine milk-derived exosomes enhance goblet cell activity and prevent the development of experimental necrotizing enterocolitis. *PLOS ONE* **2019**, *14*, e0211431. [CrossRef] [PubMed]
33. Valpacos, M.; Arni, D.; Keir, A.; Aspirot, A.; Wilde, J.C.; Beasley, S.; De Luca, D.; Pfister, R.E.; Karam, O. Diagnosis and Management of Necrotizing Enterocolitis: An International Survey of Neonatologists and Pediatric Surgeons. *Neonatology* **2018**, *113*, 170–176. [CrossRef] [PubMed]
34. Hock, A.M.; Chen, Y.; Miyake, H.; Koike, Y.; Seo, S.; Pierro, A. Initiation of Enteral Feeding After Necrotizing Enterocolitis. *Eur. J. Pediatr. Surg.* **2018**, *28*, 44–50.
35. Bohnhorst, B.; Müller, S.; Dördelmann, M.; Peter, C.S.; Petersen, C.; Poets, C.F. Early feeding after necrotizing enterocolitis in preterm infants. *J. Pediatr.* **2003**, *143*, 484–487. [CrossRef]
36. Kuik, S.J.; Kalteren, W.S.; Mebius, M.J.; Bos, A.F.; Hulscher, J.B.F.; Kooi, E.M.W. Predicting intestinal recovery after necrotizing enterocolitis in preterm infants. *Pediatr. Res.* **2019**, 1–9. [CrossRef]
37. Heath, M.; Buckley, R.; Gerber, Z.; Davis, P.; Linneman, L.; Gong, Q.; Barkemeyer, B.; Fang, Z.; Good, M.; Penn, D.; et al. Association of Intestinal Alkaline Phosphatase With Necrotizing Enterocolitis Among Premature Infants. *JAMA Netw. Open* **2019**, *2*, e1914996. [CrossRef]
38. Neu, J. Neonatal necrotizing enterocolitis: An update. *Acta Paediatr.* **2005**, *94*, 100–105. [CrossRef]
39. Ibrahim, H.; Jeroudi, M.A.; Baier, R.J.; Dhanireddy, R.; Krouskop, R.W. Aggressive Early Total Parental Nutrition in Low-Birth-Weight Infants. *J. Perinatol.* **2004**, *24*, 482–486. [CrossRef]
40. Can, E.; Bulbul, A.; Uslu, S.; Cömert, S.; Bolat, F.; Nuhoğlu, A.; Nuhoğlu, A. Effects of aggressive parenteral nutrition on growth and clinical outcome in preterm infants. *Pediatr. Int.* **2012**, *54*, 869–874. [CrossRef]
41. Akinkuotu, A.C.; Nuthakki, S.; Sheikh, F.; Cruz, S.M.; Welty, S.E.; Olutoye, O.O. The effect of supplemental parenteral nutrition on outcomes of necrotizing enterocolitis in premature, low birth weight neonates. *Am. J. Surg.* **2015**, *210*, 1045–1050. [CrossRef]
42. Christian, V.; Polzin, E.; Welak, S.R. Nutrition Management of Necrotizing Enterocolitis. *Nutr. Clin. Pr.* **2018**, *33*, 476–482. [CrossRef]
43. Goulet, O.; Ruemmele, F. Causes and Management of Intestinal Failure in Children. *Gastroenterol.* **2006**, *130*, S16–S28. [CrossRef]
44. Buchman, A.L.; Scolapio, J.; Fryer, J. AGA technical review on short bowel syndrome and intestinal transplantation. *Gastroenterology* **2003**, *124*, 1111–1134. [CrossRef]
45. Welters, C.F.M.; DeJong, C.H.C.; Deutz, N.E.; Heineman, E. Intestinal adaptation in short bowel syndrome. *ANZ J. Surg.* **2002**, *72*, 229–236. [CrossRef]
46. Ksiazyk, J.; Piena, M.; Kierkus, J.; Lyszkowska, M. Hydrolyzed versus nonhydrolyzed protein diet in short bowel syndrome in children. *J. Pediatr. Gastroenterol. Nutr.* **2002**, *35*, 615–618. [CrossRef]
47. Grabinger, T.; Garzon, J.F.G.; Hausmann, M.; Geirnaert, A.; Lacroix, C.; Hennet, T. Alleviation of Intestinal Inflammation by Oral Supplementation With 2-Fucosyllactose in Mice. *Front. Microbiol.* **2019**, *10*, 1385. [CrossRef]
48. Bartholome, A.; Albin, D.; Baker, D.; Holst, J.J.; Tappenden, K. Supplementation of total parenteral nutrition with butyrate acutely increases structural aspects of intestinal adaptation after an 80% jejunoileal resection in neonatal piglets. *J. Parenter. Enter. Nutr.* **2004**, *28*, 210–222. [CrossRef]
49. Barclay, A.R.; Paxton, C.E.; Gillett, P.; Hoole, D.; Livingstone, J.; Young, D.; Wilson, D.C.; Menon, G.; Munro, F. Regionally acquired intestinal failure data suggest an underestimate in national service requirements. *Arch. Dis. Child.* **2009**, *94*, 938–943. [CrossRef]
50. Quirós-Tejeira, R.E.; Ament, M.E.; Reyen, L.; Herzog, F.; Merjanian, M.; Olivares-Serrano, N.; Vargas, J.H. Long-term parenteral nutritional support and intestinal adaptation in children with short bowel syndrome: A 25-year experience. *J. Pediatr.* **2004**, *145*, 157–163. [CrossRef]

51. Goulet, O.; Baglin-Gobet, S.; Talbotec, C.; Fourcade, L.; Colomb, V.; Sauvat, F.; Jais, J.-P.; Michel, J.-L.; Jan, D.; Ricour, C. Outcome and Long-Term Growth After Extensive Small Bowel Resection in the Neonatal Period: A Survey of 87 Children. *Eur. J. Pediatr. Surg.* **2005**, *15*, 95–101. [CrossRef]
52. Spencer, A.U.; Neaga, A.; West, B.; Safran, J.; Brown, P.; Btaiche, I.; Kuzma-O'Reilly, B.; Teitelbaum, D.H. Pediatric short bowel syndrome: redefining predictors of success. *Ann. Surg.* **2005**, *242*, 403. [CrossRef]
53. Squires, R.H.; Duggan, C.; Teitelbaum, D.H.; Wales, P.W.; Balint, J.; Venick, R.; Rhee, S.; Sudan, D.; Mercer, D.; Martinez, J.A.; et al. Natural history of pediatric intestinal failure: initial report from the Pediatric Intestinal Failure Consortium. *J. Pediatr.* **2012**, *161*, 723–728. [CrossRef]
54. Khan, F.A.; Squires, R.H.; Litman, H.J.; Balint, J.; Carter, B.A.; Fisher, J.G.; Horslen, S.; Kocoshis, S.; Martinez, J.A.; Mercer, D.; et al. Predictors of Enteral Autonomy in Children with Intestinal Failure: A Multicenter Cohort Study. *J. Pediatr.* **2015**, *167*, 29–34. [CrossRef]
55. Tappenden, K.A. Pathophysiology of short bowel syndrome: considerations of resected and residual anatomy. *JPEN J. Parenter. Enteral Nutr.* **2014**, *38*, 14S–22S. [CrossRef]
56. Amin, S.C.; Pappas, C.; Iyengar, H.; Maheshwari, A. Short bowel syndrome in the NICU. *Clin. Perinatol.* **2013**, *40*, 53–68. [CrossRef]
57. Serrano, M.-S.; Schmidt-Sommerfeld, E. Nutrition support of infants with short bowel syndrome. *Nutr.* **2002**, *18*, 966–970. [CrossRef]
58. Kocoshis, S.A. Medical management of pediatric intestinal failure. *Semin. Pediatr. Surg.* **2010**, *19*, 20–26. [CrossRef]
59. Batra, A.; Beattie, R. Management of short bowel syndrome in infancy. *Early Hum. Dev.* **2013**, *89*, 899–904. [CrossRef]
60. Tappenden, K.A. Intestinal Adaptation Following Resection. *J. Parenter. Enter. Nutr.* **2014**, *38*, 23S–31S. [CrossRef]
61. Choi, P.M.; Sun, R.C.; Guo, J.; Erwin, C.R.; Warner, B.W. High-fat diet enhances villus growth during the adaptation response to massive proximal small bowel resection. *J. Gastrointest. Surg.* **2014**, *18*, 286–294. [CrossRef] [PubMed]
62. Sukhotnik, I.; Shiloni, E.; Krausz, M.M.; Yakirevich, E.; Sabo, E.; Mogilner, J.; Coran, A.G.; Harmon, C.M. Low-fat diet impairs postresection intestinal adaptation in a rat model of short bowel syndrome. *J. Pediatr. Surg.* **2003**, *38*, 1182–1187. [CrossRef]
63. Chen, W.-J.; Yang, C.-L.; Lai, H.-S.; Chen, K.-M. Effects of Lipids on Intestinal Adaptation Following 60% Resection in Rats. *J. Surg. Res.* **1995**, *58*, 253–259. [CrossRef] [PubMed]
64. Vanderhoof, J.A.; Park, J.H.; Herrington, M.K.; Adrian, T.E. Effects of dietary menhaden oil on mucosal adaptation after small bowel resection in rats. *Gastroenterol.* **1994**, *106*, 94–99. [CrossRef]
65. Kollman, K.A.; Lien, E.L.; Vanderhoof, J.A. Dietary lipids influence intestinal adaptation after massive bowel resection. *J. Pediatr. Gastroenterol. Nutr.* **1999**, *28*, 41–45. [CrossRef]
66. Choi, P.M.; Sun, R.C.; Sommovilla, J.; Diaz-Miron, J.; Khil, J.; Erwin, C.R.; Guo, J.; Warner, B.W. The role of enteral fat as a modulator of body composition after small bowel resection. *Surg.* **2014**, *156*, 412–418. [CrossRef]
67. Weale, A.R.; Edwards, A.G.; Bailey, M.; Lear, P. Intestinal adaptation after massive intestinal resection. *Postgrad. Med J.* **2005**, *81*, 178–184. [CrossRef] [PubMed]
68. Welters, C.F.; DeJong, C.H.; Deutz, N.E.; Heineman, E. Intestinal function and metabolism in the early adaptive phase after massive small bowel resection in the rat. *J. Pediatr. Surg.* **2001**, *36*, 1746–1751. [CrossRef]
69. Bines, J.; Francis, D.; Hill, D. Reducing parenteral requirement in children with short bowel syndrome: impact of an amino acid-based complete infant formula. *J. Pediatr. Gastroenterol. Nutr.* **1998**, *26*, 123–128. [CrossRef]
70. Schaart, M.W.; De Bruijn, A.C.J.M.; Tibboel, D.; Renes, I.B.; Van Goudoever, J.B. Dietary Protein Absorption of the Small Intestine in Human Neonates. *J. Parenter. Enter. Nutr.* **2007**, *31*, 482–486. [CrossRef]
71. Kim, M.-H.; Kim, H. The Roles of Glutamine in the Intestine and Its Implication in Intestinal Diseases. *Int. J. Mol. Sci.* **2017**, *18*, 1051. [CrossRef] [PubMed]
72. Scolapio, J.S.; McGreevy, K.; Tennyson, G.; Burnett, O. Effect of glutamine in short-bowel syndrome. *Clin. Nutr.* **2001**, *20*, 319–323. [CrossRef] [PubMed]

73. Koruda, M.J.; Rolandelli, R.H.; Settle, R.G.; Saul, S.H.; Rombeau, J.L. The Effect of a Pectin-Supplemented Elemental Diet on Intestinal Adaptation to Massive Small Bowel Resection. *J. Parenter. Enter. Nutr.* **1986**, *10*, 343–350. [CrossRef] [PubMed]
74. Allin, B.S.R.; Long, A.M.; Gupta, A.; Lakhoo, K.; Knight, M. One-year outcomes following surgery for necrotising enterocolitis: a UK-wide cohort study. *Arch. Dis. Child. Fetal Neonatal. Ed.* **2018**, *103*, F461–F466. [CrossRef] [PubMed]
75. Abi Nader, E.; Lambe, C.; Talbotec, C.; Dong, L.; Pigneur, B.; Goulet, O.A. New Concept to Achieve Optimal Weight Gain in Malnourished Infants on Total Parenteral Nutrition. *JPEN J. Parenter. Enteral Nutr.* **2018**, *42*, 78–86. [PubMed]
76. Engelstad, H.J.; Barron, L.; Moen, J.; Wylie, T.N.; Wylie, K.; Rubin, D.C.; Davidson, N.; Cade, W.T.; Warner, B.B.; Warner, B.W. Remnant Small Bowel Length in Pediatric Short Bowel Syndrome and the Correlation with Intestinal Dysbiosis and Linear Growth. *J. Am. Coll. Surg.* **2018**, *227*, 439–449. [CrossRef]
77. Andorsky, D.J.; Lund, D.P.; Lillehei, C.W.; Jaksic, T.; DiCanzio, J.; Richardson, D.S.; Collier, S.B.; Lo, C.; Duggan, C. Nutritional and other postoperative management of neonates with short bowel syndrome correlates with clinical outcomes. *J. Pediatr.* **2001**, *139*, 27–33. [CrossRef]
78. Belza, C.; Fitzgerald, K.; de Silva, N.; Avitzur, Y.; Steinberg, K.; Courtney-Martin, G.; Wales, P.W. Predicting Intestinal Adaptation in Pediatric Intestinal Failure: A Retrospective Cohort Study. *Ann. Surg.* **2019**, *269*, 988–993. [CrossRef]
79. Linseisen, J.; Hoffmann, J.; Lienhard, S.; Jauch, K.W.; Wolfram, G. Antioxidant status of surgical patients receiving TPN with an omega-3-fatty acid-containing lipid emulsion supplemented with alpha-tocopherol. *Clin. Nutr.* **2000**, *19*, 177–184. [CrossRef]
80. Cotogni, P.; Muzio, G.; Trombetta, A.; Ranieri, V.M.; Canuto, R.A. Impact of the omega-3 to omega-6 polyunsaturated fatty acid ratio on cytokine release in human alveolar cells. *JPEN J. Parenter. Enteral Nutr.* **2011**, *35*, 114–121. [CrossRef]
81. Wang, Y.; Feng, Y.; Lu, L.-N.; Wang, W.-P.; He, Z.-J.; Xie, L.-J.; Hong, L.; Tang, Q.-Y.; Cai, W.; Information, P.E.K.F.C. The effects of different lipid emulsions on the lipid profile, fatty acid composition, and antioxidant capacity of preterm infants: A double-blind, randomized clinical trial. *Clin. Nutr.* **2016**, *35*, 1023–1031. [CrossRef] [PubMed]
82. Hukkinen, M.; Mutanen, A.; Nissinen, M.; Merras-Salmio, L.; Gylling, H.; Pakarinen, M.P. Parenteral Plant Sterols Accumulate in the Liver Reflecting Their Increased Serum Levels and Portal Inflammation in Children With Intestinal Failure. *JPEN J. Parenter. Enteral Nutr.* **2017**, *41*, 1014–1022. [CrossRef] [PubMed]
83. Kurvinen, A.; Nissinen, M.J.; Andersson, S.; Korhonen, P.; Ruuska, T.; Taimisto, M.; Kalliomäki, M.; Lehtonen, L.; Sankilampi, U.; Arikoski, P.; et al. Parenteral Plant Sterols and Intestinal Failure–associated Liver Disease in Neonates. *J. Pediatr. Gastroenterol. Nutr.* **2012**, *54*, 803–811. [CrossRef] [PubMed]
84. El Kasmi, K.C.; Anderson, A.L.; Devereaux, M.W.; Vue, P.M.; Zhang, W.; Setchell, K.D.R.; Karpen, S.J.; Sokol, R.J. Phytosterols Promote Liver Injury and Kupffer Cell Activation in Parenteral Nutrition-Associated Liver Disease. *Sci. Transl. Med.* **2013**, *5*, 206ra137. [CrossRef] [PubMed]
85. Cober, M.P.; Killu, G.; Brattain, A.; Welch, K.B.; Kunisaki, S.M.; Teitelbaum, D.H. Intravenous Fat Emulsions Reduction for Patients with Parenteral Nutrition–Associated Liver Disease. *J. Pediatr.* **2012**, *160*, 421–427. [CrossRef]
86. Nehra, D.; Fallon, E.M.; Carlson, S.J.; Potemkin, A.K.; Hevelone, N.D.; Mitchell, P.D.; Gura PharmD, K.M.; Puder, M. Provision of a soy-based intravenous lipid emulsion at 1 g/kg/d does not prevent cholestasis in neonates. *JPEN J. Parenter. Enteral Nutr.* **2013**, *37*, 498–505. [CrossRef]
87. Kalish, B.T.; Le, H.D.; Fitzgerald, J.M.; Wang, S.; Seamon, K.; Gura, K.M.; Gronert, K.; Puder, M. Intravenous fish oil lipid emulsion promotes a shift toward anti-inflammatory proresolving lipid mediators. *Am. J. Physiol. Liver Physiol.* **2013**, *305*, G818–G828. [CrossRef]
88. Wanten, G.; Beunk, J.; Naber, A.; Swinkels, D. Tocopherol isoforms in parenteral lipid emulsions and neutrophil activation. *Clin. Nutr.* **2002**, *21*, 417–422. [CrossRef]
89. Soden, J.S.; Lovell, M.A.; Brown, K.; Partrick, D.A.; Sokol, R.J. Failure of Resolution of Portal Fibrosis during Omega-3 Fatty Acid Lipid Emulsion Therapy in Two Patients with Irreversible Intestinal Failure. *J. Pediatr.* **2010**, *156*, 327–331. [CrossRef]

90. Mercer, D.F.; Hobson, B.D.; Fischer, R.T.; Talmon, G.A.; Perry, D.A.; Gerhardt, B.K.; Grant, W.J.; Botha, J.F.; Langnas, A.N.; Quirós-Tejeira, R.E. Hepatic Fibrosis Persists and Progresses Despite Biochemical Improvement in Children Treated With Intravenous Fish Oil Emulsion. *J. Pediatr. Gastroenterol. Nutr.* **2013**, *56*, 364–369. [CrossRef]
91. Calkins, K.L.; Dunn, J.C.; Shew, S.B.; Reyen, L.; Farmer, D.G.; Devaskar, S.U.; Venick, R.S. Pediatric intestinal failure-associated liver disease is reversed with 6 months of intravenous fish oil. *JPEN J. Parenter. Enteral Nutr.* **2014**, *38*, 682–692. [CrossRef] [PubMed]
92. Nandivada, P.; Fell, G.L.; Mitchell, P.D.; Potemkin, A.K.; O'Loughlin, A.A.; Gura, K.M.; Puder, M. Long-Term Fish Oil Lipid Emulsion Use in Children With Intestinal Failure–Associated Liver Disease. *J. Parenter. Enter. Nutr.* **2016**, *41*, 930–937. [CrossRef] [PubMed]
93. Najm, S.; Löfqvist, C.; Hellgren, G.; Engström, E.; Lundgren, P.; Hård, A.-L.; Lapillonne, A.; Savman, K.; Nilsson, A.K.; Andersson, M.X.; et al. Effects of a lipid emulsion containing fish oil on polyunsaturated fatty acid profiles, growth and morbidities in extremely premature infants: A randomized controlled trial. *Clin. Nutr. ESPEN* **2017**, *20*, 17–23. [CrossRef] [PubMed]
94. Muhammed, R.; Bremner, R.; Protheroe, S.; Johnson, T.; Holden, C.; Murphy, M.S. Resolution of Parenteral Nutrition–associated Jaundice on Changing From a Soybean Oil Emulsion to a Complex Mixed-Lipid Emulsion. *J. Pediatr. Gastroenterol. Nutr.* **2012**, *54*, 797–802. [CrossRef] [PubMed]
95. Mundi, M.S.; Martindale, R.G.; Hurt, R.T. Emergence of Mixed-Oil Fat Emulsions for Use in Parenteral Nutrition. *J. Parenter. Enter. Nutr.* **2017**, *41*, 3S–13S. [CrossRef]

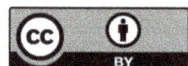

© 2020 by the authors. Licensee MDPI, Basel, Switzerland. This article is an open access article distributed under the terms and conditions of the Creative Commons Attribution (CC BY) license (http://creativecommons.org/licenses/by/4.0/).

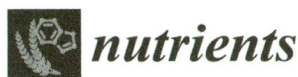 

*Review*

# Role of Nutrition in Prevention of Neonatal Spontaneous Intestinal Perforation and Its Complications: A Systematic Review

**Oluwabunmi Olaloye [1,2,†], Matthew Swatski [3,†] and Liza Konnikova [1,2,4,5,\*]**

1. Division of Newborn Medicine, University of Pittsburgh Medical Center Children's Hospital of Pittsburgh, Pittsburgh, PA 15224, USA; olaloyeoo@upmc.edu
2. Department of Pediatrics, Yale Medical School, New Haven, CT 06520, USA
3. School of Medicine, University of Pittsburgh, Pittsburgh, PA 15213, USA; swatski.matthew@medstudent.pitt.edu
4. Department of Immunology, University of Pittsburgh, Pittsburgh, PA 15213, USA
5. Department of Developmental Biology, University of Pittsburgh, Pittsburgh, PA 15213, USA
\* Correspondence: liza.konnikova@yale.edu; Tel.: +1-203-688-2896
† These authors contributed equally.

Received: 22 March 2020; Accepted: 28 April 2020; Published: 8 May 2020

**Abstract:** *Background*: Spontaneous intestinal perforation (SIP) is a devastating complication of prematurity, and extremely low birthweight (ELBW < 1000 g) infants born prior to 28 weeks are at highest risk. The role of nutrition and feeding practices in prevention and complications of SIP is unclear. The purpose of this review is to compile evidence to support early nutrition initiation in infants at risk for and after surgery for SIP. *Methods*: A search of PubMed, EMBASE and Medline was performed using relevant search terms according to Preferred Reporting Items for Systematic Reviews and Meta-Analyses (PRISMA) guidelines. Abstracts and full texts were reviewed by co-first authors. Studies with infants diagnosed with SIP that included information on nutrition/feeding practices prior to SIP and post-operatively were included. Primary outcome was time to first feed. Secondary outcomes were incidence of SIP, time to full enteral feeds, duration of parenteral nutrition, length of stay, neurodevelopmental outcomes and mortality. *Results*: Nineteen articles met inclusion criteria—nine studies included feeding/nutrition data prior to SIP and ten studies included data on post-operative nutrition. Two case series, one cohort study and sixteen historical control studies were included. Three studies showed reduced incidence of SIP with initiation of enteral nutrition in the first three days of life. Two studies showed reduced mortality and neurodevelopmental impairment in infants with early feeding. *Conclusions*: Available data suggest that early enteral nutrition in ELBW infants reduces incidence of SIP without increased mortality.

**Keywords:** spontaneous intestinal perforation; prematurity; feeding; nutrition

## 1. Introduction

Spontaneous intestinal perforation (SIP) is a devastating gastrointestinal complication of prematurity that occurs within the first week of life in infants born prior to 28 weeks of gestational age (GA) and with extremely low birthweight (ELBW < 1000 g) [1]. The incidence of SIP is highest in the most vulnerable preterm infants [2,3] with high frequency of long-term complications and high economic burden. Necrotizing enterocolitis (NEC), another gastrointestinal complication of prematurity that occurs slightly later, is a separate clinical entity. Both NEC and SIP can present with abdominal distension, temperature and hemodynamic instability [4,5]. NEC is distinguished by the presence of a thickened abdominal wall, distended loops and presence of pneumatosis intestinalis [5], while more patients with SIP present with a bluish discoloration of the abdominal wall and pneumoperitoneum on radiographs [5]. Infants with SIP typically present with isolated intestinal perforation diagnosed as free abdominal air [6,7] and on histology there is evidence of hemorrhagic necrosis primarily in the antimesenteric border of the terminal ileum [5]. On the contrary, NEC is characterized by severe inflammation and bacterial translocation resulting in intraluminal air and intestinal perforation in severe cases [8].

Currently, SIP is thought to be secondary to ischemia [9,10] and involves a deficiency of muscularis propria in about a quarter of cases [11]. SIP often occurs in the terminal ileum, a watershed region prone to local ischemia that can be compounded by regional intestinal ischemia, secondary to hypotension, the presence of an umbilical arterial catheter (UAC), patent ductus arteriosus (PDA) and birth asphyxia [9,12]. Local ischemia, impaired collagen synthesis from early steroid use, birth trauma and abnormal embryologic development can result in muscularis propria deficiency that can similarly lead to SIP [10,13,14]. Likewise, antenatal and postnatal factors (outlined in Table 1) can increase the risk of SIP occurrence in infants at greatest risk.

Table 1. Risk factors associated with increased incidence of SIP in preterm neonates.

| Prenatal | Postnatal |
| --- | --- |
| Maternal preeclampsia | Medications |
| Chorioaminoitis | -   Indomethacin |
| Syncytial knots | -   Inotropes |
| Multiple gestation | -   Early steroids |
| Cytomegalovirus | Fresh frozen plasma |
| In utero growth restriction | Intraventricular Hemorrhage |

An understanding of preventative strategies for developing SIP is critical as early complications such as intestinal failure [15] can be severe, resulting in a prolonged neonatal intensive care unit (NICU) stay and long-term complications [16–18]. Similarly, data on any protective factors that are crucial in SIP prevention are limited. While there is extensive data on the relationship between early nutrition and the incidence of NEC [19,20], studies on feeding practices prior to and after the development of SIP are limited. Given the high morbidity and mortality related to SIP, insight into risk factor modification, specifically nutrition, is essential. We sought to systematically identify and review literature on early feeding prior to and after surgery for SIP to assess safety and potential benefits.

## 2. Materials and Methods

This review was conducted according to the Preferred Reporting Items for Systematic Reviews and Meta-Analyses (PRISMA) guidelines.

### 2.1. Search Strategy

An electronic search of online databases—PubMed, Medlin and Embase—was conducted January to March 2020 using the following search terms: "spontaneous intestinal perforation," "neonate," "newborn" and "nutrition." Reference lists from resulting articles were also reviewed for additional studies.

### 2.2. Inclusion and Exclusion Criteria

Studies were included if pre- and post-operative characteristics of infants with SIP were provided, specifically if nutrition (enteral feeds prior to surgery and post-operative total parenteral nutrition (TPN)) data was recorded (Figure 1). Analysis of studies in languages other than English on non-human subjects and review articles were excluded. Case reports where no data on survival or length of hospital stay was reported were also excluded.

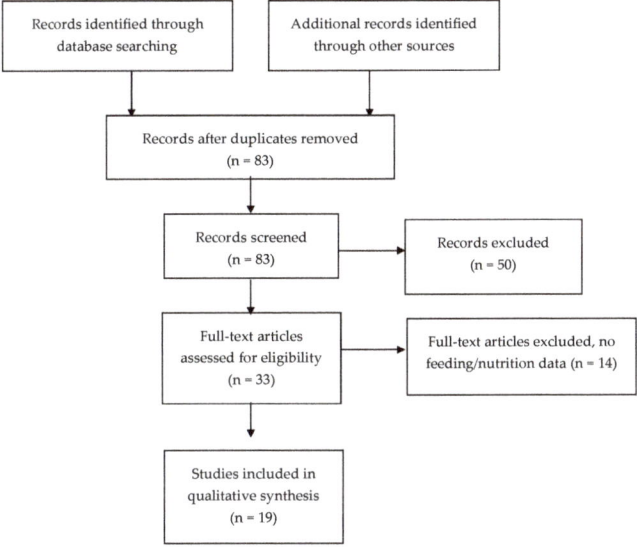

**Figure 1.** Flowchart of systematic review results.

*2.3. Study Selection*

All abstracts and titles identified using the search criteria were independently reviewed by the first two authors (O.O. and M.S.) and irrelevant studies were removed. The full text of relevant articles was reviewed by O.O. and M.S. for inclusion criteria until a consensus was reached. Screening reference lists was performed by O.O.

*2.4. Data Collection Process*

Selected articles were classified by study type and divided into two groups based on reporting of nutrition data prior to SIP (enteral nutrition) and post-operatively. Variables extracted included patient demographics/characteristics (gestational age, weight) and feeding characteristics (route, type of feeding, timing). Outcomes extracted included length of stay (LOS), time to full enteral nutrition, duration of TPN and mortality/survival as well as long-term neurodevelopmental outcomes when reported. For the meta-analysis, retrospective cohort studies that reported timing of early enteral nutrition as well as relative risk of outcomes were included.

## 3. Results

*3.1. Inclusio*

There were 33 full text articles that met criteria for full-text review. Of these, 14 were subsequently excluded because no information on enteral nutrition prior to SIP or TPN data post-operatively were reported. A total of 19 articles (Tables 2–4) were included in the analysis (Figure 1). Included articles are summarized according to category of nutritional data—studies with nutrition prior to SIP in Table 2; studies with data after surgery in Table 3; outcomes reported are outlined in Table 4. There were no randomized control trials (RCTs) in neonates examining the impact of early enteral nutrition on SIP progression and outcomes after surgery. However, 12 studies retrospective cohort studies (III-2), two studies with historical controls (III-3) and one case series [9] were included (Tables 2 and 3).

Table 2. Studies with documentation on feeding regimen prior to spontaneous intestinal perforation (SIP) diagnosis.

| Authors | Institution(s), Country | Type of Study | Patients in Study (n) | Patients with SIP (n) | Mean GA (wks) | Feeding Regimen Prior to SIP | Comments |
|---|---|---|---|---|---|---|---|
| Buchheit [4] | University of Louisville, United States | R | 42 | 21 | 29 | Unknown | 38% enteral feedings in the SIP, 86% in the NEC group ($p < 0.005$). |
| Kelleher [21] | Neonatal Research Network, United States | R | 15751 | 652 | | Total Parenteral Nutrition ± Enteral Feeding | |
| Holland [11] | The Royal Alexandria Hospital for Children Australia | R | 23 | 23 | 27 | Enteral Formula Feeds | 6 (26%) of the 23 patients received enteral feeds prior to development of SIP |
| Kawase [22] | Toho University Perinatal Center, Japan | R | 556 | 10 | 26.3 | Unknown | |
| Maas [23] | Tübingen University Children's Hospital, Germany | R | 77 | 9 | 26.7 | Enteral feeds were initiated at 20 mL/kg/day of preterm formula on day 1. | Rates of NEC were low, whereas that of SIP was rather high at 9.4%. |
| Meyer [9] | Minneapolis Children's Medical Center, United States | C | 250 | 7 | | No enteral nutrition | |
| Shah, J [3] | The Canadian Neonatal Network, Canada | R | 17426 | 178 | | Unknown | |
| Stavel [24] | The Canadian Neonatal Network, Canada | R | 4268 | 129 | SIP: 25 All: 34 | DOL 0–2 | |
| Varma [25] | Johns Hopkins University School of Medicine, United States | R | 111 | 18 | | | SIP (n = 18) Age at First Feed: 4 d. Mother's Milk: 14 (78%) Donor's Milk: 2 (11%) Cow's Milk: 1 (6%) Hydrolysate: 0 Amino Acid: 0 Unknown: 1 (6%) |
| **Total:** | | | 38504 | 1047 | | | |

R—retrospective chart review, C—case report, wks—weeks, GA—gestational age.

**Table 3.** Studies with documentation on post-operative nutrition in SIP patients.

| Authors | Institution(s) Country | Type of Study | Patients in Study (n) | Patients with SIP (n) | GA (wks) | TPN Duration (after SIP) | Time to EN (Days) | Time to Full EN (Days) |
|---|---|---|---|---|---|---|---|---|
| Vongbhavit [26] | University of California at Davis, United States | R | 60 | 30 | PNAC: 25.5 Without PNAC: 25.9 | Omegavan after 4 wks. w/DB > 2 mg/dL | PNAC: 20 Without PNAC: 10 | PNAC: 46 Without PNAC: 25 |
| Cass [27] | Texas Children's Hospital, United States | R | 21 | 10 | SIP: 25.5 NEC: 27.5 | Unknown | SIP: 26.3 NEC: 73.5 | SIP: 41.6 NEC: 98 |
| Chiu [28] | Children's Memorial Hospital, United States | R | 46 | 15 | SIP: 26.7 NEC: 28.4 | SIP: 24 NEC: 46 | SIP: 16 NEC: 21 | Unknown |
| Eicher [29] | Tübingen University Children's Hospital in Tübingen, Germany | R | 280 | 19 | 25 | SIP: 21.0 | SIP: 6 | SIP: 15 |
| Gollin [30] | Loma Linda University Children's Hospital, United States | R | 29 | 29 | 25.0 ± 1.5 | 68.8 | Unknown | 68.8 |
| Jakaitis [31] | Children's Healthcare of Atlanta at Egleston, United States | R | 89 | 89 | PD:25.1 PD + Lap: 25.8 | PD: 62.7 PD + Lap: 94.3 | PD: 20.1 PD + Lap: 26.1 | PD: 60.4 PD + Lap: 25.9 |
| Karila [16] | University of Helsinki Children's Hospital and University of Tampere Children's Hospital, Finland | R | 225 | 83 | 27 | Unknown | Unknown | Unknown |
| Kelleher [21] | Neonatal Research Network, United States | R | 15751 | 652 | I+E+: 26 I+E−: 25 I−E+: 27 I−E−: 26 | I+E+: 19 I+E−: 28.5 I−E+: 17 I−E−: 29 | Unknown | I+E+: 19 I+E−: 27 I−E+: 16 I−E−: 26 |
| Shah B [32] | Women & Infants Hospital of Rhode Island, United States | CC | 53 | 13 | SIP: 25.8 NEC: 27.1 Control: 29.5 | SIP: 76 NEC: 46 Control: 27 | SIP: 10 NEC: 6 Control: 3 | Unknown |
| Varma [25] | Johns Hopkins University School of Medicine, United States | R | 111 | 18 | SIP: 25 All: 34 | SIP: 33.5 All: 51.5 | SIP: 12.5 All: 12.5 | Unknown |
| Wadhawan [33] | Neonatal Research Network, United States | R | 11960 | 280 | SIP: 26.3 No SIP: 26.9 | SIP: 28.1 No SIP: 49.6 | SIP: 14.7 No SIP: 7.3 | Unknown |
| Total: | | | 28625 | 1238 | | | | |

R—retrospective chart review, C—case report, CC—case control, wks—weeks, d—days, S.D.—standard deviation.

Table 4. Outcomes of studies that document feeding regimens prior to SIP diagnosis and those that document post-operative nutrition in SIP patients.

| Authors | | LOS (Days) | Enteral Feeds Prior to Perforation (Days) | Time to Begin Enteral Feeds (Days) | Time to Full Enteral Feeds (Days) | Length of TPN (Days) | Mortality | Risk of Bias |
|---|---|---|---|---|---|---|---|---|
| Buchheit [4] | SIP | 82 | 8 | X | X | X | 5/21 (24%) | Low |
| | NEC | 107 | 18 | X | X | X | 12/21 (57%) | |
| Cass [27] | SIP | X | 3/10 (30%) * | 26.3 * | 41.6 * | X | 1/10 (10%) * | Low |
| | NEC | X | 10/11 (91%) | 73.5 | 98 | X | 8/11 (73%) | |
| Chiu [28] | SIP | X | 5/13 (38%) * | 16 * | X | 24 * | 15% * | Low |
| | NEC | X | 17/20 (85%) | 21 | X | 46 | 45% | |
| Eicher [29] | SIP | 128 | X | 6 | 15 | 21.0 * | 3/19 (16%) | Low |
| | NEC | 121 | X | 8 | 18 | 34.5 * | 2/9 (22%) | |
| Gollin [30] | SIP & NEC | 111 | 10/29 (34%) | X | 68.8 | 68.8 | 38% | Low |
| Holland [11] | SIP | X | 7/23 (30%) | X | X | X | 26% | Moderate (convenience sample) |
| Jakaitis [31] | PD | 120.3 | 36/67 (53.7%) | 20.1 * | 60.4 * | 62.7 * | 18% | Moderate (criteria for groups unclear) |
| | PD + LAP | 144.5 | 10/22 (45.5%) | 26.1 * | 95.5 * | 94.3 * | 5% | |
| Karila [16] | SIP | X | X | X | X | 25 | 23% | Low |
| | NEC | X | X | X | X | 27 | 27% | |
| Kawase [22] | Perf. | X | X | X | X | X | 82/541 (15.2%) | Moderate (definition for groups unclear) |
| Kelleher [21] | I+E+ | X | DOL 0-3 | X | 19 ˆ | 19 ˆ | 146/1185 (12%) | Low |
| | I+E- | X | X | X | 27 | 28.5 | 742/4674 (16%) | |
| | I-E+ | X | DOL 0-3 | X | 16 ˆ | 17 ˆ | 287/3119 (9%) | |
| | I-E- | X | X | X | 26 | 29 | 1037/6714 (16%) | |
| Maas [23] | ELGANs | 90 | 96/96 (100%) | X | 7 | 7 | 24% | Low |
| Meyer [9] | SIP | X | X | X | X | X | 3/7 (43%) | Low |
| Pumberger [5] | SIP | X | 13/13 (100%) | X | X | X | X | Low |
| | NEC | X | 16/16 (100%) | X | X | X | X | |
| B. Shah [32] | SIP | 110 | 100% | 10 * | X | 76 * | 1/13 (8%) | Low |
| | NEC | 98 | 100% | 6 * | X | 46 * | 1/14 (7%) | |
| | Control | 94 | 100% | 3 | X | 27 | 2/26 (8%) | |
| J. Shah [3] | SIP | X | X | X | X | X | 44/178 (24.7%) | Low |
| | NEC perf. | X | X | X | X | X | 124/246 (50.4%) | |
| | NEC no perf. | X | X | X | X | X | 101/538 (18.8%) | |
| | No NEC/perf. | X | X | X | X | X | 902/16464 (5.5%) | |

Table 4. Cont.

| Authors | | LOS (Days) | Enteral Feeds Prior to Perforation (Days) | Time to Begin Enteral Feeds (Days) | Time to Full Enteral Feeds (Days) | Length of TPN (Days) | Mortality | Risk of Bias |
|---|---|---|---|---|---|---|---|---|
| Vongbhavit [26] | PNAC | 123 * | X | 20 * | 46 * | 82 * | 4/17 (24%) | Low |
| | w/o PNAC | 77 * | X | 10 * | 25 * | 32 * | 14/43 (33%) | |
| Stavel [24] | I+E+ | 80 ^ | DOL 0-2 | X | 23 ^ | 18 ^ | 35/285 (12.3%) | Low |
| | I+E− | 99 ^ | X | X | 35 ^ | 28 ^ | 39/213 (18.3%) | |
| | I−E− | 86 ^ | X | X | 29 ^ | 26 ^ | 223/1941 (11.5%) | |
| | I−E+ | 74 | DOL 0-2 | X | 21 | 18 | 201/1829 (11.0%) | |
| Varma [25] | SIP | 119.5 * | 100% | 12.5 * | 17/18 (94%) | 51.5 * | X | Low |
| | All | 63 | 100% | 10 | 103/111 (93%) | 33.5 * | X | |
| Wadhawan [33] | SIP | X | X | 14.7 * | X | 48.1 * | 198/249 (79.5%)* 5568/9987 (55.8%)* (NDI & Death) | Low |
| | No SIP | X | X | 7.4 * | X | 29.6 * | | |

X: no available data, I: indomethacin, E: early feeding * $p < 0.05$, ^ $p < 0.05$ compared to reference group (I−/E−).

*3.2. Risk of Bias*

Most of the studies were retrospective cohort studies conducted at single centers, including Buchheit [4], Eicher [29], and Gollin [30] who reported characteristics and outcomes in infants with SIP and NEC. This study design has an inherent risk of selection bias, and inherent differences between the pathogenesis and complications associated with NEC can skew results, especially given the retrospective nature of these studies. Additionally, only two studies by Stavel et al. [24] and J Shah [3] et al. included data on control infants without NEC or SIP. There is a risk of detection bias as it is not possible to blind outcomes in these studies.

Data from the case series by Meyer et al. [9] was confounded by potential information and reporting bias given the retrospective nature and lack of a control group.

*3.3. Grouping According to Nutrition Data*

Articles fell broadly into three groups: studies that included feeding or nutrition data prior to SIP diagnosis [4,5,9,11,22–24], studies with data post-operative nutrition [3,16,21,26,29–33] and studies that listed any outcomes of interest (LOS, time to full feeds, length of TPN, mortality, neurodevelopmental outcomes; Table 4).

Data on timing, type and volume of feeding prior to SIP was limited. In the study by Meyer et al. [9], no patients with SIP had been fed prior to disease onset. Two studies documented the proportion of patients receiving enteral nutrition (EN) before SIP: Buchheit [4] reported 38% (8/21) and Holland [11] 23% (6/23). Maas et al. [23] reported a rate of SIP of 9.4% after implementation of a feeding protocol for early transition to full EN. The only study evaluating the direct impact of early EN (within 72 h of life) on SIP was by Stavel et al. [24]. A total of eight additional studies [16,21,26,29–33] reported TPN data after surgery for SIP.

*3.4. Outcomes*

3.4.1. Early Enteral Nutrition (EEN)

Varma [25] retrospectively reviewed the use of breast milk in infants who had surgery prior to six months of age. Eighteen out of 111 infants required surgery for SIP and 16/18 (89%) received human milk, and the median age at first feed was four (IQR 3–8) days. Maas et al. [23] described the feasibility of an EEN protocol in extremely low gestational age neonates (ELGANs, <28 weeks) with the initiation of 20 mL/kg/day of preterm formula or human milk within 24 h of life and advances of 25–30 mL/kg/day. Forty-three out of 96 (50%) infants received full EN by seven days of life. SIP was reported in 9/96 (9.4%) of infants. No data on timing of SIP was noted. While the incidence of SIP is comparable to similar European centers (8.2% by Bassler [34]), Maas did not report rates of SIP at their institution prior to initiation of this protocol. The study was not designed to evaluate the EEN as a protective factor for SIP but suggests that an EEN protocol is feasible in ELGANs.

Stavel [24] from the Canadian Neonatal Network (CNN, tertiary NICUs) published a retrospective cohort study of 4268 ELBW infants born prior to 30 weeks evaluating the effect of exposure to prophylactic indomethacin and early feeding on the incidence of SIP [24]. EEN was initiated within the first two days [24]. There was a notable—although not significant—reduction in the incidence of SIP in the early feeding group (EF+, 54/2114, 2.5%) compared to the no EF group (EF-, 75/2154, 3.5%) with an adjusted odds ratio (aOR 1.32, 95% CI [0.88–1.99]) of SIP in the EF- group. However, there was no documentation about volume or type of EN provided. Kelleher from the Neonatal Research Network (NRN) performed a similar retrospective study of over 15,000 ELBW infants [21]. They reported data on four groups based on exposure to indomethacin (I+/−) and early feeding (first two days, E+/−). A significant reduction in relative risk (%, aRR [95%CI]) of SIP in the first 14 days of life was documented in the E+ groups (I+/E+: 3%, 0.58 [0.37–0.90] $p < 0.05$, I−/E+ 1%, 0.53 [0.36–0.77], $p < 0.0001$) compared to the reference group (I−/E−: 3%). Overall, when these studies were combined there was a significant reduction in relative risk of SIP in infants receiving early enteral nutrition (0.58 [0.38–0.88], $p = 0.01$, Figure 2A). Therefore, early enteral nutrition reduces the incidence of SIP in ELBW infants.

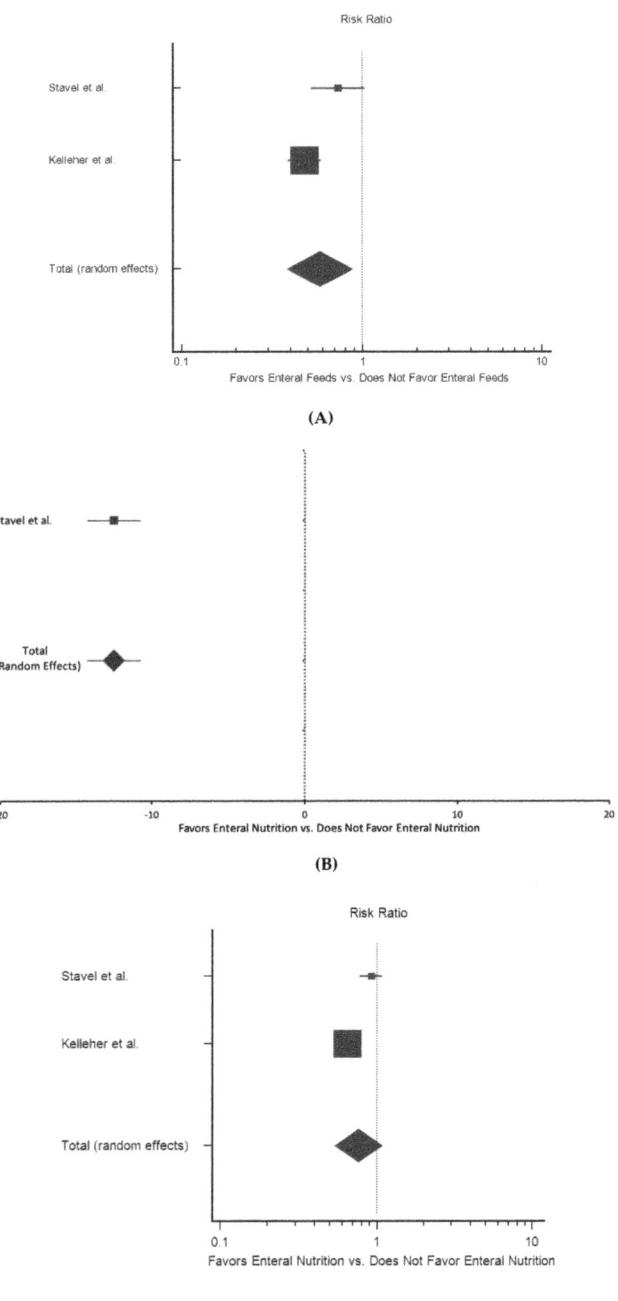

**Figure 2.** Relative risk and outcomes reported in selected studies. (**A**) Early Nutrition and SIP Incidence; (**B**) Early Nutrition and LOS; (**C**) Early Nutrition and overall mortality.

3.4.2. Time to Full Enteral Feeds after SIP

Eicher [29], Jakaitis [31], B Shah [32], Vongbhavit [26], Varma [25], Cass [27] and Wadhawan [33] reported time to initiation of EN (range from 6 to 21 days) and time to full EN (range from 15 to 95.5 days) after SIP (Table 3). Varma [25] reported days to first post-operative feed (median 12.5, IQR (10–20)) and the majority of SIP infants received human milk (16/18, 88%) and bolus feeding (15/18, 83%). Cass [27] reported shorter time from peritoneal drain (PD) placement to feeding initiation in infants with SIP (26.3 ± 9.9 days) compared to infants with NEC (73.5 ± 3.5 d $p < 0.05$). Eicher [29] reported the shortest time to initiation of EN with mean of six (range 4–9) days and full EN mean of 15 days after surgery. On the contrary, Jakaitis [31] documented the longest time to initiation of EN (20.1 days in peritoneal drain (PD) only, 26.1 days in PD and laparotomy (LAP) group, $p < 0.05$) and full EN (60.4 days in PD, 95.5 days in PD + LAP, $p < 0.05$). No defined protocol for initiation and advancement was described in either study. Vongbhavit [26] noted that differences in delay in initiation of post-operative EN increased the risk of parenteral nutrition-associated cholestasis (PNAC), defined as a conjugated bilirubin ≥ 2 mg/dL. Initiation of EN and full EN was shorter in SIP infants without PNAC (10 days, 25 days) compared to those with PNAC (20 days, 46 days $p < 0.05$). Institutional differences and type of surgery as reported by [31] resulted in variations in timing of EN. However, delay in initiation of EN increased the risk of PNAC.

3.4.3. Parenteral Nutrition Duration

Current management of SIP involves surgery (or drain placement), cessation of feeds, and a course of antibiotics [27,35]. Nutrition during recovery is exclusively provided by total parenteral nutrition (TPN), similar to infants being treated for NEC [36]. The most prevalent risk associated with prolonged TPN exposure is cholestasis [37]. Eleven studies ([21,24–26,28–32,36,38] Table 3) reported data on duration of TPN after surgery with a range in SIP patients of (21–94.3 days). TPN duration was shortest in Eicher [29], with an average of 21 days in infants with SIP likely due to early initiation of EN by six days post-op. Jakaitis [31] reported the longest duration of TPN use in the PD only (62.7 days) and PD + LAP group (94.3 days). This suggests that earlier initiation of EN appears to correlate with shorter duration of TPN. Stavel [24] evaluated the role of early indomethacin (I) and early feeding (E) on TPN duration. Number of days of TPN was shorter in both EN groups (I+/E+, mean(range): 18 (12–32) and I−/E+ 18 (12–29)) compared to no EN (I+/E− 28 (19–40, $p < 0.01$) and I−/E− 26 (16–39, $p < 0.01$)). EN initiated within the first two days of life decreased the duration of TPN in ELBW infants <30 weeks [24].

3.4.4. Length of Stay

Eight studies [4,24–26,29–32] documented length of stay (LOS) in SIP and controls with a range from 72 days in I−/E+ group in the Stavel [24] study to 144.5 days in the PD + LAP group in the Jakaitis [31] study. In those studies where data on both NEC and SIP was available, no significant differences in LOS were noted in Buchheit [4] (82 days vs. 107 days), Eicher [29] (128 days vs. 121 days) and B Shah [32] (110 days vs. 98 days) in patients with SIP compared to NEC. Jakaitis [31] reported longest LOS with no significant differences between the two surgical options available, PD and PD + LAP (120.3 days vs 144.5 days). In Vongbhavit [26], patients without PNAC had significantly shorter LOS compared to the PNAC group (77 days vs. 123 days $p < 0.05$) likely due to earlier EN and shorter TPN duration. Stavel [24] reported shorter median (IQR) LOS in early feeding groups (I+/E+, 80 (50,118), I−/E+ 74 (45, 103)) when compared to no early feeding groups (I+/E− 99 (66, 124), I−/E− 86 (55, 112), Figure 2B) for all infants in the study. Data on the impact of EN on LOS in infants with SIP was not reported.

3.4.5. Neurodevelopmental Outcomes

Wadhawan et al. [33] retrospectively identified ELBW infants with SIP in the Neonatal Research Network database (1998–2005) and is the only study that reported neurodevelopmental impairment (NDI) in patients with SIP. NDI among survivors was defined as at least one of the following: cerebral palsy, bilateral blindness, bilateral deafness, Bayley Mental Developmental Index (MDI) or Psychomotor Development Index (PDI) less than 70 [33] at 18–22 months. Overall NDI among survivors was higher in SIP infants compared to no SIP (86/137 (62.8%) vs. 2614/7033 (37.2%) $p < 0.0001$). Similarly, MDI < 70 (72/134 (53.7%) vs. 2177/6953 (31.3%) $p < 0.0001$), PDI < 70 (65/133 (48.9%) vs. 1476/6892 (21.4%) $p < 0.0001$), and cerebral palsy (24/140 (17.1%) vs. 486/7418 (6.6%) $p < 0.0001$) were higher in infants with SIP [33]. However, these findings could be confounded by the increased incidence of severe IVH (grade 3 or 4) in patients with SIP (95/277 (34.3%) vs. 1942/11233 (17.3%) $p < 0.05$). The authors of the study did not perform a regression analysis that adjusted for potential confounders. Additionally, while age at first feeds was significantly later in infants with SIP (14.7 ± 15.1 vs. 7.4 ± 6.8 $p < 0.05$) no comparisons between feeding and outcomes were documented [33].

Kelleher [21] reported severe NDI at 18–22 months in four groups based on exposure to indomethacin (I+/−) and early (first two days) feeding (E+/−), with a significant reduction in severe NDI in E+ groups (I+/E+ %, aRR [95% CI] 25%, 0.72 [0.61-0.83], $p < 0.0001$, I−/E+ 20%, 0.76 [0.68–0.84], $p < 0.0001$) compared to the reference group I−/E− (34%) [33]. The median days (IQR) to full EN was also significantly shorter in the E+ groups (I+/E+: 19 (14,29) $p < 0.001$, I−/E+ 16 (11,25) $p < 0.001$) compared to the reference group (I−/E− 26 (18,38)) [21]. This suggests a protective effect of early nutrition on improved neurodevelopmental outcomes overall in ELBW infants; it is possible that this is similarly protective in infants with SIP.

3.4.6. Mortality

Mortality alone or in combination with NDI was reported in 17 studies (Table 4) [3,4,9,11,16,21,22,24,26,29–32] with a range of 8%–32% in infants with SIP. Shah [3] reported an almost three-fold increased mortality in infants with SIP compared to infants without NEC or SIP (aOR 2.78, 95% CI [1.8, 4.28] $p < 0.05$). Wadhawan [33] reported a significant and large increase in NDI or death in infants with SIP compared to ELBW infants without SIP (198/249 (79.5%) vs. 5568/9987 (55.8%) $p < 0.001$).

However, mortality in ELBW infants is dependent on numerous factors, some of which can be modified by early enteral nutrition. Stavel et al. [24] and Kelleher [21] reported overall mortality in four groups based on one's exposure to indomethacin (I) and/or early feeding (E) (Figure 2C). Stavel [24] noted a reduction in the overall mortality in the early feeding group (236/2114 (11.2%)) compared to the late feeding group (262/2154 (12.2%)) with an adjusted OR of 0.89 (95% CI [0.71, 1.12]). Although the reduction in mortality was not statistically significant, it suggests a possible protective effect of early enteral nutrition. In the Kelleher [21] study, there was a large and significant relative risk (RR) reduction in either death or NDI in the early feeding groups (I+/E+: 37%, aRR 0.83, 95% CI [0.75–0.91] $p < 0.001$, I−/E+: 31%, aRR 0.82, 95% CI [0.76–0.89], $p < 0.0001$) compared to the reference group (I−/E−: 48%). Overall, when these studies were combined, early enteral nutrition was not associated with increased mortality but rather has a trend towards decreased mortality (RR [95% CI], 0.764 [0.54–1.08], $p = 0.13$, Figure 2B). Thus, early feeding in the presence or absence of indomethacin is not associated with increased mortality.

3.5. Other Complications

Shah [3] reported an increase (aOR) in major morbidity: bronchopulmonary dysplasia (2.78, 95% CI [1.93–4.20] $p < 0.05$), periventricular leukomalacia (1.62, 95% CI [0.85–3.07] NS), severe retinopathy of prematurity (3.14, 95% CI [1.88–5.2])) and nosocomial infections (3.54, 95% CI [2.54, 4.94] $p < 0.05$)) in infants with SIP vs. those without NEC or SIP (OR 4.23, 95% CI [2.88, 6.20], $p < 0.05$). No other studies reported on risk of short- and long-term complications relative to early nutrition or occurrence of SIP.

## 4. Discussion

Although there are no randomized trials evaluating early nutrition in decreasing rates of SIP or SIP associated morbidities, the available data summarized in this review suggest that initiation of early enteral nutrition in ELBW infants decreases the incidence of SIP, duration of total parenteral nutrition, risk of parenteral nutrition-associated cholestasis and length of stay, all without being associated with increased mortality. Furthermore, evidence from a large cohort [21] suggests that ELBW infants receiving early enteral nutrition (with or without prophylactic indomethacin) have a lower incidence of neurodevelopmental impairment and mortality. Moreover, the overall growth improved in ELGANs who were fed using an early enteral nutrition protocol [23]. Consistent with existing data, introduction of early enteral nutrition using a standardized protocol has been associated with improved weight gain [39] and reduced incidence of NEC [40] and death.

There were limited data on initiating early enteral nutrition post-operatively in SIP patients, so optimal timing for initiation and impact of post-operative EEN remains unclear. However, data from a systematic review in pediatric patients (including neonates) undergoing abdominal surgery suggests that introduction of EEN post-operatively resulted in a significant decrease in time to full EN with a trend towards reduced LOS and no increase in complications [41].

Timing and type of enteral nutrition provided after birth in neonates impacts intestinal health and immune function [42]. After delivery, enteral nutrition is crucial for intestinal adaptation, and lack of luminal nutrients can impede appropriate intestinal development (as reviewed in [42]). Enteral nutrition components that promote intestinal health include: (1) arginine, which improves structure and function, (2) glutamine for increased protein synthesis, (3) threonine, which promotes mucin synthesis, and (4) polyunsaturated fatty acids that enrich enterocyte phospholipids [42,43] (Figure 3). Early bovine colostrum feeds in animal models resulted in higher first-pass threonine utilization, increased protein synthesis and mucosal growth in the distal small intestine [43], as well as improved immune and digestive functions [44]. Similarly, in neonates who received human milk in the first 24 h of life, Shimizu et al. [45] reported an increase in plasma concentration of glicentin (a component of enteroglucagon that promotes mucin secretion and improved intestinal growth compared to delayed enteral nutrition). Human milk, specifically colostrum, is considered optimal enteral nutrition in preterm neonates as it results in decreased inflammatory response [46], stimulates neutrophil recruitment [44], selectively targets T cells and granulocyte [47], and resulted in reduction of SIP incidence (6% to 3%) in a small, single center study [48]. This suggests that in the absence of early enteral nutrition (as reported in [21,24]) there is likely reduced protein synthesis, decreased mucin production, impaired enterocyte phospholipids, inadequate mucosal growth and a predisposition to intestinal injury and subsequent SIP development.

Currently, clinical studies do not provide adequate information on the timing or type of post-operative enteral nutrition in infants with SIP. However, in neonates who required surgery for congenital anomalies, post-operative early enteral nutrition resulted in decreased time to full enteral nutrition and a trend towards decreased hospital stays without increased complications [49–51]. Furthermore, post-operative implementation of a human milk-based feeding protocol resulted in reduced time to full feed and decreased incidence of intestinal failure-associated liver disease [52]. In animal models, post-operative early enteral nutrition resulted in improved healing [53], likely through conservation of collagen [54] and improved weight gain. It is possible that early initiation of enteral feeds after surgery in SIP patients is similarly beneficial, however additional studies are needed.

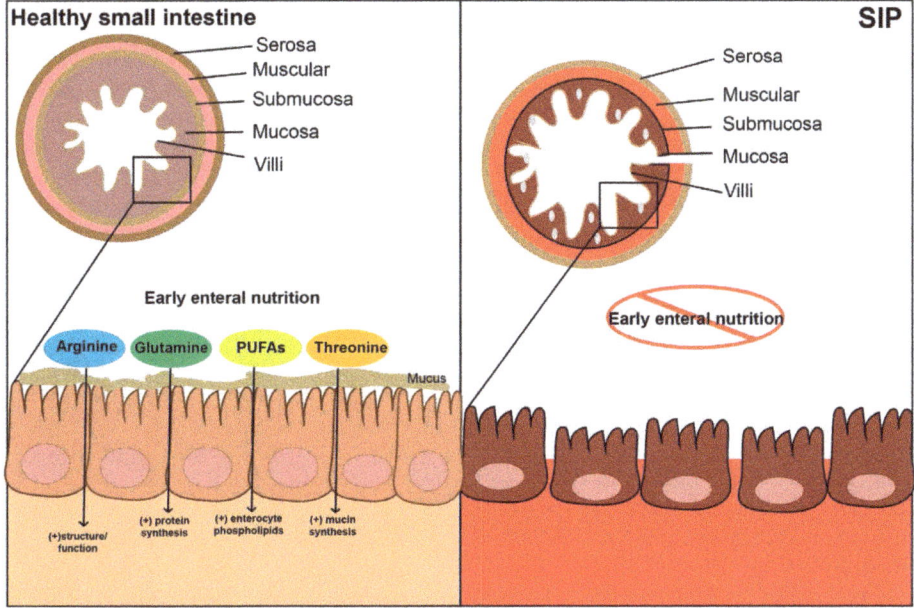

**Figure 3.** Relationship of early enteral nutrition to SIP. Early enteral nutrition provides arginine, threonine, glutamine and polyunsaturated fats (PUFAs) that result in improved gut structure/function, mucin synthesis and production of enterocyte phospholipids. Delayed enteral nutrition results in increased SIP susceptibility.

## 5. Future Directions

Data from existing clinical studies show that early enteral nutrition in ELBW infants is feasible and beneficial. In the future, larger scale, multicenter studies dedicated specifically to patients with SIP evaluating the time to first feed, type of feeds (breast milk/formula) and feeding advancement schedules would be beneficial. In post-operative SIP cases, information regarding timing of first feeds as it relates to short-term outcomes (duration of hospital stay [44], parenteral nutrition dependence) and long-term outcomes (gastrointestinal complications, growth and neurodevelopment) would be important to collect. These data would inform us on best nutritional practices to reduce the incidence and severity of SIP.

## 6. Conclusions

The retrospective nature of studies that include the pre- and post-operative feeding and nutrition regimen of infants with SIP present a challenge in delineating the role of nutrition in disease prevention and improvement of outcomes. There is some evidence to suggest that initiation of feeds within the first 72 h in infants at the highest risk of SIP (ELBW, <28 weeks GA) could be protective. The potentially protective role of early feeding has been shown in both small and large retrospective studies [23,24,55,56].

**Author Contributions:** Conceptualization O.O. and L.K.; data curation, O.O. and M.S.; writing—original draft preparation, O.O. and M.S. writing—review and editing, O.O., M.S., L.K. All authors have read and agreed to the published version of the manuscript.

**Funding:** This research received no external funding.

**Conflicts of Interest:** The authors declare no conflict of interest.

## References

1. Gordon, P.V. Understanding intestinal vulnerability to perforation in the extremely low birth weight infant. *Pediatr. Res.* **2009**, *65*, 138–144. [CrossRef] [PubMed]
2. Singh, R.; Shah, B.; Allred, E.N.; Grzybowski, M.; Martin, C.R.; Leviton, A. ELGAN Study co-investigators The antecedents and correlates of necrotizing enterocolitis and spontaneous intestinal perforation among infants born before the 28th week of gestation. *J. Neonatal. Perinatal. Med.* **2016**, *9*, 159–170. [CrossRef] [PubMed]
3. Shah, J.; Singhal, N.; da Silva, O.; Rouvinez-Bouali, N.; Seshia, M.; Lee, S.K.; Shah, P.S. Canadian Neonatal Network Intestinal perforation in very preterm neonates: Risk factors and outcomes. *J. Perinatol.* **2015**, *35*, 595–600. [CrossRef] [PubMed]
4. Buchheit, J.Q.; Stewart, D.L. Clinical comparison of localized intestinal perforation and necrotizing enterocolitis in neonates. *Pediatrics* **1994**, *93*, 32–36. [PubMed]
5. Pumberger, W.; Mayr, M.; Kohlhauser, C.; Weninger, M. Spontaneous localized intestinal perforation in very-low-birth-weight infants: A distinct clinical entity different from necrotizing enterocolitis. *J. Am. Coll. Surg.* **2002**, *195*, 796–803. [CrossRef]
6. Kubota, A.; Yamanaka, H.; Okuyama, H.; Shiraishi, J.; Kawahara, H.; Hasegawa, T.; Ueno, T.; Kitajima, H.; Kuwae, Y.; Nakayama, M. Focal intestinal perforation in extremely-low-birth-weight neonates: Etiological consideration from histological findings. *Pediatr. Surg. Int.* **2007**, *23*, 997–1000. [CrossRef]
7. Okuyama, H.; Kubota, A.; Oue, T.; Kuroda, S.; Ikegami, R.; Kamiyama, M. A comparison of the clinical presentation and outcome of focal intestinal perforation and necrotizing enterocolitis in very-low-birth-weight neonates. *Pediatr. Surg. Int.* **2002**, *18*, 704–706. [CrossRef]
8. Chen, A.-C.; Chung, M.-Y.; Chang, J.H.; Lin, H.-C. Pathogenesis implication for necrotizing enterocolitis prevention in preterm very-low-birth-weight infants. *J. Pediatr. Gastroenterol. Nutr.* **2014**, *58*, 7–11. [CrossRef]
9. Meyer, C.L.; Payne, N.R.; Roback, S.A. Spontaneous, isolated intestinal perforations in neonates with birth weight less than 1,000 g not associated with necrotizing enterocolitis. *J. Pediatr. Surg.* **1991**, *26*, 714–717. [CrossRef]
10. Aschner, J.L.; Deluga, K.S.; Metlay, L.A.; Emmens, R.W.; Hendricks-Munoz, K.D. Spontaneous focal gastrointestinal perforation in very low birth weight infants. *J. Pediatr.* **1988**, *113*, 364–367. [CrossRef]
11. Holland, A.J.A.; Shun, A.; Martin, H.C.O.; Cooke-Yarborough, C.; Holland, J. Small bowel perforation in the premature neonate: Congenital or acquired? *Pediatr. Surg. Int.* **2003**, *19*, 489–494. [CrossRef] [PubMed]
12. Spadone, D.; Clark, F.; James, E.; Laster, J.; Hoch, J.; Silver, D. Heparin-induced thrombocytopenia in the newborn. *J. Vasc. Surg.* **1992**, *15*, 306–311; discussion 311. [CrossRef]
13. Gordon, P.; Rutledge, J.; Sawin, R.; Thomas, S.; Woodrum, D. Early postnatal dexamethasone increases the risk of focal small bowel perforation in extremely low birth weight infants. *J. Perinatol.* **1999**, *19*, 573–577. [CrossRef]
14. Alawadhi, A.; Chou, S.; Carpenter, B. Segmental agenesis of intestinal muscularis: A case report. *J. Pediatr. Surg.* **1989**, *24*, 1089–1090. [CrossRef]
15. Houben, C.H.; Feng, X.-N.; Chan, K.W.E.; Mou, J.W.C.; Tam, Y.H.; Lee, K.H. Spontaneous Intestinal Perforation: The Long-Term Outcome. *Eur. J. Pediatr. Surg.* **2017**, *27*, 346–351. [CrossRef] [PubMed]
16. Karila, K.; Anttila, A.; Iber, T.; Pakarinen, M.; Koivusalo, A. Outcomes of surgery for necrotizing enterocolitis and spontaneous intestinal perforation in Finland during 1986-2014. *J. Pediatr. Surg.* **2018**, *53*, 1928–1932. [CrossRef]
17. Berry, M.J.; Port, L.J.; Gately, C.; Stringer, M.D. Outcomes of infants born at 23 and 24 weeks' gestation with gut perforation. *J. Pediatr. Surg.* **2019**, *54*, 2092–2098. [CrossRef]
18. Shin, S.H.; Kim, E.-K.; Yoo, H.; Choi, Y.H.; Kim, S.; Lee, B.K.; Jung, Y.H.; Kim, H.-Y.; Kim, H.-S.; Choi, J.-H. Surgical Necrotizing Enterocolitis versus Spontaneous Intestinal Perforation in White Matter Injury on Brain Magnetic Resonance Imaging. *Neonatology* **2016**, *110*, 148–154. [CrossRef]
19. Cacho, N.T.; Parker, L.A.; Neu, J. Necrotizing enterocolitis and human milk feeding: A systematic review. *Clin. Perinatol.* **2017**, *44*, 49–67. [CrossRef]
20. Wang, K.; Tao, G.; Sylvester, K.G. Recent advances in prevention and therapies for clinical or experimental necrotizing enterocolitis. *Dig. Dis. Sci.* **2019**, 1–8. [CrossRef]

21. Kelleher, J.; Salas, A.A.; Bhat, R.; Ambalavanan, N.; Saha, S.; Stoll, B.J.; Bell, E.F.; Walsh, M.C.; Laptook, A.R.; Sánchez, P.J.; et al. GDB Subcommittee, Eunice Kennedy Shriver National Institute of Child Health and Human Development Neonatal Research Network Prophylactic indomethacin and intestinal perforation in extremely low birth weight infants. *Pediatrics* **2014**, *134*, e1369–e1377. [CrossRef] [PubMed]
22. Kawase, Y.; Ishii, T.; Arai, H.; Uga, N. Gastrointestinal perforation in very low-birthweight infants. *Pediatr. Int.* **2006**, *48*, 599–603. [CrossRef]
23. Maas, C.; Franz, A.R.; von Krogh, S.; Arand, J.; Poets, C.F. Growth and morbidity of extremely preterm infants after early full enteral nutrition. *Arch. Dis. Child. Fetal Neonatal Ed.* **2018**, *103*, F79–F81. [CrossRef]
24. Stavel, M.; Wong, J.; Cieslak, Z.; Sherlock, R.; Claveau, M.; Shah, P.S. Effect of prophylactic indomethacin administration and early feeding on spontaneous intestinal perforation in extremely low-birth-weight infants. *J. Perinatol.* **2017**, *37*, 188–193. [CrossRef] [PubMed]
25. Varma, S.; Bartlett, E.L.; Nam, L.; Shores, D.R. Use of breast milk and other feeding practices following gastrointestinal surgery in infants. *J. Pediatr. Gastroenterol. Nutr.* **2019**, *68*, 264–271. [CrossRef] [PubMed]
26. Vongbhavit, K.; Underwood, M.A. Predictive Value of the Aspartate Aminotransferase to Platelet Ratio Index for Parenteral Nutrition-Associated Cholestasis in Premature Infants With Intestinal Perforation. *JPEN J. Parenter Enteral Nutr.* **2018**, *42*, 797–804. [CrossRef]
27. Cass, D.L.; Brandt, M.L.; Patel, D.L.; Nuchtern, J.G.; Minifee, P.K.; Wesson, D.E. Peritoneal drainage as definitive treatment for neonates with isolated intestinal perforation. *J. Pediatr. Surg.* **2000**, *35*, 1531–1536. [CrossRef]
28. Chiu, B.; Pillai, S.B.; Almond, P.S.; Beth Madonna, M.; Reynolds, M.; Luck, S.R.; Arensman, R.M. To drain or not to drain: A single institution experience with neonatal intestinal perforation. *J. Perinat Med.* **2006**, *34*, 338–341. [CrossRef]
29. Eicher, C.; Seitz, G.; Bevot, A.; Moll, M.; Goelz, R.; Arand, J.; Poets, C.; Fuchs, J. Surgical management of extremely low birth weight infants with neonatal bowel perforation: A single-center experience and a review of the literature. *Neonatology* **2012**, *101*, 285–292. [CrossRef]
30. Gollin, G.; Abarbanell, A.; Baerg, J.E. Peritoneal drainage as definitive management of intestinal perforation in extremely-low-birth-weight infants. *J. Pediatr. Surg.* **2003**, *38*, 1814–1817. [CrossRef]
31. Jakaitis, B.M.; Bhatia, A.M. Definitive peritoneal drainage in the extremely low birth weight infant with spontaneous intestinal perforation: Predictors and hospital outcomes. *J. Perinatol.* **2015**, *35*, 607–611. [CrossRef] [PubMed]
32. Shah, B.A.; Migliori, A.; Kurihara, I.; Sharma, S.; Lim, Y.-P.; Padbury, J. Blood Level of Inter-Alpha Inhibitor Proteins Distinguishes Necrotizing Enterocolitis From Spontaneous Intestinal Perforation. *J. Pediatr.* **2017**, *180*, 135.e1–140.e1. [CrossRef] [PubMed]
33. Wadhawan, R.; Oh, W.; Vohr, B.R.; Saha, S.; Das, A.; Bell, E.F.; Laptook, A.; Shankaran, S.; Stoll, B.J.; Walsh, M.C.; et al. Spontaneous intestinal perforation in extremely low birth weight infants: Association with indometacin therapy and effects on neurodevelopmental outcomes at 18-22 months corrected age. *Arch. Dis. Child. Fetal Neonatal Ed.* **2013**, *98*, F127–F132. [CrossRef] [PubMed]
34. Bassler, D.; Plavka, R.; Shinwell, E.S.; Hallman, M.; Jarreau, P.-H.; Carnielli, V.; Van den Anker, J.N.; Meisner, C.; Engel, C.; Schwab, M.; et al. NEUROSIS Trial Group Early inhaled budesonide for the prevention of bronchopulmonary dysplasia. *N. Engl. J. Med.* **2015**, *373*, 1497–1506. [CrossRef] [PubMed]
35. Gébus, M.; Michel, J.L.; Samperiz, S.; Harper, L.; Alessandri, J.L.; Ramful, D. Management of neonatal spontaneous intestinal perforation by peritoneal needle aspiration. *J. Perinatol.* **2018**, *38*, 159–163. [CrossRef] [PubMed]
36. Karila, K.; Anttila, A.; Iber, T.; Pakarinen, M.; Koivusalo, A. Intestinal failure associated cholestasis in surgical necrotizing enterocolitis and spontaneous intestinal perforation. *J. Pediatr. Surg.* **2019**, *54*, 460–464. [CrossRef]
37. Beath, S.V.; Kelly, D.A. Total Parenteral Nutrition-Induced Cholestasis: Prevention and Management. *Clin. Liver Dis.* **2016**, *20*, 159–176. [CrossRef]
38. Wadhawan, R.; Oh, W.; Hintz, S.R.; Blakely, M.L.; Das, A.; Bell, E.F.; Saha, S.; Laptook, A.R.; Shankaran, S.; Stoll, B.J.; et al. NICHD Neonatal Research Network Neurodevelopmental outcomes of extremely low birth weight infants with spontaneous intestinal perforation or surgical necrotizing enterocolitis. *J. Perinatol.* **2014**, *34*, 64–70. [CrossRef]
39. Manea, A.; Boia, M.; Iacob, D.; Dima, M.; Iacob, R.E. Benefits of early enteral nutrition in extremely low birth weight infants. *Singapore Med. J.* **2016**, *57*, 616–618. [CrossRef]

40. Viswanathan, S.; McNelis, K.; Super, D.; Einstadter, D.; Groh-Wargo, S.; Collin, M. Standardized slow enteral feeding protocol and the incidence of necrotizing enterocolitis in extremely low birth weight infants. *JPEN J. Parenter Enteral Nutr.* **2015**, *39*, 644–654. [CrossRef]
41. Greer, D.; Karunaratne, Y.G.; Karpelowsky, J.; Adams, S. Early Enteral Feeding after Pediatric Abdominal Surgery: A Systematic Review of the Literature. *J. Pediatr. Surg.* **2019**. [CrossRef] [PubMed]
42. Jacobi, S.K.; Odle, J. Nutritional factors influencing intestinal health of the neonate. *Adv. Nutr.* **2012**, *3*, 687–696. [CrossRef]
43. Puiman, P.J.; Jensen, M.; Stoll, B.; Renes, I.B.; de Bruijn, A.C.J.M.; Dorst, K.; Schierbeek, H.; Schmidt, M.; Boehm, G.; Burrin, D.G.; et al. Intestinal threonine utilization for protein and mucin synthesis is decreased in formula-fed preterm pigs. *J. Nutr.* **2011**, *141*, 1306–1311. [CrossRef] [PubMed]
44. Li, Y.; Pan, X.; Nguyen, D.N.; Ren, S.; Moodley, A.; Sangild, P.T. Bovine colostrum before or after formula feeding improves systemic immune protection and gut function in newborn preterm pigs. *Front. Immunol.* **2019**, *10*, 3062. [CrossRef] [PubMed]
45. Shimizu, T.; Tadokoro, R.; Kaneko, N.; Suzuki, M.; Tanaka, K.; Shinohara, K.; Shiga, S.; Yamashiro, Y. Effects of extremely early enteral feeding on plasma glicentin levels in very-low-birthweight infants. *J. Paediatr. Child. Health* **2006**, *42*, 636–639. [CrossRef]
46. Walker, A. Breast milk as the gold standard for protective nutrients. *J. Pediatr.* **2010**, *156*, S3–S7. [CrossRef]
47. Perri, M.; Lucente, M.; Cannataro, R.; De Luca, I.F.; Gallelli, L.; Moro, G.; De Sarro, G.; Caroleo, M.C.; Cione, E. Variation in Immune-Related microRNAs Profile in Human Milk Amongst Lactating Women. *Microrna* **2018**, *7*, 107–114. [CrossRef]
48. Snyder, R.; Herdt, A.; Mejias-Cepeda, N.; Ladino, J.; Crowley, K.; Levy, P. Early provision of oropharyngeal colostrum leads to sustained breast milk feedings in preterm infants. *Pediatr. Neonatol.* **2017**, *58*, 534–540. [CrossRef]
49. Ekingen, G.; Ceran, C.; Guvenc, B.H.; Tuzlaci, A.; Kahraman, H. Early enteral feeding in newborn surgical patients. *Nutrition* **2005**, *21*, 142–146. [CrossRef]
50. Jiang, W.; Lv, X.; Xu, X.; Geng, Q.; Zhang, J.; Tang, W. Early enteral nutrition for upper digestive tract malformation in neonate. *Asia Pac. J. Clin. Nutr.* **2015**, *24*, 38–43. [CrossRef]
51. Walter-Nicolet, E.; Rousseau, V.; Kieffer, F.; Fusaro, F.; Bourdaud, N.; Oucherif, S.; Benachi, A.; Sarnacki, S.; Mitanchez, D. Neonatal outcome of gastroschisis is mainly influenced by nutritional management. *J. Pediatr. Gastroenterol. Nutr.* **2009**, *48*, 612–617. [CrossRef]
52. Shores, D.R.; Alaish, S.M.; Aucott, S.W.; Bullard, J.E.; Haney, C.; Tymann, H.; Nonyane, B.A.S.; Schwarz, K.B. Postoperative Enteral Nutrition Guidelines Reduce the Risk of Intestinal Failure-Associated Liver Disease in Surgical Infants. *J. Pediatr.* **2018**, *195*, 140.e1–147.e1. [CrossRef]
53. Tadano, S.; Terashima, H.; Fukuzawa, J.; Matsuo, R.; Ikeda, O.; Ohkohchi, N. Early postoperative oral intake accelerates upper gastrointestinal anastomotic healing in the rat model. *J. Surg. Res.* **2011**, *169*, 202–208. [CrossRef]
54. Kiyama, T.; Onda, M.; Tokunaga, A.; Yoshiyuki, T.; Barbul, A. Effect of early postoperative feeding on the healing of colonic anastomoses in the presence of intra-abdominal sepsis in rats. *Dis. Colon Rectum* **2000**, *43*, S54–S58. [CrossRef] [PubMed]
55. Dako, J.; Buzzard, J.; Jain, M.; Pandey, R.; Groh-Wargo, S.; Shekhawat, P. Slow enteral feeding decreases risk of transfusion associated necrotizing enterocolitis. *J. Neonatal. Perinatal. Med.* **2018**, *11*, 231–239. [CrossRef] [PubMed]
56. Ramani, M.; Ambalavanan, N. Feeding practices and necrotizing enterocolitis. *Clin. Perinatol* **2013**, *40*, 1–10. [CrossRef] [PubMed]

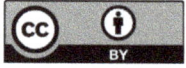

© 2020 by the authors. Licensee MDPI, Basel, Switzerland. This article is an open access article distributed under the terms and conditions of the Creative Commons Attribution (CC BY) license (http://creativecommons.org/licenses/by/4.0/).

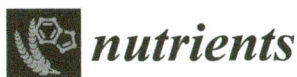 

Review

# Understanding the Elements of Maternal Protection from Systemic Bacterial Infections during Early Life

Sierra A. Kleist and Kathryn A. Knoop *

Department of Immunology, Mayo Clinic, Rochester, MN 55905, USA; Kleist.Sierra@mayo.edu
* Correspondence: Knoop.Kathryn@mayo.edu; Tel.: +507-422-6536

Received: 12 March 2020; Accepted: 8 April 2020; Published: 10 April 2020

**Abstract:** Late-onset sepsis (LOS) and other systemic bloodstream infections are notable causes of neonatal mortality, particularly in prematurely born very low birth weight infants. Breastfeeding in early life has numerous health benefits, impacting the health of the newborn in both the short-term and in the long-term. Though the known benefits of an exclusive mother's own milk diet in early life have been well recognized and described, it is less understood how breastfed infants enjoy a potential reduction in risk of LOS and other systemic infections. Here we review how gut residing pathogens within the intestinal microbiota of infants can cause a subset of sepsis cases and the components of breastmilk that may prevent the dissemination of pathogens from the intestine.

**Keywords:** breastmilk; late onset sepsis; bloodstream infections; enteric pathogens

## 1. Introduction

Bloodstream infections (BSIs) resulting from bacterial dissemination can be extremely harmful to neonates, particularly preterm and very low birth weight (VLBW, <1500 g) newborns. Late-onset neonatal sepsis (LOS) is defined as sepsis occurring 72 h after delivery. LOS has an incidence rate of 10% in preterm infants and is associated with long-term neurological development deficiencies [1,2]. Cases resulting from bacterial BSIs account for 26% of all deaths in preterm infants. LOS will continue to be an important issue among preterm infants as there is a constant reduction of the age of viability resulting from increased medical technology for treating babies born extremely preterm and at a VLBW, those that are most at risk for neonatal BSIs [3,4].

Antibiotics are currently the first line of defense against LOS, but are possibly causing more harm than good. Empirical antibiotics are given to a majority of preterm neonates, regardless of if the infant has a positive blood culture or not, as a preemptive measure of reducing sepsis [2]. This practice may have the opposite intended effect as multiple studies [5,6] have shown an association between prolonged empirical antibiotic administration in premature babies and increased likelihood of developing LOS, necrotizing enterocolitis (NEC), and/or death. Central line placement, used for administration of parenteral nutrition and antibiotics, risks the introduction of pathogens to the bloodstream and is the likely cause of many BSIs. As such, increased hygienic practices implemented in hospitals have resulted in a stark decrease in LOS caused by normal skin commensals [7]. However, despite these efforts, LOS rates in neonates remain unchanged among cases caused by gut commensals, suggesting the bacteria are entering the bloodstream through another mechanism [7].

## 2. Breastfeeding and LOS

A preterm infant's diet plays a crucial role in disease development or avoidance. Parenteral feedings are often the only option for delivering nutrients to VLBW infants in the days immediately following birth, but long term use is strongly associated with increased risk of LOS development [8,9]. When an infant's organs become mature enough to handle partial or full enteral nutrition, mother's own milk (MOM) is the preferred source of nutrition [10], though preterm infants once were formula-fed at higher rates compared to newborns delivered at term. It is logical to hypothesize ailing infants physically unable to be enterally-fed are more likely to develop LOS in connection with a frail condition [8]. When MOM is unavailable, human donor milk and/or formula are given to infants instead. A number of clinical studies have demonstrated a clear connection between feeding with MOM and protection against LOS in premature infants, in addition to the benefits of a faster transition to enteral feedings, decreased likelihood of mortality, and reduced length of hospital stay [11,12]. Further, a historical clinical observation showed an LOS incidence of 57% amongst the formula-fed infants compared to an LOS incidence of 7% in MOM-fed infants, which included partial-MOM fed infants [13]. Reduced risk of LOS was correlated with increased consumption of human milk, with the odds of LOS in a NICU cohort decreasing 19% for every 10 mL/kg dose per day of human milk [11]. While this cohort pooled infants receiving donor milk with those receiving MOM into a single human milk- fed group, more than 90% of the infants in that cohort were given MOM exclusively [11]. Recent systemic data analysis suggested a possible, though not-significant, 23% risk reduction in developing LOS among exclusively breastfed infants as compared to exclusively formula-fed infants [14]. Additional clinical observations showed similar significant results where 25% of formula-fed infants developed LOS compared to 14% of MOM-fed infants [12], supporting an initiative to promote exclusive breastfeeding as the preferred protective diet in early days of life of any enterally-fed infant. To date, use of donor milk has not shown a reduction of risk of LOS, in contrast to MOM diets [15], though mechanisms of protection unique to MOM remain unclear. More clinical data should be gathered comparing the outcomes of MOM-fed infants to those fed donor milk or fortified formula as better alternatives become available to those infants unable to be fed MOM. In extremely rare cases, LOS may be the result of contaminated breast milk [16], but in the vast majority of cases, MOM-fed infants have overall better outcomes than those who require parenteral nutrition, or other enteral diets.

## 3. Enteric Origin of Pathogens

### 3.1. Pathogens in LOS

The potential mechanism of how breastmilk may protect from bacterial BSIs and LOS initially became elucidated around 10 years ago when multiple groups observed the pathogens residing in the gastrointestinal (GI) tract prior to sepsis events [17–20]. Following birth, the gastrointestinal tract becomes colonized by commensal bacteria in a dynamic process that is initially pioneered by facultative anaerobic proteobacteria and lactobacilli [21–25]. Common causative pathogens of LOS can be found residing in the gut, including Gram-positive members of the lactobacillales order such as Group B *Streptococcus* (GBS) or *Enterococcus faecalis*; and Gram-negative bacilli (GNB) of the gammaproteobacteria class such as *Klebsiella pneumonia* [18], *Escherichia coli* [18], *Pseudomonas aeruginosa* [26], or *Enterobacteriaceae* species [27]. Due to the low density of the commensal flora in neonates, such pathobionts [28], bacterial species that can reside in the gut microbiota as a commensal but also have the potential to become pathogenic, can colonize the GI tract [29]. By acting as a reservoir for potential pathogens, the gut microbiota poses a risk to the neonate if it becomes dysbiotic, resulting in pathogen expansion [30,31].

Preventing enteric bacterial dissemination of pathobionts may prove to be more difficult than preventing intravenous dissemination, where increased hygienic practices have reduced LOS rates [7,32]. Additionally, animal work suggests the enteral route of infection may contribute to the virulence of sepsis pathogens when compared to the intraperitoneal route of infection [33], underlining the importance of developing therapeutics preventing enteric dissemination. Prophylactic use of oral antibiotics rarely target only potential pathogens, but also disrupts the normal developing microbiota contributing to dysbiosis in the microbial community [34–36]. Dysbiosis, in turn, can result in enteric infection and dissemination as pathobionts gain an increased foothold in the microbial community [30].

Antibiotic resistance is a growing concern in neonatal sepsis cases, and as such, dependence and overuse of antibiotics should be avoided [37,38].

*3.2. Modification of the Infant Gut Microbiota*

Introduction of probiotic strains of commensal bacteria has been proposed as a therapeutic strategy to treat or prevent dysbiosis of the gut microbiota and prevent a number of diseases including enteric infections and LOS [39]. Live strains of commensal bacteria such as *Lactobacillus* and *Bifidobacterium* species may improve gut health by preventing pathogen colonization and promoting the development of a healthy microbiota [40,41]. Modest improvements in gut health following single probiotic strains such as *Saccharomyces bourlardii*, *Lactobacillus reuteri*, *Lactobacillus acidophilus* and *Bifidobacterium lactis* have been observed [42], including a reduction in the time needed for progression to full enteral feeding in preterm infants given *Saccharomyces boulardii* or *B. lactis*, though this effect is less pronounced in exclusively formula-fed infants [43].

Probiotic mixes containing multiple strains have shown the most success in reducing the risk of LOS in enterally-fed infants [44]. Such formulations can range from a mix of three strains: *L. acidophilus*, *E. faecium* and *Bifidobacterium infantum* [45] to a mix of eight strains: *Streptococcus thermophilus*, *Bifidobacterium breve*, *Bifidobacterium longum*, *Bifidobacterium infantis*, *L. acidophilus*, *Lactobacillus plantarum*, *Lactobacillus paracasei* and *Lactobacillus delbrueckii spp bulgaricus* [46], suggesting multiple strains may have complementary roles in combination to restore intestinal health and provide protection. However, probiotics such as *Lactobacillus rhamnosus GG*, *S. boulardii*, *L. reuteri*, *Lactobacillus sporogenes*, or *B. breve* as single strains, or even mixes of multiple strains show a limited effect in reducing LOS in formula-fed infants [47]. This apparent limitation of probiotics in improving outcomes in formula-fed infants as compared to breastfed infants suggests a greater deficit in the gut health of formula-fed infants that is harder to overcome with therapeutic interventions [48,49].

The shaping of the gut microbiome by breastmilk has been repeatedly observed and formula-fed infants have a gut microbiota distinct from the community found in the GI tract of breastfed infants [50–53]. Diet during early life can influence bacterial translocation as intestinal permeability was found to be significantly decreased [54] and barrier function matured quicker in breastfed preterm infants [55] when compared to formula-fed preterm infants. In animal models, formula feeding resulted in increased bacterial translocation [56–58]. VLBW babies in intensive care units, those most at risk of developing sepsis, often lack access to breastmilk. Therefore, identification of protective components of breastmilk that prevent dissemination represents fertile ground for the development of therapeutics to prevent bacterial infections and LOS.

## 4. Components of Breastmilk

Breastmilk is a complex formulation of nutrients, proteins, and growth factors providing neonates with benefits beyond the incomparable nourishment. Figure 1 shows maternal protection against intestinal pathogens. Several biologically active factors promote gut health and confer protection from enteric infections to the neonate. Breastmilk changes substantially throughout lactation from colostrum in the days initially following delivery to transitional milk and then mature milk approximately two weeks following delivery. Proteins such as antibodies and growth factors are present in higher concentrations in colostrum and transitional milk compared to mature milk [59,60]. Given the biological role for such proteins, breastmilk is therefore considered one component of the "mother-breastmilk-infant triad" [61] and perhaps synchronized between mother and child to afford age-appropriate nutrition and protection to neonates provided with MOM in the first weeks of life. Such factors and proteins present in breastmilk are discussed in this section. The key components of breastmilk reviewed here all can be found in higher concentrations in colostrum and transitional milk early in lactation, asking the question that for breastmilk to have protective effects in neonates, is timing everything?

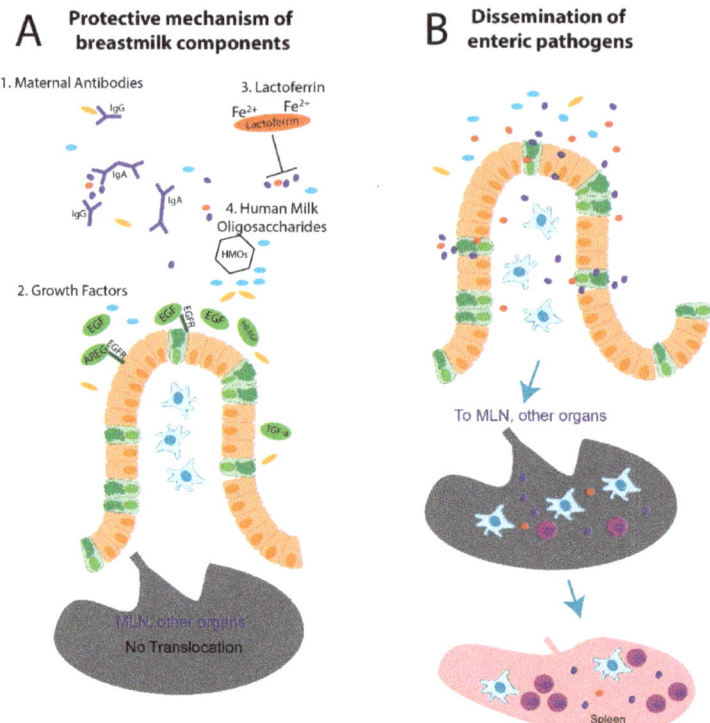

**Figure 1.** Maternal protection from enteric pathogens. (**A**) Components in breastmilk can limit enteric pathogen dissemination. (1) Maternal antibodies (IgG, IgA) can bind bacteria and directly inhibit pathogen adherence and invasion [62]. (2) Growth factors [epidermal growth factor (EGF), amphiregulin (AREG), heparin-binding epidermal growth factor-like factor (HB-EGF), and tumor-growth factor-alpha (TGF-α)] bind the epidermal growth factor receptor (EGFR) on epithelial cells to promote barrier function by cell proliferation and growth [63], and by limiting translocation via goblet cells [64]. (3) Lactoferrin sequesters iron which limits pathogen growth [65]. (4) Human milk oligosaccharides (HMOs) promote the development of the intestinal microbiota [66], which can offer colonization resistance to enteric pathogens [30]. (**B**) In the absence of these factors, pathogens can colonize the intestine lumen, cross the epithelium potentially through goblet cells [64], and disseminate to organs through the system, including the mesenteric lymph node (MLN) and spleen, resulting in late-onset sepsis (LOS).

### 4.1. Antibodies

Maternal antibodies, including IgM, IgG, and IgA subtypes, offer superior protection to neonates both within the intestinal lumen, and systemically. These antibodies can provide passive immunity within the neonate to any potential systemic infections [67]. Within the lumen of the neonatal GI tract, IgA is particularly important in providing protection from invasive enteric pathogens by directly binding and preventing adherence and evasion [62,67]. Beyond protection from pathogen translocation from the intestinal lumen, maternal IgG antibodies transferred to the neonates also offered protection from E. coli within the circulation [62]. There has been modest clinical evidence that IgM administration may offer systemic protection from bacterial infections [68], though neither IgM nor IgG administration reduced LOS mortality [69]. Animal work has shown maternal antibodies educate the neonatal immune responses by dampening T cell-mediated responses in early life [70], potentially quieting inflammatory responses that may precede or accompany LOS [71–73]. Thus, maternal antibodies protect the neonate by preventing enteric pathogens from translocating from the intestinal lumen, and potentially limiting systemic infections and intestinal inflammation.

*4.2. Growth Factors*

Growth factors present in the breastmilk include a family of ligands that neonates can sense through the epidermal growth factor receptor (EGFR) expressed on intestinal epithelial cells [25,63,64]: epidermal growth factor (EGF), amphiregulin (AREG), heparin-binding epidermal growth factor-like factor (HB-EGF), and tumor-growth factor-alpha (TGF-α) [74]. All are found in temporal gradients, with the highest concentration in colostrum [74–78]. EGF is one of the most abundantly concentrated growth factors in breastmilk, though EGFR ligands perform redundant functions [79], suggesting these ligands have a necessary role in early life. EGF passes through the digestive tract resisting low pH and enzymatic degradation [80,81] and can be measured in the stool of breastfed children [64], suggesting it has a biological effect throughout the intestines. EGFR activation in the neonate results in epithelial cell division, nutrient uptake, improved intestinal barrier function, reduced bacterial translocation, and reduced Toll-like receptor signaling [63,80–83]. Recent animal work modeling decreased EGFR ligands within the GI tract of neonatal mice observed translocation of enteric pathogens resulting in a systemic infection in a model of LOS, which was reversed by oral administration of recombinant EGF [64]. Thus growth factors, through the activation of EGFR on neonatal epithelial cells can limit enteric pathogens from disseminating and potentially prevent systemic infections.

*4.3. Lactoferrin*

Lactoferrin, also present in increased concentrations in the first weeks of lactation, can remain a significant component of breastmilk for months after lactation begins [84–86]. The primary function of lactoferrin is to bind iron for transfer to the neonate through epithelial cell absorption, which the growing neonate utilizes as an important nutrient. Therefore, lactoferrin has anti-microbial properties primarily through the iron-binding capacity as iron sequestration can limit the amount of free iron available for bacterial growth [65,87,88]. Lactoferricin, a derivative of lactoferrin, may be directly bacteriostatic and can bind bacterial wall components, potentially limiting luminal pathogens [89,90]. Lactoferrin may also promote the development of the mucosal immune system by stimulating dendritic cells that shape intestinal immune responses and enhancing IgA production in Peyer's patches [91]. Lactoferrin has been the target of several clinical trials as a supplement to enteral diets to protect against enteric infections and LOS [92]. While therapeutic lactoferrin may have beneficial effects on modifying the neonatal microbiome and reducing potential pathobionts [93], the efficacy of lactoferrin in reducing LOS mortality remains controversial [94–96]. Thus, lactoferrin protects the neonate with direct anti-microbial effects, potentially limiting pathogen colonization within the microbiota.

*4.4. Human Milk Oligosaccharides*

Oligosaccharides in breastmilk, known as human milk oligosaccharides (HMOs), support the maturation of the normal infant microbiota, which in turn provides colonization resistance to enteric pathogens [66,97–100]. These glycans are dynamically produced in the first weeks of lactation [101,102] and are essentially undigested by the infant [103], but instead utilized by the developing microbiota [52]. HMOs can be utilized as a nutrient source by commensal members of the microbiota, and also probiotic strains such as *B. breve*, as colonization of the intestinal tract of infants was associated with HMO concentration and fucosylation [104]. HMOs may also modulate the growth of potential pathogens, and have been shown to have a direct effect against the formation of GBS biofilms [105]. Additionally, observations suggest HMOs may have a direct impact on infant's epithelial cells by increasing mucus expression [106] and promoting goblet cell maturation [107], both of which can improve barrier function by enhancing the mucus layer covering the intestinal epithelium that can prevent bacterial encroachment and translocation. Finally HMOs may have an impact on the infant's immune system by binding c-type lectins, siglecs, galectins and selectins expressed by phagocytic and antigen-presenting cells, such as dendritic cells, monocytes and neutrophils [108–110]. These interactions could modulate immune responses through regulating leukocyte trafficking, influencing cytokine responses and inhibiting TLR-mediated inflammation, all of which could affect LOS development and outcomes [66,111,112]. Clinically, infants born to mothers unable to produce some forms of HMOs trended toward an increased risk of LOS [113]. Similarly, a low diversity of HMOs from mothers was associated with an increase in NEC, though was not significantly associated with an increase is LOS cases [114]. These clinical data suggest more work needs to be compiled regarding supplementation of infant diets with HMOs to potentially improve gut function and sepsis outcomes [115]. Thus, HMOs may protect the neonate by shaping the microbiota, which may protect from pathogen colonization.

## 5. Future Directions

### 5.1. Supplements and MOM Alternatives

Donor milk represents a worthy alternative when MOM is unavailable, though reports have shown the processing of donor milk, including pasteurization and potentially multiple freeze-thaw cycles, may reduce the concentrations of the beneficial proteins, particularly immunoglobulins and lactoferrin [74,116]. Pasteurization of MOM showed a non-significant trend of increased infectious LOS morbidity [117], suggesting the reduction of these beneficial components in MOM could lead to an increased risk of LOS. Pasteurization is an imperative step in donor milk processing to prevent potential transmission of pathogens through contaminated breast milk [16], and work optimizing pasteurization processes to remove pathogenic threat while maintaining beneficial factors is currently being completed [118,119]. The Holder pasteurization method, the recommended pasteurization method of donor milk, sterilizes bacteria present in the milk, and does not degrade growth factors such as EGF and TGF-β [119]. Immunoglobulins and lactoferrin are reduced following Holder pasteurization, though may be protected following high temperature short time (HTST) treatments, an experimental pasteurization method [120,121]. Additionally, the increased concentrations of these proteins early in lactation suggests age-matched donor milk or supplements containing a combination of immunoglobulins, growth factors, lactoferrin, and HMOs at concentrations found in colostrum may represent the next steps in the progression toward an appropriate alternative when MOM cannot be provided.

### 5.2. Animal Modeling

While clinical interventions are quickly being brought to the NICU, animal models are revealing potential mechanisms of acquisition and protection against LOS. Therefore, the development and use of animal models that represent how LOS is clinically acquired is essential [30,62,64]. Traditional models of LOS have been limited to intravenous injection of cecal contents or single bacterial components, such as lipopolysaccharide. While these models may help elucidate how neonates respond to systemic bacterial insults, these models lack insight into the enteric route of entry pathogens may utilize. Injection of cecal contents may introduce too many bacterial elements as most LOS patients are infected with only one bacterial species at a time. Similarly, intravenous injection of lipopolysaccharide, a component of some bacterial cell walls, may reduce relevance as there can be strain variation in LOS pathology within the same bacterial species [64]. As increased hygienic practices reduce the number of intravenous-acquired LOS cases, similar interest should be placed on reducing the number of LOS cases resulting from an enteric route of origin, with animal work modeling the oral route of pathogen entry. Understanding how MOM and the developing microbiota protect the neonate from enteric pathogens will provide clear directions for future therapeutics.

## 6. Conclusions

While the clinical connection between breastfeeding and reduced LOS risk is currently a potential, though logical, correlation, the many components within breastmilk offer observable benefits to the developing neonate, particularly within the intestinal environment. If enteric pathogens continue to threaten infants and cause a substantial portion of LOS cases, factors present in breastmilk may provide exceptional protection to the neonate, representing strong candidates for supplementation of breast milk that could prevent of translocating pathogens. Clinical measures such as the reduction of unnecessary antibiotics to protect the intestinal microbiome, promotion of an exclusive MOM diet when available, and sophistication of supplements combining immunoglobulins, growth factors, lactoferrin, and HMOs to formula or donor milk could result in further reduction of LOS cases by focusing on protection from enteric pathogens.

**Author Contributions:** Conceptualization, original draft preparation, review and editing, S.A.K., K.A.K.; funding acquisition, K.A.K. All authors have read and agreed to the published version of the manuscript.

**Funding:** Supported by grants: DK109006-K.A.K., AI144721-K.A.K., AI095542 MIST Scholars Award–K.A.K.

**Acknowledgments:** The authors wish to acknowledge Kara Greenfield, Kathryn Lin, and Lila Yokanovich for their advice with this manuscript.

**Conflicts of Interest:** K.A.K. is an inventor on U.S. Nonprovisional Application Serial No. 15/880,658 Compositions and Methods for Modulation of Dietary and Microbial Exposure.

## References

1. Cortese, F.; Scicchitano, P.; Gesualdo, M.; Filaninno, A.; De Giorgi, E.; Schettini, F.; Laforgia, N.; Ciccone, M.M. Early and late infections in newborns: Where do we stand? A review. *Pediatr. Neonatol.* **2016**, *57*, 265–273. [CrossRef]
2. Raymond, S.L.; Rincon, J.C.; Wynn, J.L.; Moldawer, L.L.; Larson, S.D. Impact of early-life exposures to infections, antibiotics, and vaccines on perinatal and long-term health and disease. *Front. Immunol.* **2017**, *8*. [CrossRef]
3. Stoll, B.J.; Gordon, T.; Korones, S.B.; Shankaran, S.; Tyson, J.E.; Bauer, C.R.; Fanaroff, A.A.; Lemons, J.A.; Donovan, E.F.; Oh, W.; et al. Late-onset sepsis in very low birth weight neonates: A report from the National Institute of Child Health and Human Development Neonatal Research Network. *J. Pediatr.* **1996**, *129*, 63–71. [CrossRef]
4. Stoll, B.J.; Hansen, N.; Fanaroff, A.A.; Wright, L.L.; Carlo, W.A.; Ehrenkranz, R.A.; Lemons, J.A.; Donovan, E.F.; Stark, A.R.; Tyson, J.E.; et al. Late-onset sepsis in very low birth weight neonates: The experience of the NICHD neonatal research network. *Pediatrics* **2002**, *110*, 285. [CrossRef]
5. Cotten, C.M.; Taylor, S.; Stoll, B.; Goldberg, R.N.; Hansen, N.I.; Sánchez, P.J.; Ambalavanan, N.; Benjamin, D.K., Jr.; Network, N.N.R. Prolonged duration of initial empirical antibiotic treatment is associated with increased rates of necrotizing enterocolitis and death for extremely low birth weight infants. *Pediatrics* **2009**, *123*, 58–66. [CrossRef]
6. Kuppala, V.S.; Meinzen-Derr, J.; Morrow, A.L.; Schibler, K.R. Prolonged initial empirical antibiotic treatment is associated with adverse outcomes in premature infants. *J. Pediatr.* **2011**, *159*, 720–725. [CrossRef]
7. Pharande, P.; Lindrea, K.B.; Smyth, J.; Evans, M.; Lui, K.; Bolisetty, S. Trends in late-onset sepsis in a neonatal intensive care unit following implementation of infection control bundle: A 15-year audit. *J. Paediatr. Child Health* **2018**, *54*, 1314–1320. [CrossRef]
8. el Manouni el Hassani, S.; Berkhout, D.J.C.; Niemarkt, H.J.; Mann, S.; de Boode, W.P.; Cossey, V.; Hulzebos, C.V.; van Kaam, A.H.; Kramer, B.W.; van Lingen, R.A.; et al. Risk factors for late-onset sepsis in preterm infants: A multicenter case-control study. *Neonatology* **2019**, *116*, 42–51. [CrossRef]
9. Kung, Y.-H.; Hsieh, Y.-F.; Weng, Y.-H.; Lien, R.-I.; Luo, J.; Wang, Y.; Huang, Y.-C.; Chen, C.-L.; Chen, C.-J. Risk factors of late-onset neonatal sepsis in Taiwan: A matched case-control study. *J. Microbiol. Immunol. Infect.* **2016**, *49*, 430–435. [CrossRef]
10. Moro, G.E.; Arslanoglu, S.; Bertino, E.; Corvaglia, L.; Montirosso, R.; Picaud, J.-C.; Polberger, S.; Schanler, R.J.; Steel, C.; van Goudoever, J.; et al. XII. Human milk in feeding premature infants: Consensus statement. *J. Pediatr. Gastroenterol. Nutr.* **2015**, *61*, S16–S19. [CrossRef]
11. Patel, A.L.; Johnson, T.J.; Engstrom, J.L.; Fogg, L.F.; Jegier, B.J.; Bigger, H.R.; Meier, P.P. Impact of early human milk on sepsis and health-care costs in very low birth weight infants. *J. Perinatol.* **2013**, *33*, 514–519. [CrossRef]

12. Cortez, J.; Makker, K.; Kraemer, D.F.; Neu, J.; Sharma, R.; Hudak, M.L. Maternal milk feedings reduce sepsis, necrotizing enterocolitis and improve outcomes of premature infants. *J. Perinatol.* **2018**, *38*, 71–74. [CrossRef]
13. Ashraf, R.N.; Jalil, F.; Zaman, S.; Karlberg, J.; Khan, S.R.; Lindblad, B.S.; Hanson, L.A. Breast feeding and protection against neonatal sepsis in a high risk population. *Arch. Dis. Child.* **1991**, *66*, 488–490. [CrossRef]
14. Miller, J.; Tonkin, E.; Damarell, A.R.; McPhee, J.A.; Suganuma, M.; Suganuma, H.; Middleton, F.P.; Makrides, M.; Collins, T.C. A systematic review and meta-analysis of human milk feeding and morbidity in very low birth weight infants. *Nutrients* **2018**, *10*, 707. [CrossRef]
15. Meier, P.; Patel, A.; Esquerra-Zwiers, A. Donor human milk update: Evidence, mechanisms, and priorities for research and practice. *J. Pediatr.* **2017**, *180*, 15–21. [CrossRef]
16. Widger, J.; O'Connell, N.H.; Stack, T. Breast milk causing neonatal sepsis and death. *Clin. Microbiol. Infect.* **2010**, *16*, 1796–1798. [CrossRef]
17. Carl, M.A.; Ndao, I.M.; Springman, A.C.; Manning, S.D.; Johnson, J.R.; Johnston, B.D.; Burnham, C.A.; Weinstock, E.S.; Weinstock, G.M.; Wylie, T.N.; et al. Sepsis from the gut: The enteric habitat of bacteria that cause late-onset neonatal bloodstream infections. *Clin. Infect. Dis.* **2014**, *58*, 1211–1218. [CrossRef]
18. Almuneef, M.A.; Baltimore, R.S.; Farrel, P.A.; Reagan-Cirincione, P.; Dembry, L.M. Molecular typing demonstrating transmission of gram-negative rods in a neonatal intensive care unit in the absence of a recognized epidemic. *Clin. Infect. Dis.* **2001**, *32*, 220–227. [CrossRef]
19. Graham, P.L., 3rd; Della-Latta, P.; Wu, F.; Zhou, J.; Saiman, L. The gastrointestinal tract serves as the reservoir for Gram-negative pathogens in very low birth weight infants. *Pediatr. Infect. Dis. J.* **2007**, *26*, 1153–1156. [CrossRef]
20. Smith, A.; Saiman, L.; Zhou, J.; Della-Latta, P.; Jia, H.; Graham, P.L., 3rd. Concordance of gastrointestinal tract colonization and subsequent bloodstream infections with gram-negative bacilli in very low birth weight infants in the neonatal intensive care unit. *Pediatr. Infect. Dis. J.* **2010**, *29*, 831–835. [CrossRef]
21. Eckburg, P.B.; Bik, E.M.; Bernstein, C.N.; Purdom, E.; Dethlefsen, L.; Sargent, M.; Gill, S.R.; Nelson, K.E.; Relman, D.A. Diversity of the Human Intestinal Microbial Flora. *Science (N. Y.)* **2005**, *308*, 1635–1638. [CrossRef] [PubMed]
22. Koenig, J.E.; Spor, A.; Scalfone, N.; Fricker, A.D.; Stombaugh, J.; Knight, R.; Angenent, L.T.; Ley, R.E. Succession of microbial consortia in the developing infant gut microbiome. *Proc. Natl. Acad. Sci. USA* **2011**, *108*, 4578–4585. [CrossRef] [PubMed]
23. Yatsunenko, T.; Rey, F.E.; Manary, M.J.; Trehan, I.; Dominguez-Bello, M.G.; Contreras, M.; Magris, M.; Hidalgo, G.; Baldassano, R.N.; Anokhin, A.P.; et al. Human gut microbiome viewed across age and geography. *Nature* **2012**, *486*, 222–227. [CrossRef] [PubMed]
24. Azad, M.B.; Konya, T.; Persaud, R.R.; Guttman, D.S.; Chari, R.S.; Field, C.J.; Sears, M.R.; Mandhane, P.J.; Turvey, S.E.; Subbarao, P.; et al. Impact of maternal intrapartum antibiotics, method of birth and breastfeeding on gut microbiota during the first year of life: A prospective cohort study. *BJOG* **2016**, *123*, 983–993. [CrossRef]
25. Knoop, K.A.; Gustafsson, J.K.; McDonald, K.G.; Kulkarni, D.H.; Coughlin, P.E.; McCrate, S.; Kim, D.; Hsieh, C.S.; Hogan, S.P.; Elson, C.O.; et al. Microbial antigen encounter during a preweaning interval is critical for tolerance to gut bacteria. *Sci. Immunol.* **2017**, *2*. [CrossRef]
26. Foca, M.; Jakob, K.; Whittier, S.; Latta, P.D.; Factor, S.; Rubenstein, D.; Saiman, L. Endemic Pseudomonas aeruginosa Infection in a Neonatal Intensive Care Unit. *N. Engl. J. Med.* **2000**, *343*, 695–700. [CrossRef]
27. Chen, H.N.; Lee, M.L.; Yu, W.K.; Lin, Y.W.; Tsao, L.Y. Late-onset Enterobacter cloacae sepsis in very-low-birth-weight neonates: Experience in a medical center. *Pediatr. Neonatol.* **2009**, *50*, 3–7. [CrossRef]
28. Hornef, M. Pathogens, commensal symbionts, and pathobionts: discovery and functional effects on the host. *ILAR J.* **2015**, *56*, 159–162. [CrossRef]
29. Kolter, J.; Henneke, P. Codevelopment of microbiota and innate immunity and the risk for Group B streptococcal disease. *Front. Immunol.* **2017**, *8*, 1497. [CrossRef]
30. Singer, J.R.; Blosser, E.G.; Zindl, C.L.; Silberger, D.J.; Conlan, S.; Laufer, V.A.; DiToro, D.; Deming, C.; Kumar, R.; Morrow, C.D.; et al. Preventing dysbiosis of the neonatal mouse intestinal microbiome protects against late-onset sepsis. *Nat. Med.* **2019**, *25*, 1772–1782. [CrossRef]
31. Sanidad, K.Z.; Zeng, M.Y. LOS in the dysbiotic gut. *Cell Host Microbe* **2020**, *27*, 11–13. [CrossRef] [PubMed]
32. Bizzarro, M.J.; Raskind, C.; Baltimore, R.S.; Gallagher, P.G. Seventy-Five years of neonatal sepsis at Yale: 1928–2003. *Pediatrics* **2005**, *116*, 595. [CrossRef] [PubMed]

33. Cole, B.K.; Scott, E.; Ilikj, M.; Bard, D.; Akins, D.R.; Dyer, D.W.; Chavez-Bueno, S. Route of infection alters virulence of neonatal septicemia Escherichia coli clinical isolates. *PLoS ONE* **2017**, *12*, e0189032. [CrossRef]
34. Sekirov, I.; Tam, N.M.; Jogova, M.; Robertson, M.L.; Li, Y.; Lupp, C.; Finlay, B.B. Antibiotic-induced perturbations of the intestinal microbiota alter host susceptibility to enteric infection. *Infect. Immun.* **2008**, *76*, 4726–4736. [CrossRef]
35. Deshmukh, H.S.; Liu, Y.; Menkiti, O.R.; Mei, J.; Dai, N.; O'Leary, C.E.; Oliver, P.M.; Kolls, J.K.; Weiser, J.N.; Worthen, G.S. The microbiota regulates neutrophil homeostasis and host resistance to Escherichia coli K1 sepsis in neonatal mice. *Nat. Med.* **2014**, *20*, 524–530. [CrossRef]
36. Vangay, P.; Ward, T.; Gerber, J.S.; Knights, D. Antibiotics, pediatric dysbiosis, and disease. *Cell Host Microbe* **2015**, *17*, 553–564. [CrossRef]
37. Bizzarro, M.J.; Dembry, L.-M.; Baltimore, R.S.; Gallagher, P.G. Changing patterns in neonatal *Escherichia coli*; sepsis and ampicillin resistance in the era of intrapartum antibiotic prophylaxis. *Pediatrics* **2008**, *121*, 689. [CrossRef]
38. Mohsen, L.; Ramy, N.; Saied, D.; Akmal, D.; Salama, N.; Abdel Haleim, M.M.; Aly, H. Emerging antimicrobial resistance in early and late-onset neonatal sepsis. *Antimicrob. Resist. Infect. Control* **2017**, *6*, 63. [CrossRef]
39. Panigrahi, P.; Parida, S.; Nanda, N.C.; Satpathy, R.; Pradhan, L.; Chandel, D.S.; Baccaglini, L.; Mohapatra, A.; Mohapatra, S.S.; Misra, P.R.; et al. A randomized synbiotic trial to prevent sepsis among infants in rural India. *Nature* **2017**, *548*, 407. [CrossRef]
40. Garrido, D.; Barile, D.; Mills, D.A. A Molecular basis for bifidobacterial enrichment in the infant gastrointestinal tract. *Adv. Nutr.* **2012**, *3*, 415S–421S. [CrossRef]
41. Sassone-Corsi, M.; Raffatellu, M. No vacancy: How beneficial microbes cooperate with immunity to provide colonization resistance to pathogens. *J. Immunol.* **2015**, *194*, 4081. [CrossRef]
42. Mugambi, M.N.; Musekiwa, A.; Lombard, M.; Young, T.; Blaauw, R. Probiotics, prebiotics infant formula use in preterm or low birth weight infants: A systematic review. *Nutr. J.* **2012**, *11*, 58. [CrossRef]
43. Aceti, A.; Gori, D.; Barone, G.; Callegari, M.L.; Fantini, M.P.; Indrio, F.; Maggio, L.; Meneghin, F.; Morelli, L.; Zuccotti, G.; et al. Probiotics and time to achieve full enteral feeding in human milk-fed and formula-fed preterm infants: systematic review and meta-analysis. *Nutrients* **2016**, *8*, 471. [CrossRef]
44. Rao, S.C.; Athalye-Jape, G.K.; Deshpande, G.C.; Simmer, K.N.; Patole, S.K. Probiotic supplementation and late-onset sepsis in preterm infants: A meta-analysis. *Pediatrics* **2016**, *137*, e20153684. [CrossRef]
45. Kanic, Z.; Micetic Turk, D.; Burja, S.; Kanic, V.; Dinevski, D. Influence of a combination of probiotics on bacterial infections in very low birthweight newborns. *Wien. Klin. Wochenschr.* **2015**, *127*, 210–215. [CrossRef]
46. Sinha, A.; Gupta, S.S.; Chellani, H.; Maliye, C.; Kumari, V.; Arya, S.; Garg, B.S.; Gaur, S.D.; Gaind, R.; Deotale, V.; et al. Role of probiotics VSL#3 in prevention of suspected sepsis in low birthweight infants in India: A randomised controlled trial. *BMJ Open* **2015**, *5*, e006564. [CrossRef]
47. Aceti, A.; Maggio, L.; Beghetti, I.; Gori, D.; Barone, G.; Callegari, M.L.; Fantini, M.P.; Indrio, F.; Meneghin, F.; Morelli, L.; et al. Probiotics prevent late-onset sepsis in human milk-fed, very low birth weight preterm infants: Systematic review and meta-analysis. *Nutrients* **2017**, *9*, 904. [CrossRef]
48. Jakaitis, B.M.; Denning, P.W. Human breast milk and the gastrointestinal innate immune system. *Clin. Perinatol.* **2014**, *41*, 423–435. [CrossRef]
49. Yeruva, L.; Spencer, N.E.; Saraf, M.K.; Hennings, L.; Bowlin, A.K.; Cleves, M.A.; Mercer, K.; Chintapalli, S.V.; Shankar, K.; Rank, R.G.; et al. Formula diet alters small intestine morphology, microbial abundance and reduces VE-cadherin and IL-10 expression in neonatal porcine model. *BMC Gastroenterol.* **2016**, *16*, 40. [CrossRef]
50. Guaraldi, F.; Salvatori, G. Effect of breast and formula feeding on gut microbiota shaping in newborns. *Front. Cell. Infect. Microbiol.* **2012**, *2*, 94. [CrossRef]
51. Goldsmith, F.; O'Sullivan, A.; Smilowitz, J.T.; Freeman, S.L. Lactation and intestinal microbiota: How early diet shapes the infant gut. *J. Mammary Gland Biol. Neoplasia* **2015**, *20*, 149–158. [CrossRef]
52. Davis, J.C.C.; Lewis, Z.T.; Krishnan, S.; Bernstein, R.M.; Moore, S.E.; Prentice, A.M.; Mills, D.A.; Lebrilla, C.B.; Zivkovic, A.M. Growth and morbidity of gambian infants are influenced by maternal milk oligosaccharides and infant gut microbiota. *Sci. Rep.* **2017**, *7*, 40466. [CrossRef]
53. Baumann-Dudenhoeffer, A.M.; D'Souza, A.W.; Tarr, P.I.; Warner, B.B.; Dantas, G. Infant diet and maternal gestational weight gain predict early metabolic maturation of gut microbiomes. *Nat. Med.* **2018**, *24*, 1822–1829. [CrossRef]

54. Taylor, S.N.; Basile, L.A.; Ebeling, M.; Wagner, C.L. Intestinal permeability in preterm infants by feeding type: Mother's milk versus formula. *Breastfeed. Med.* **2009**, *4*, 11–15. [CrossRef]
55. Saleem, B.; Okogbule-Wonodi, A.C.; Fasano, A.; Magder, L.S.; Ravel, J.; Kapoor, S.; Viscardi, R.M. Intestinal barrier maturation in very low birthweight infants: Relationship to feeding and antibiotic exposure. *J. Pediatr.* **2017**, *183*, 31–36.e31. [CrossRef]
56. Go, L.L.; Albanese, C.T.; Watkins, S.C.; Simmons, R.L.; Rowe, M.I. Breast milk protects the neonate from bacterial translocation. *J. Pediatr. Surg.* **1994**, *29*, 1059–1064. [CrossRef]
57. Yajima, M.; Nakayama, M.; Hatano, S.; Yamazaki, K.; Aoyama, Y.; Yajima, T.; Kuwata, T. Bacterial translocation in neonatal rats: The relation between intestinal flora, translocated bacteria, and influence of milk. *J. Pediatr. Gastroenterol. Nutr.* **2001**, *33*, 592–601. [CrossRef]
58. Nakayama, M.; Yajima, M.; Hatano, S.; Yajima, T.; Kuwata, T. Intestinal adherent bacteria and bacterial translocation in breast-fed and formula-fed rats in relation to susceptibility to infection. *Pediatr. Res.* **2003**, *54*, 364. [CrossRef]
59. Goldsmith, S.J.; Dickson, J.S.; Barnhart, H.M.; Toledo, R.T.; Eiten-Miller, R.R. IgA, IgG, IgM and lactoferrin contents of human milk during early lactation and the effect of processing and storage. *J. Food Prot.* **1983**, *46*, 4–7. [CrossRef]
60. Castellote, C.; Casillas, R.; Ramírez-Santana, C.; Pérez-Cano, F.J.; Castell, M.; Moretones, M.G.; López-Sabater, M.C.; Franch, À. Premature delivery influences the immunological composition of colostrum and transitional and mature human milk. *J. Nutr.* **2011**, *141*, 1181–1187. [CrossRef]
61. Bode, L.; Raman, A.S.; Murch, S.H.; Rollins, N.C.; Gordon, J.I. Understanding the mother-breastmilk-infant "triad". *Science* **2020**, *367*, 1070. [CrossRef] [PubMed]
62. Zheng, W.; Zhao, W.; Wu, M.; Song, X.; Caro, F.; Sun, X.; Gazzaniga, F.; Stefanetti, G.; Oh, S.; Mekalanos, J.J.; et al. Microbiota-targeted maternal antibodies protect neonates from enteric infection. *Nature* **2020**, *577*, 543–548. [CrossRef] [PubMed]
63. Miettinen, P.J.; Berger, J.E.; Meneses, J.; Phung, Y.; Pedersen, R.A.; Werb, Z.; Derynck, R. Epithelial immaturity and multiorgan failure in mice lacking epidermal growth factor receptor. *Nature* **1995**, *376*, 337–341. [CrossRef]
64. Knoop, K.A.; Coughlin, P.E.; Floyd, A.N.; Ndao, I.M.; Hall-Moore, C.; Shaikh, N.; Gasparrini, A.J.; Rusconi, B.; Escobedo, M.; Good, M.; et al. Maternal activation of the EGFR prevents translocation of gut-residing pathogenic Escherichia coli in a model of late-onset neonatal sepsis. *Proc. Natl. Acad. Sci. USA* **2020**. [CrossRef]
65. Vogel, H.J. Lactoferrin, a bird's eye view. *Biochem. Cell Biol.* **2012**, *90*, 233–244. [CrossRef] [PubMed]
66. Smilowitz, J.T.; Lebrilla, C.B.; Mills, D.A.; German, J.B.; Freeman, S.L. Breast milk oligosaccharides: structure-function relationships in the neonate. *Annu. Rev. Nutr.* **2014**, *34*, 143–169. [CrossRef]
67. Van de Perre, P. Transfer of antibody via mother's milk. *Vaccine* **2003**, *21*, 3374–3376. [CrossRef]
68. Capasso, L.; Borrelli, A.; Cerullo, J.; Pisanti, R.; Figliuolo, C.; Izzo, F.; Paccone, M.; Ferrara, T.; Lama, S.; Raimondi, F. Role of immunoglobulins in neonatal sepsis. *Transl. Med. Unisa* **2014**, *11*, 28–33.
69. Li, Y.; Yang, S.; Wang, G.; Liu, M.; Zhang, Z.; Liu, H.; Yu, K.; Wang, C. Effects of immunotherapy on mortality in neonates with suspected or proven sepsis: A systematic review and network meta-analysis. *BMC Pediatr.* **2019**, *19*, 270. [CrossRef]
70. Koch Meghan, A.; Reiner Gabrielle, L.; Lugo Kyler, A.; Kreuk Lieselotte, S.M.; Stanbery Alison, G.; Ansaldo, E.; Seher Thaddeus, D.; Ludington William, B.; Barton Gregory, M. Maternal IgG and IgA antibodies dampen mucosal t helper cell responses in early life. *Cell* **2016**, *165*, 827–841. [CrossRef]
71. Collins, A.; Weitkamp, J.-H.; Wynn, J.L. Why are preterm newborns at increased risk of infection? *Arch. Dis. Child. Fetal Neonatal Ed.* **2018**, *103*, F391–F394. [CrossRef]
72. Raymond, S.L.; López, M.C.; Baker, H.V.; Larson, S.D.; Efron, P.A.; Sweeney, T.E.; Khatri, P.; Moldawer, L.L.; Wynn, J.L. Unique transcriptomic response to sepsis is observed among patients of different age groups. *PLoS ONE* **2017**, *12*, e0184159. [CrossRef]
73. Wynn, J.L.; Guthrie, S.O.; Wong, H.R.; Lahni, P.; Ungaro, R.; Lopez, M.C.; Baker, H.V.; Moldawer, L.L. Postnatal age is a critical determinant of the neonatal host response to sepsis. *Mol. Med.* **2015**, *21*, 496–504. [CrossRef] [PubMed]
74. Ballard, O.; Morrow, A.L. Human milk composition: Nutrients and bioactive factors. *Pediatr. Clin. N. Am.* **2013**, *60*, 49–74. [CrossRef] [PubMed]

75. Kobata, R.; Tsukahara, H.; Ohshima, Y.; Ohta, N.; Tokuriki, S.; Tamura, S.; Mayumi, M. High levels of growth factors in human breast milk. *Early Hum. Dev.* **2008**, *84*, 67–69. [CrossRef] [PubMed]
76. Michalsky, M.P.; Lara-Marquez, M.; Chun, L.; Besner, G.E. Heparin-binding EGF-like growth factor is present in human amniotic fluid and breast milk. *J. Pediatr. Surg.* **2002**, *37*, 1–6. [CrossRef]
77. Nojiri, T.; Yoshizato, T.; Fukami, T.; Obama, H.; Yagi, H.; Yotsumoto, F.; Miyamoto, S. Clinical significance of amphiregulin and epidermal growth factor in colostrum. *Arch. Gynecol. Obs.* **2012**, *286*, 643–647. [CrossRef]
78. Matsuoka, Y.; Idota, T. The concentration of epidermal growth factor in Japanese mother's milk. *J. Nutr. Sci. Vitaminol.* **1995**, *41*, 241–251. [CrossRef]
79. Luetteke, N.C.; Qiu, T.H.; Fenton, S.E.; Troyer, K.L.; Riedel, R.F.; Chang, A.; Lee, D.C. Targeted inactivation of the EGF and amphiregulin genes reveals distinct roles for EGF receptor ligands in mouse mammary gland development. *Development* **1999**, *126*, 2739.
80. Read, L.C.; Upton, F.M.; Francis, G.L.; Wallace, J.C.; Dahlenberg, G.W.; Ballard, F.J. Changes in the growth-promoting activity of human milk during lactation. *Pediatr. Res.* **1984**, *18*, 133–139. [CrossRef]
81. Chang, C.-J.; Chao, J.C.-J. Effect of human milk and epidermal growth factor on growth of human intestinal Caco-2 cells. *J. Pediatr. Gastroenterol. Nutr.* **2002**, *34*, 394–401. [CrossRef] [PubMed]
82. Okuyama, H.; Urao, M.; Lee, D.; Drongowski, R.A.; Coran, A.G. The effect of epidermal growth factor on bacterial translocation in newborn rabbits. *J. Pediatr. Surg.* **1998**, *33*, 225–228. [CrossRef]
83. Good, M.; Sodhi, C.P.; Egan, C.E.; Afrazi, A.; Jia, H.; Yamaguchi, Y.; Lu, P.; Branca, M.F.; Ma, C.; Prindle, T., Jr.; et al. Breast milk protects against the development of necrotizing enterocolitis through inhibition of Toll-like receptor 4 in the intestinal epithelium via activation of the epidermal growth factor receptor. *Mucosal Immunol.* **2015**. [CrossRef] [PubMed]
84. Villavicencio, A.; Rueda, M.S.; Turin, C.G.; Ochoa, T.J. Factors affecting lactoferrin concentration in human milk: How much do we know? *Biochem. Cell Biol.* **2017**, *95*, 12–21. [CrossRef] [PubMed]
85. Yang, Z.; Jiang, R.; Chen, Q.; Wang, J.; Duan, Y.; Pang, X.; Jiang, S.; Bi, Y.; Zhang, H.; Lönnerdal, B.; et al. Concentration of lactoferrin in human milk and its variation during lactation in different Chinese populations. *Nutrients* **2018**, *10*, 1235. [CrossRef] [PubMed]
86. Czosnykowska-Łukacka, M.; Orczyk-Pawiłowicz, M.; Broers, B.; Królak-Olejnik, B. Lactoferrin in human milk of prolonged lactation. *Nutrients* **2019**, *11*, 2350. [CrossRef] [PubMed]
87. Bullen, J.J.; Rogers, H.J.; Leigh, L. Iron-binding proteins in milk and resistance to Escherichia coli infection in infants. *Br. Med. J.* **1972**, *1*, 69–75. [CrossRef]
88. Sherman, M.P.; Miller, M.M.; Sherman, J.; Niklas, V. Lactoferrin and necrotizing enterocolitis. *Curr. Opin. Pediatr.* **2014**, *26*, 146–150. [CrossRef]
89. Elass-Rochard, E.; Roseanu, A.; Legrand, D.; Trif, M.; Salmon, V.; Motas, C.; Montreuil, J.; Spik, G. Lactoferrin-lipopolysaccharide interaction: Involvement of the 28-34 loop region of human lactoferrin in the high-affinity binding to Escherichia coli 055B5 lipopolysaccharide. *Biochem. J.* **1995**, *312*, 839–845. [CrossRef]
90. Dijkshoorn, L.; Brouwer, C.P.; Bogaards, S.J.; Nemec, A.; Van Den Broek, P.J.; Nibbering, P.H. The synthetic N-terminal peptide of human lactoferrin, hLF (1-11), is highly effective against experimental infection caused by multidrug-resistant Acinetobacter baumannii. *Antimicrob. Agents Chemother.* **2004**, *48*, 4919–4921. [CrossRef]
91. Sherman, M.P.; Adamkin, D.H.; Radmacher, P.G.; Sherman, J.; Niklas, V. Protective Proteins in mammalian milks. *NeoReviews* **2012**, *13*, e293. [CrossRef]
92. He, Y.; Cao, L.; Yu, J. Prophylactic lactoferrin for preventing late-onset sepsis and necrotizing enterocolitis in preterm infants: A PRISMA-compliant systematic review and meta-analysis. *Med. (Baltim.)* **2018**, *97*, e11976. [CrossRef] [PubMed]
93. Sherman, M.P.; Sherman, J.; Arcinue, R.; Niklas, V. Randomized control trial of human recombinant lactoferrin: A substudy reveals effects on the fecal microbiome of very low birth weight infants. *J. Pediatr.* **2016**, *173*, S37–S42. [CrossRef] [PubMed]
94. Ochoa, T.J.; Zegarra, J.; Bellomo, S.; Carcamo, C.P.; Cam, L.; Castañeda, A.; Villavicencio, A.; Gonzales, J.; Rueda, M.S.; Turin, C.G.; et al. Randomized controlled trial of bovine lactoferrin for prevention of sepsis and neurodevelopment impairment in infants weighing less than 2000 grams. *J. Pediatr.* **2020**. [CrossRef] [PubMed]

95. Manzoni, P.; Militello, M.A.; Rizzollo, S.; Tavella, E.; Messina, A.; Pieretto, M.; Boano, E.; Carlino, M.; Tognato, E.; Spola, R.; et al. Is lactoferrin more effective in reducing late-onset sepsis in preterm neonates fed formula than in those receiving mother's own milk? Secondary analyses of two multicenter randomized controlled trials. *Am. J. Perinatol.* **2019**, *36*, S120–S125. [CrossRef] [PubMed]
96. Doyle, L.W.; Cheong, J.L.Y. Does bovine lactoferrin prevent late-onset neonatal sepsis? *Lancet* **2019**, *393*, 382–384. [CrossRef]
97. Blanton, L.V.; Charbonneau, M.R.; Salih, T.; Barratt, M.J.; Venkatesh, S.; Ilkaveya, O.; Subramanian, S.; Manary, M.J.; Trehan, I.; Jorgensen, J.M.; et al. Gut bacteria that prevent growth impairments transmitted by microbiota from malnourished children. *Science* **2016**, *351*. [CrossRef]
98. Kim, Y.-G.; Sakamoto, K.; Seo, S.-U.; Pickard, J.M.; Gillilland, M.G.; Pudlo, N.A.; Hoostal, M.; Li, X.; Wang, T.D.; Feehley, T.; et al. Neonatal acquisition of Clostridiaspecies protects against colonization by bacterial pathogens. *Science* **2017**, *356*, 315. [CrossRef]
99. Feng, L.; Raman, A.S.; Hibberd, M.C.; Cheng, J.; Griffin, N.W.; Peng, Y.; Leyn, S.A.; Rodionov, D.A.; Osterman, A.L.; Gordon, J.I. Identifying determinants of bacterial fitness in a model of human gut microbial succession. *Proc. Natl. Acad. Sci. USA* **2020**, *117*, 2622. [CrossRef]
100. Moossavi, S.; Atakora, F.; Miliku, K.; Sepehri, S.; Robertson, B.; Duan, Q.L.; Becker, A.B.; Mandhane, P.J.; Turvey, S.E.; Moraes, T.J.; et al. Integrated analysis of human milk microbiota with oligosaccharides and fatty acids in the child cohort. *Front. Nutr.* **2019**, *6*. [CrossRef]
101. Thurl, S.; Munzert, M.; Henker, J.; Boehm, G.; Müller-Werner, B.; Jelinek, J.; Stahl, B. Variation of human milk oligosaccharides in relation to milk groups and lactational periods. *Br. J. Nutr.* **2010**, *104*, 1261–1271. [CrossRef] [PubMed]
102. Kunz, C.; Meyer, C.; Collado, M.C.; Geiger, L.; García-Mantrana, I.; Bertua-Ríos, B.; Martínez-Costa, C.; Borsch, C.; Rudloff, S. Influence of gestational age, secretor, and lewis blood group status on the oligosaccharide content of human milk. *J. Pediatr. Gastroenterol. Nutr.* **2017**, *64*, 789–798. [CrossRef] [PubMed]
103. Engfer, M.B.; Stahl, B.; Finke, B.; Sawatzki, G.; Daniel, H. Human milk oligosaccharides are resistant to enzymatic hydrolysis in the upper gastrointestinal tract. *Am. J. Clin. Nutr.* **2000**, *71*, 1589–1596. [CrossRef] [PubMed]
104. Underwood, M.A.; Davis, J.C.C.; Kalanetra, K.M.; Gehlot, S.; Patole, S.; Tancredi, D.J.; Mills, D.A.; Lebrilla, C.B.; Simmer, K. Digestion of human milk oligosaccharides by bifidobacterium breve in the premature infant. *J. Pediatr. Gastroenterol. Nutr.* **2017**, *65*, 449–455. [CrossRef] [PubMed]
105. Ackerman, D.L.; Doster, R.S.; Weitkamp, J.-H.; Aronoff, D.M.; Gaddy, J.A.; Townsend, S.D. Human milk oligosaccharides exhibit antimicrobial and antibiofilm properties against group b streptococcus. *ACS Infect. Dis.* **2017**, *3*, 595–605. [CrossRef] [PubMed]
106. Wu, R.Y.; Li, B.; Koike, Y.; Määttänen, P.; Miyake, H.; Cadete, M.; Johnson-Henry, K.C.; Botts, S.R.; Lee, C.; Abrahamsson, T.R.; et al. Human milk oligosaccharides increase mucin expression in experimental necrotizing enterocolitis. *Mol. Nutr. Food Res.* **2019**, *63*, 1800658. [CrossRef]
107. Cheng, L.; Kong, C.; Walvoort, M.T.C.; Faas, M.M.; de Vos, P. Human milk oligosaccharides differently modulate goblet cells under homeostatic, proinflammatory conditions and ER stress. *Mol. Nutr. Food Res.* **2020**, *64*, e1900976. [CrossRef]
108. Bode, L.; Kunz, C.; Muhly-Reinholz, M.; Mayer, K.; Seeger, W.; Rudloff, S. Inhibition of monocyte, lymphocyte, and neutrophil adhesion to endothelial cells by human milk oligosaccharides. *Thromb. Haemost.* **2004**, *92*, 1402–1410. [CrossRef]
109. Bode, L.; Rudloff, S.; Kunz, C.; Strobel, S.; Klein, N. Human milk oligosaccharides reduce platelet-neutrophil complex formation leading to a decrease in neutrophil beta 2 integrin expression. *J. Leukoc. Biol.* **2004**, *76*, 820–826. [CrossRef]
110. Noll, A.J.; Yu, Y.; Lasanajak, Y.; Duska-McEwen, G.; Buck, R.H.; Smith, D.F.; Cummings, R.D. Human DC-SIGN binds specific human milk glycans. *Biochem. J.* **2016**, *473*, 1343–1353. [CrossRef]
111. Donovan, S.M.; Comstock, S.S. Human milk oligosaccharides influence neonatal mucosal and systemic immunity. *Ann. Nutr. Metab.* **2016**, *69* (Suppl. 2), 42–51. [CrossRef] [PubMed]
112. Triantis, V.; Bode, L.; van Neerven, R.J.J. Immunological effects of human milk oligosaccharides. *Front. Pediatr.* **2018**, *6*, 190. [CrossRef] [PubMed]

113. Morrow, A.L.; Meinzen-Derr, J.; Huang, P.; Schibler, K.R.; Cahill, T.; Keddache, M.; Kallapur, S.G.; Newburg, D.S.; Tabangin, M.; Warner, B.B.; et al. Fucosyltransferase 2 non-secretor and low secretor status predicts severe outcomes in premature infants. *J. Pediatr.* **2011**, *158*, 745–751. [CrossRef] [PubMed]
114. Wejryd, E.; Martí, M.; Marchini, G.; Werme, A.; Jonsson, B.; Landberg, E.; Abrahamsson, T.R. Low diversity of human milk oligosaccharides is associated with necrotising enterocolitis in extremely low birth weight infants. *Nutrients* **2018**, *10*, 1556. [CrossRef] [PubMed]
115. Bering, S.B. Human milk oligosaccharides to prevent gut dysfunction and necrotizing enterocolitis in preterm neonates. *Nutrients* **2018**, *10*, 1461. [CrossRef]
116. Demers-Mathieu, V.; Huston, R.K.; Markell, A.M.; McCulley, E.A.; Martin, R.L.; Spooner, M.; Dallas, D.C. Differences in maternal immunoglobulins within mother's own breast milk and donor breast milk and across digestion in preterm infants. *Nutrients* **2019**, *11*, 920. [CrossRef]
117. Cossey, V.; Cossey, V.; Vanhole, C.; Eerdekens, A.; Rayyan, M.; Fieuws, S.; Schuermans, A. Pasteurization of mother's own milk for preterm infants does not reduce the incidence of late-onset sepsis. *Neonatology* **2013**, *103*, 170–176. [CrossRef]
118. Czank, C.; Prime, D.K.; Hartmann, B.; Simmer, K.; Hartmann, P.E. Retention of the immunological proteins of pasteurized human milk in relation to pasteurizer design and practice. *Pediatr. Res.* **2009**, *66*, 374–379. [CrossRef]
119. Peila, C.; Moro, G.E.; Bertino, E.; Cavallarin, L.; Giribaldi, M.; Giuliani, F.; Cresi, F.; Coscia, A. The effect of holder pasteurization on nutrients and biologically-active components in donor human milk: A review. *Nutrients* **2016**, *8*, 477. [CrossRef]
120. Baro, C.; Giribaldi, M.; Arslanoglu, S.; Giuffrida, M.G.; Dellavalle, G.; Conti, A.; Tonetto, P.; Biasini, A.; Coscia, A.; Fabris, C.; et al. Effect of two pasteurization methods on the protein content of human milk. *Front. Biosci. (Elite Ed.)* **2011**, *3*, 818–829. [CrossRef]
121. Escuder-Vieco, D.; Espinosa-Martos, I.; Rodríguez, J.M.; Fernández, L.; Pallás-Alonso, C.R. Effect of HTST and holder pasteurization on the concentration of immunoglobulins, growth factors, and hormones in donor human milk. *Front. Immunol.* **2018**, *9*, 2222. [CrossRef] [PubMed]

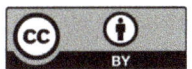

© 2020 by the authors. Licensee MDPI, Basel, Switzerland. This article is an open access article distributed under the terms and conditions of the Creative Commons Attribution (CC BY) license (http://creativecommons.org/licenses/by/4.0/).

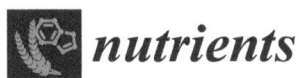 

Article

# Oropharyngeal Colostrum Positively Modulates the Inflammatory Response in Preterm Neonates

Estefanía Martín-Álvarez [1], Javier Diaz-Castro [2,3,*], Manuela Peña-Caballero [1], Laura Serrano-López [1], Jorge Moreno-Fernández [2,3], Belen Sánchez-Martínez [1], Francisca Martín-Peregrina [1], Mercedes Alonso-Moya [1], José Maldonado-Lozano [4,5], Jose A. Hurtado-Suazo [1] and Julio J. Ochoa [2,3]

[1] Unit of Neonatology, Pediatric Service, Hospital Universitario Materno-Infantil Virgen de las Nieves, 18014 Granada, Spain; estenia.martin.alvarez@gmail.com (E.M.-Á.); mapeca06@yahoo.es (M.P.-C.); lserranolopez@hotmail.com (L.S.-L.); belensamar@gmail.com (B.S.-M.); paquimarpe@gmail.com (F.M.-P.); malonsomo@gmail.com (M.A.-M.); jahsuazo@yahoo.es (J.A.H.-S.)
[2] Department of Physiology, University of Granada, 18071 Granada, Spain; jorgemf@ugr.es (J.M.-F.); jjoh@ugr.es (J.J.O.)
[3] Institute of Nutrition and Food Technology "José Mataix Verdú", University of Granada, 18071 Granada, Spain
[4] Pediatrics Department, Virgen de las Nieves University Hospital, University of Granada, 18071 Granada, Spain; jmaldon@ugr.es
[5] Institute of Biosanitary Research of Granada, Maternal and Child Health Network, Carlos III Institute, 28020 Madrid, Spain
* Correspondence: javierdc@ugr.es; Tel.: +34-958-241-000 (ext. 20303)

Received: 16 December 2019; Accepted: 1 February 2020; Published: 5 February 2020

**Abstract:** During the first days of life, premature infants have physiological difficulties swallowing, thereby missing out on the benefits of breastfeeding. The aim of this study is to assess the effects of oropharyngeal mother's milk administration in the inflammatory signaling of extremely premature infants. Neonates ($n = 100$) (<32 week's gestation and/or <1500 g) were divided into two groups: mother's milk group ($n = 48$), receiving 0.2 mL of oropharyngeal mother's milk every 4 h for the first 15 days of life, and a control group ($n = 52$), not receiving oropharyngeal mother's milk. Serum concentrations of interleukin (IL) IL-6, IL-8, IL-10, IL-1ra, tumor necrosis factor alpha (TNF-$\alpha$), and interferón gamma (IFN-$\gamma$) were assessed at 1, 3, 15, and 30 days of postnatal life. Maternal and neonatal outcomes were collected. The rate of common neonatal morbidities in both groups was similar. The mother's milk group achieved full enteral feeding earlier, and showed a decrease in Il-6 on days 15 and 30, in IL-8 on day 30, and in TNF-$\alpha$ and INF-$\gamma$ on day 15, as well as an increase in IL-1ra on days 3 and 15 and in IL-10 on day 30. Oropharyngeal mother's milk administration for 15 days decreases the pro-inflammatory state of preterm neonates and provides full enteral nutrition earlier, which could have a positive influence on the development of the immune system and inflammatory response, thereby positively influencing other developmental outcomes.

**Keywords:** colostrum administration; premature neonates; inflammation; clinical outcomes

---

## 1. Introduction

Inflammation is implicated in a high proportion of preterm births [1], and is associated with fetal inflammatory response syndrome (FIRS). This syndrome is characterized by systemic inflammation and is associated with the development of long-term sequelae by multifunctional organic failures such as sepsis neonatal, bronchopulmonary dysplasia, intraventricular hemorrhage, and necrotizing enterocolitis (NEC), thereby increasing perinatal and neonatal mortality and morbidity [2]. During pregnancy, especially in preterm neonates, several developing tissues are especially vulnerable and are profoundly affected by cytokines that circulate rapidly through fetal blood, potentially causing inflammatory signaling, which can trigger intracellular signaling cascades that result in organ damage and neonatal morbidity [3]. Under these conditions, the most vulnerable tissues are lung, brain, and intestine [4,5]. Taking into account the importance of inflammation regarding morbidity and/or neonatal mortality, it is important to obtain all possible information about inflammatory signaling in newborns [6–9].

Mother's milk is the best first immune stimulator in infants, featuring the perfect species-specific nutrition, because it contains many types of protective agents and enhances neurodevelopmental outcomes [10,11]. These effects are attributed to a multitude of protective (immune and trophic) biofactors [11–13]. Milk biofactors protect against infection, providing antimicrobial, anti-inflammatory, and immunomodulatory functions, preventing adherence to the gastrointestinal mucosa of pathogens, improving gastrointestinal microbiota, keeping the integrity of the intestinal barrier and repairing injured areas, promoting intestinal motility and maturation, and providing antioxidant defense [10,12,13].

Despite the importance of breastfeeding in the development of the newborn's immune system, in some cases, this feeding is not possible in the first days of life, especially in premature infants, due, among others causes, to the existence of physiological difficulties in swallowing. Therefore, it is of great interest to search for noninvasive mechanisms that allow these neonates to receive the advantages of breast milk; the administration of oropharyngeal mother's milk is a safe and well tolerated intervention with many clinical benefits. In this clinical intervention, with even extremely preterm babies [14,15], small volumes of mother's milk, especially colostrum, are directly dropped onto the oropharyngeal mucosa [16]. Although many studies support the clinical implications of this safe clinical intervention, there is scarce evidence of its effects on inflammatory signaling and/or its clinical benefits. It is therefore necessary to increase the study population in order to draw more reliable conclusions [15,17,18]. In addition, to date, published studies have supplied colostrum only during the first days of life and in preterm infants of less than 28 weeks' gestation. For to these reasons, it is necessary to deepen our understanding and clarify the clinical implications related to this practice; therefore, the aim of this study is to assess the effects of oropharyngeal administration of mother's milk. This is the first study to characterize the serum pro- and anti-inflammatory biomarker profiles of extremely premature infants.

## 2. Methods

### 2.1. Experimental Design and Subjects

Informed consent was obtained from the parents before they participated in the study. The study was conducted in accordance with the Declaration of Helsinki, and the protocol was approved by the Ethics Committee of the University Hospital "Virgen de las Nieves" (PI-0374-2014). Inclusion criteria were extremely preterm infants in the Neonatal Intensive Care Unit with <32 weeks' gestation and/or with a weight below 1500 g at birth. Exclusion criteria were chromosomopathies or congenital abnormalities, consumption or intake more than 10 mcg/kg/min of vasoconstrictive drugs, and/or HIV-positive mother. Neonates ($n = 100$) were divided into two groups: the mother's milk group ($n = 48$) receiving mother's milk via oropharynx, and the control group ($n = 52$), which did not receive oropharyngeal mother's milk, because it was not available in the first 24 h of life. Figure 1 shows the flowchart of the infants involved in this study and the reasons for the dropouts.

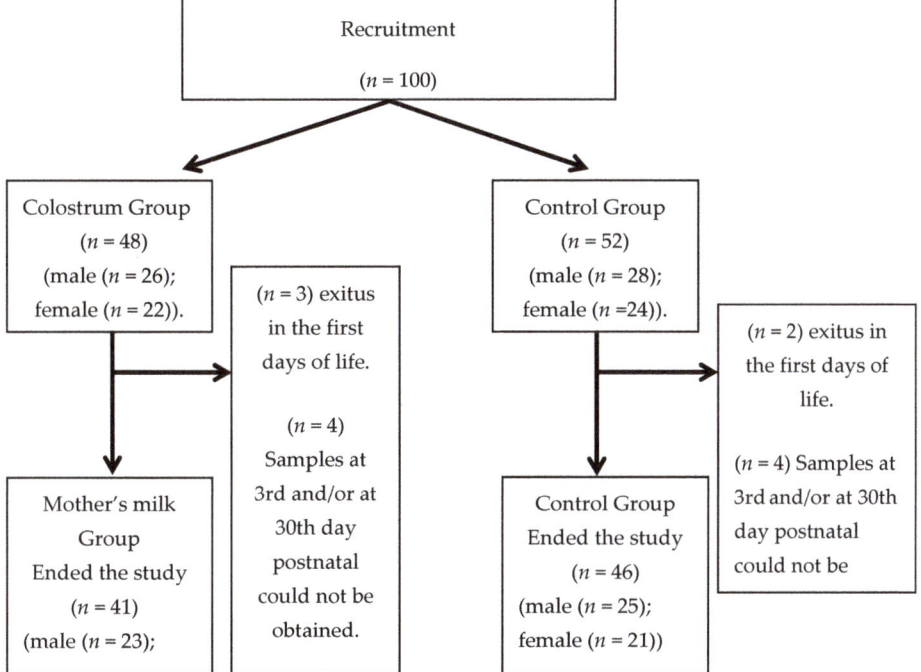

**Figure 1.** Flowchart showing participant progress and dropouts in the study.

*2.2. Milk Sampling and Administration*

The protocol for obtaining and administering breast milk has been previously described [19]. After being informed by the researchers in the first 24 h postpartum, the mothers had to obtain mother's milk every 2 to 3 h by electric pumping (Mendela, Baar, Switzerland) (at least eight times every 24 h). Mother's milk was collected in prelabeled, sterile vials, and then a trained nurse administered the milk to the neonates through sterile syringes (BD, Franklin Lakes, NJ, USA) via the oropharyngeal route. Each day, syringes were prepared with 0.2 mL mother's milk, labelled, and stored at 4 °C in labelled plastic cups. Prior to the administration of the milk, the syringe was heated for 5 min in the infant's incubator. For at least 2 min, the nurse administered 100 µL of the mother's milk on one side of the oral mucosa, and then another 100 µL on the other side in order to maximize oropharynx absorption (a total of 200 µL). The intervention was repeated every 4 h for the next 15 days. During the intervention, neonatal welfare was monitored, controlling any sign of discomfort (tachycardia, bradycardia, tachypnoea, bradypnea, $PO_2$, and changes in blood pressure), and in case of alterations, the procedure stopped. The enteral nutrition of each patient, regardless of the assigned group, was decided by the medical team responsible for their care. The trophic enteral nutrition began in the first 24–48 h, i.e., as soon as possible, if there were no contraindications.

*2.3. Sample Collection and Analysis*

Four blood samples were obtained during the first 30 days of postnatal life to evaluate the influence on the inflammatory signaling: at enrolment (M1), on the 3rd day (M2), on the 15th day (M3) and on the 30th day (M4). The serum was stored after being aliquoted at −80 °C until further use.

*2.4. Maternal and Neonatal Outcomes*

Mother variables comprised type of birth, prenatal corticosteroids, prenatal antibiotics, prenatal amniotic infection risk, preterm outcomes (sex, Apgar score, weight, height and head circumference at birth, weight gaining first month and Clinical Risk Index for Babies (CRIB)), time to achieve enteral feeding (at least 100–120 mL/kg/day), volume of enteral feeding, volume of parenteral feeding, and modifications in cerebral ultrasound (classification by de Vries et al. [20]), NEC grade greater or equal to II according to the modified Bell' staging classification [21], or proven sepsis [22].

*2.5. Inflammatory Parameters Measurement*

The pro- and anti-inflammatory parameters studied (IL-6, IL-8, IL-10, IL-1ra, TNF-α, and IFN-γ) were determined using a Multiplex panel (Human Sepsis Magnetic Bead Panel 3, HTH17MAG- 14K) based on the luminex xMAP technology (Merck Millipore, Boston, MA, USA). Cytokine concentrations in plasma samples were determined by comparing the mean of duplicate samples with the standard curve for each assay.

*2.6. Statistical Analysis*

The results are presented as the mean ± standard error of mean (SEM). The sample size calculation has been previously described [19]. The Kolmogorov-Smirnoff's and Levene's tests were used to check the normality and homogeneity of variance, respectively. To compare the baseline characteristics between the case and control groups, the Student $t$ test for independent samples or Mann-Whitney test were used for the numerical variables in case of nonnormality. Categorical variables were checked using the chi-square Pearson or Fisher test when the conditions of applicability were not met. To assess the effect of the oropharyngeal administration and the time evolution for each variable studied in each group, a general linear model for repeated measures procedure was applied, with Bonferroni correction for multiple comparisons (the $p$-values were corrected considering six possible comparisons). A Bonferrini's test allowed us to determine the intra- and inter- subject differences. A value of $p < 0.05$ was considered significant. The SPSS version 21.0 (SPSS Statistics for Windows, SPSS INC., Chicago, IL, USA) software was used for data analysis.

## 3. Results

*3.1. Maternal and Neonatal General Characteristics*

Neonatal and maternal general characteristics are shown in Table 1. No differences were recorded in the different period of the study for the mothers or neonates, including volumes of enteral and parenteral feeding supplied in the different periods of study. Regarding sex differences, there were no significant differences between groups. In relation to smoking, we have no record that mothers smoked during pregnancy, according to the records in the anamnesis of the mothers.

**Table 1.** Maternal and neonatal general characteristics.

| Maternal and Neonatal Characteristics | Units | Mother's Milk Group | Control Group | p-Value |
|---|---|---|---|---|
| Type of birth | Vaginal (%) | 47.5 | 34.8 | 0.33 |
|  | Cesarean (%) | 52.5 | 65.2 |  |
| Prenatal corticosteroids | No (%) | 12.5 | 10.9 | 0.47 |
|  | Yes (%) | 89.1 | 87.5 |  |
| Prenatal antibiotics | No (%) | 20.5 | 15.2 | 0.49 |
|  | Yes (%) | 76.9 | 84.8 |  |
| Prenatal amniotic infection risk * | No (%) | 32.5 | 39.1 | 0.41 |
|  | Yes (%) | 67.5 | 60.9% |  |
| Gestational age (weeks) |  | 29.9 ± 0.4 | 29.5 ± 0.3 | 0.34 |
| Sex | Male (%) | 60.0 | 56.5% | 0.91 |
|  | Female (%) | 40.0 | 43.5% |  |
| Apgar 1 | min | 6.4 ± 0.3 | 6.6 ± 0.3 | 0.65 |
| Apgar 5 | min | 8.1 ± 0.2 | 8.1 ± 0.2 | 0.83 |
| Weight | g | 1230.1 ± 48.2 | 1267.6 ± 52.4 | 0.60 |
| Height | cm | 38.6 ± 0.5 | 38.4 ± 0.7 | 0.69 |
| Head circumference | cm | 27.1 ± 0.4 | 27.0 ± 0.4 | 0.83 |
| Weight gaining first month | g | 612.9 ± 31.7 | 527.4 ± 49.2 | 0.06 |
| CRIB Score |  | 2.2 ± 0.4 | 2.0 ± 0.4 | 0.17 |
| Enteral Feeding | mL/kg/day |  |  |  |
| M2 |  | 39.1 ± 3.8 | 34.5 ± 4.4 | 0.53 |
| M3 |  | 152.1 ± 9.9 | 162.2 ± 6.3 | 0.21 |
| M4 |  | 160.8 ± 5.7 | 166.8 ± 8.3 | 0.84 |
| Parenteral Feeding | (mL/kg/day) |  |  |  |
| M2 |  | 84.8 ± 5.6 | 82.4 ± 5.6 | 0.92 |
| M3 |  | 19.3 ± 9.0 | 12.2 ± 4.2 | 0.15 |
| M4 |  | 7.5 ± 5.2 | 6.3 ± 4.2 | 0.54 |

Values are means ± standard error of the mean. CRIB (Clinical Risk Index for Babies); * Prenatal amniotic infection risk (Chorioamnionitis, maternal colonization of group streptococci (GBS), premature rupture of membranes, maternal fever in delivery). M2: 3rd day of postnatal life, M3: 15th day of postnatal life, M4: 30th day postnatal of life.

### 3.2. Clinical Outcomes

The clinical outcomes of preterm infants are featured in Table 2. Babies receiving mother's milk achieved full enteral feeding sooner than the control group ($p < 0.05$).

**Table 2.** Clinical outcomes at the time of discharge.

| Clinical outcomes | Mother's Milk Group | Control Group | p-Value |
|---|---|---|---|
| Days to achieve full enteral feeding * | 7.2 ± 0.6 | 9.1 ± 0.7 | 0.04 |
| Volume of full enteral feeding (mL) * | 118.9 ± 5.3 | 107.8 ± 5.7 | 0.38 |
| NEC at the end of the study (Bell stage ≥ 2) | 2 (4.9%) | 2 (4.3%) | 1 |
| Proven Sepsis at the end of the study | 3 (7.3%) | 2 (4.4%) | 0.66 |
| MV during 1st month of life | 9 (21.9%) | 13 (28.2%) | 0.72 |
| Abnormalities in ultrasound brain scan at 1st month of life | 14 (34.1%) | 10 (21.7%) | 0.11 |

* Data expressed as means ± standard error of the mean. NEC: necrotizing enterecolitis, MV: mechanical ventilation.

### 3.3. Pro- and Anti-Inflammatory Interleukins

Serum pro- and anti-inflammatory interleukins are summarized in Figure 2. IL-6 was lower after 15 and 30 days of postnatal life in the mother's milk group compared to the control group ($p < 0.05$) (Figure 2A). With regard to the evolution in both groups, a decrease was observed in M3 and M4, compared to M1 and M2 ($p < 0.05$), and in the mother's milk group, a decrease in M2 with regard to M1 was also observed ($p < 0.05$). IL-8 was lower in the first month of life in the oropharyngeal mother's milk compared to the control group ($p < 0.05$). In addition, IL-8 decreased in the mother's milk group after 30 days postnatal life compared to M1 and M2 ($p < 0.05$); in the control group, this decrease was also observed in M4, but compared with M1 and M3 ($p < 0.05$) (Figure 2B).

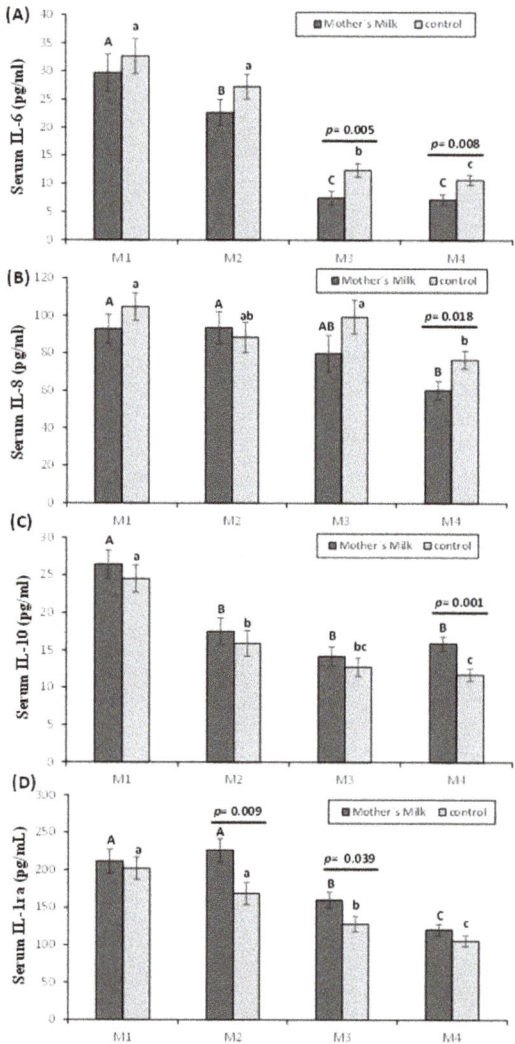

**Figure 2.** Effect of oropharyngeal mother's milk administration on the levels of IL-6 (**A**), IL-8 (**B**), IL-10 (**C**), and IL1-ra (**D**) in serum. Results are expressed as mean ± standard error of the mean. A line between bars means statistically significant differences between groups ($p < 0.05$). Different letters in every group indicate significant differences due to the time (mother's milk (A, B, C), control (a, b, c) ($p < 0.05$)). M1: Birth (basal value), M2: 3rd day of postnatal life; M3: 15th day of postnatal life, M4: 30th day of postnatal life.

The mother's milk group showed higher IL-10 levels, being statistically significant after 1 month ($p < 0.05$). IL-10 was lower in M2, M3, and M4 compared to M1 in the mother's milk group ($p < 0.05$). In the control group, a significant decrease was observed in M4 compared to M1 and M2 ($p < 0.05$), and in M3 compared to M1 ($p < 0.05$) (Figure 2C). IL-1ra levels (Figure 2D) were lower in the control group compared to the mother's milk group, being statistically significant in M2 and M3 ($p < 0.05$). IL-1ra in both groups followed the same trend, decreasing in M4 compared to M1, M2, and M3 ($p < 0.05$), and in M3 compared to M1 and M2 ($p < 0.05$).

### 3.4. Other Cytokines: TNF-α and INF-γ

Figure 3 shows the values of TNF-α (Figure 3A) and INF-γ (Figure 3B). These cytokines were higher in the control group at 15 days postpartum compared to those in the mother's milk group ($p < 0.05$). Both cytokines showed no differences in their evolution in the mother's milk group; however, in the control group, an increase in M3 was observed when comparing to M1 and M4 in both cytokines ($p < 0.05$), and in M2 compared to M1 in TNF-α ($p < 0.05$).

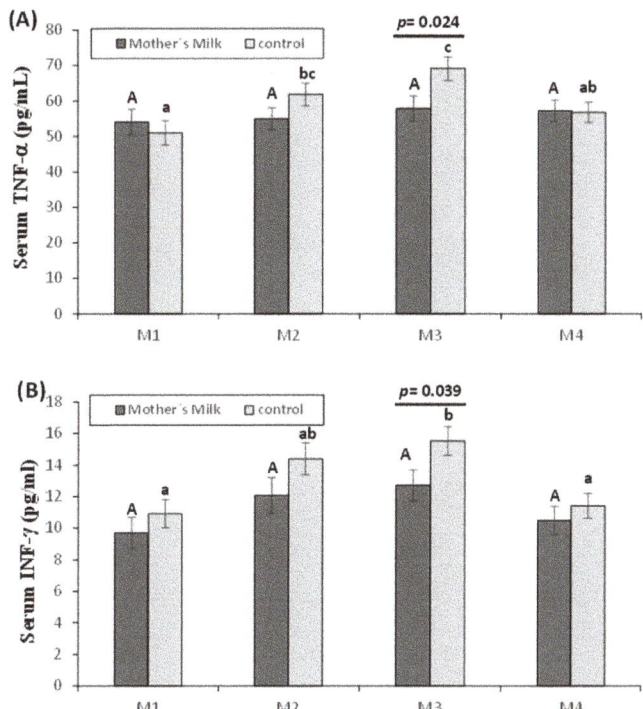

**Figure 3.** Effect of oropharyngeal mother's milk administration on the levels of TNF-α (**A**) and INF-γ (**B**) in serum. Results are expressed as mean ± standard error of the mean. A line between bars means statistically significant differences between groups ($p < 0.05$). Different letters in every group indicate significant differences due to the time (mother's milk (A, B, C), control (a, b, c) ($p < 0.05$)). M1: Birth (basal value), M2: 3rd day of postnatal life, M3: 15th day of postnatal life, M4: 30th day of postnatal life.

## 4. Discussion

Breast milk, especially mother's milk, is the perfect species-specific nutrition for preterm infants, because it has different types of bioprotective agents; however, in some cases, breastfeeding is limited, and the administration of oropharyngeal mother's milk has been shown to be a safe means of providing part of its benefits to premature newborns [19,23]. However, there are still limitations and controversies in the scientific literature, because the results are often inconclusive due to small sample sizes [14], the use of animal models [24], and the use of secretions (urine and saliva) instead of blood [14,15,17] to perform the assessments. Taking into account these limitations, together with the lack of information about inflammatory signaling, the current study was designed to include a high number of premature neonates, being the first such study to characterize the pro- and anti-inflammatory biomarker profiles of premature neonates in serum, as opposed to in other secretions such as urine and saliva after the administration of mother's milk, which strengths the results presented herein.

One of the controversies observed in the literature is focused on the time to achieve complete enteral nutrition after the administration of oropharyngeal mother's milk; in this sense, the study conducted by Rodriguez et al. [25] reports differences between groups; in contrast, Zhang et al. [15] did not observe such differences. However, in all cases, the studies were performed with a smaller population than the current study. In the current study, preterm infants receiving mother's milk achieved full enteral nutrition earlier than the control group. These results are noteworthy, because the inability to obtain enteral nutrition in the first days of life leads to villous atrophy and delayed nutrient absorption, increasing the risk of inflammation, NEC, and hospital-related infections [14]. In this sense, the oropharyngeal administration of mother's milk could be considered a potential "immune therapy" for preterm neonates during the first days of life in which they have little tolerance for enteral feeding.

In relation to inflammatory signaling, the main focus of this study, we observed that preterm neonates who received oropharyngeal mother's milk showed lower levels of pro-inflammatory cytokines (IL-6, IL-8) and higher expression of anti-inflammatory cytokines (IL-10 and IL-1ra). The only study on this topic to date with a similar number of cytokines did not show many differences between the two study groups [17], although the measurements were performed on urine and saliva, with a smaller population and a shorter administration period.

Inflammation is involved in a significant number of preterm births, despite of the presence or absence of infection [1]; it is related to the development of fetal inflammatory response syndrome, which is associated with the development to long-term sequelae due to multifunctional organ compromise such as neonatal sepsis, bronchopulmonary dysplasia, intraventricular hemorrhage, NEC, etc. [2]. Therefore, systemic inflammation in newborns could be considered an independent risk factor of morbidity, affecting several organs such as lung, intestine, and brain [2,26].

One of the most studied pro-inflammatory cytokines is IL-6, which has pleiotropic effects involving the activation of the acute phase of the immune response; it has also been used as a hallmark of the fetal inflammatory response syndrome and early neonatal sepsis [27]. This cytokine decreased progressively in all the neonates in the current study, reflecting the development of the immune system and the adaptive response of the neonate to the extrauterine conditions. However, the preterm neonates receiving oropharyngeal milk for one month showed a higher decrease of this cytokine from the 15th day of life, which could represent an advantage for preterm neonates, because inflammation is a common upstream pathway observed in major perinatal diseases [2,26].

Another early marker of neonatal sepsis is IL-8, a proinflammatory and chemotactic cytokine, which increases its expression in situations of homeostatic alterations caused by infection, trauma, and other conditions [28,29]. An important component in the inflammatory response and innate immune system is the capacity of IL-8 to attract neutrophils; therefore, the decrease recorded in preterm neonates after one month of mother's milk administration indicates a positive influence on the neonate's developing immune system and inflammatory response. Lee et al. [17] also observed a decrease in the levels of IL-8, although this was recorded in saliva and in the first 15 days of life. One of the possible causes of this lower expression is a decrease in the stimulation of this cytokine due to the increase in the Il-1ra observed in the current study, which blocks the stimulation of IL-8 by IL-1β [30].

The cytokine IL-10, as an immune-regulator, suppresses antigen-specific T-cell proliferation and inhibits Th1 responses, increasing the survival and proliferation of B cells. Although its concentration in mother's milk is not too high, its level does not decline in human milk over time [31], helping preterm neonates to cope with the inflammation that is triggered by several stressors. In addition, mother's milk from mothers delivering preterm babies is more caloric and contains higher levels of protein, fat, and bioactive factors including IL-10 [32]. Reports about this cytokine show some controversy, and in this sense, high concentrations of IL-10 in serum are related to greater severity of pathologies such as respiratory distress [33]; however, low levels of IL-10 have been associated with an increased risk of developing bronchopulmonary dysplasia [33]. In addition, it has been shown to be an important inflammatory mediator in neonatal sepsis, since it plays an important role in the prevention of excess in the inflammatory response during this life-threatening clinical condition. In our study, we observed a higher IL-10 concentration in the mother's milk group at 30 days of age, which, together with the decrease in IL-6, could have a beneficial effect, since it has been observed that a high IL-6/IL-10 ratio is found in patients with worse prognoses [29]. Similar reports to the current study did not report any effect of the administration of mother's milk on this cytokine, although the population and time of mother's milk administration were smaller [17].

Another pro-inflammatory cytokine is TNF-$\alpha$, which acts as one of the main mediators of septic shock in neonates, as well as other tissue damage. Its production is defective in term neonates [29], and its receptors in their soluble forms, TNF-RI and TNF-RII, are present in human milk [34]. In the current study, we observed an increase of TNF-$\alpha$ in the control group until day 15 of life, which could reflect the inflammatory response syndrome in the premature newborn. However, this increase was not observed in the mother's milk group, which showed a lower concentration at 15 days of age. According to Castellote et al. [35], TNF-RI levels in mother's milk can act by regulating the biological effect of TNF-$\alpha$; therefore, it is responsible for some of the anti-inflammatory effects of mother's milk.

Finally, IFN-$\gamma$ in the control group showed a similar trend to that shown by TNF-$\alpha$ with an increase until day 15 that was not observed in the mother's milk group. From the point of view of the preterm survival rate, this IFN-$\gamma$ downstream would be clearly beneficial, because in a study of ventilated preterm infants, the IFN-$\gamma$ level was higher within the first 48 h of life in infants that developed bronchopulmonary dysplasia or died [36,37].

Additionally, together with the beneficial effects on the inflammatory signaling that could be obtained by the administration of oropharyngeal mother's milk, preterm neonates receiving this clinical intervention achieved complete enteral nutrition sooner. The lower time to reach full enteral nutrition influences populations of beneficial microorganisms in the infant gut [38], improving the colonization of bacteria and the development of the preterm digestive system, resulting in a decreased release of cytokines, which may positively influence clinical outcomes.

As a secondary objective, in this study, we assessed the effect of oropharyngeal mother's milk on the incidence of NEC, proven sepsis, and other clinical outcomes. Our results show an absence of difference between the groups. We consider that this absence is due to the low prevalence of these pathologies, that would require a higher number of premature infants.

## 5. Conclusions

The current study proposes that the administration of oropharyngeal mother's milk in the first month of life contributes to decreasing the pro-inflammatory state of the preterm neonate, indicating a beneficial influence on the inflammatory response. Moreover, preterm infants receiving mother's milk via oropharynx achieved complete enteral nutrition sooner than babies who did not, representing a metabolic advantage for the underdeveloped gastrointestinal system; this could minimize comorbidities linked to nutrient absorption in this population. These findings have implications for the development of the preterm neonate, wherein inflammation plays a pathophysiological role, associated with adverse neonatal outcomes independently of the duration of gestation.

**Author Contributions:** E.M.-Á. and J.D.-C. drafted the initial manuscript and participated in the analysis. M.P.-C., L.S.-L., J.M.-L. and J.M.-F. carried out the analyses, reviewed and revised the manuscript. B.S.-M., F.M.-P. and M.A.-M. participated in data collection process. J.A.H.-S. designed the data collection instruments and coordinated and supervised data collection at Unit of Neonatology, Pediatric Service, Hospital Universitario Materno-Infantil and critically reviewed the manuscript. J.J.O. conceptualized and designed the study, coordinated and supervised data collection at Institute of Nutrition and Department of Physiology. All authors have read and agreed to the published version of the manuscript.

**Acknowledgments:** This work was supported by the Andalusian Service of Health (Public Foundation Progress and Health, grant number PI-0374–2014). The authors are grateful to the Initiative for the Humanization of Birth Assistance and Breastfeeding for the support during the study. Jorge Moreno-Fernandez was supported by fellowship from the Ministry of Education, Culture and Sport (Spain) and is grateful to the Excellence Ph.D. Program "Nutrición y Ciencias de los Alimentos" from the University of Granada. The authors are grateful to Susan Stevenson for her efficient support in the revision of the English language.

**Conflicts of Interest:** The authors have no conflict of interest to disclose.

### References

1. Romero, R.; Miranda, J.; Chaiworapongsa, T.; Korzeniewski, S.J.; Chaemsaithong, P.; Gotsch, F.; Dong, Z.; Ahmed, A.I.; Yoon, B.H.; Hassan, S.S.; et al. Prevalence and clinical significance of sterile intra-amniotic inflammation in patients with preterm labor and intact membranes. *Am. J. Reprod. Immunol.* **2014**, *72*, 458–474. [CrossRef] [PubMed]
2. Gotsch, F.; Romero, R.; Kusanovic, J.P.; Mazaki-Tovi, S.; Pineles, B.L.; Erez, O.; Espinoza, J.; Hassan, S.S. The fetal inflammatory response syndrome. *Clin. Obstet. Gynecol.* **2007**, *50*, 652–683. [CrossRef] [PubMed]
3. McAdams, R.M.; Juul, S.E. The role of cytokines and inflammatory cells in perinatal brain injury. *Neurol. Res. Int.* **2012**, *2012*, 561494. [CrossRef] [PubMed]
4. Iliodromiti, Z.; Zygouris, D.; Sifakis, S.; Pappa, K.I.; Tsikouras, P.; Salakos, N.; Daniilidis, A.; Siristatidis, C.; Vrachnis, N. Acute lung injury in preterm fetuses and neonates: Mechanisms and molecular pathways. *J. Matern-Fetal Neonatal Med.* **2013**, *26*, 1696–1704. [CrossRef]
5. Amerrican College of Obstetricians and Gynecologists. ACOG committee opinion no. 561: Nonmedically indicated early-term deliveries. *Obstet. Gynecol.* **2013**, *121*, 911–915. [CrossRef]
6. Shah, B.A.; Padbury, J.F. Neonatal sepsis: An old problem with new insights. *Virulence* **2014**, *5*, 170–178. [CrossRef]
7. Pammi, M.; Flores, A.; Leeflang, M.; Versalovic, J. Molecular assays in the diagnosis of neonatal sepsis: A systematic review and meta-analysis. *Pediatrics* **2011**, *128*, e973–e985. [CrossRef]
8. Arad, I.; Bar-Oz, B.; Ergaz, Z.; Nir, A.; Barak, V. Interleukin-6 and N-terminal pro-brain natriuretic peptide cord blood levels in premature infants: Correlations with perinatal variables. *Isr. Med. Assoc. J.* **2010**, *12*, 419–423.
9. Caldas, J.P.; Vilela, M.M.; Braghini, C.A.; Mazzola, T.N.; Marba, S.T. Antenatal maternal corticosteroid administration and markers of oxidative stress and inflammation in umbilical cord blood from very low birth weight preterm newborn infants. *J. Pediatr.* **2012**, *88*, 61–66. [CrossRef]
10. Ronnestad, A.; Abrahamsen, T.G.; Medbø, S.; Reigstad, H.; Lossius, K.; Kaaresen, P.I.; Egeland, T.; Engelund, I.E.; Irgens, L.M.; Markestad, T. Late-onset septicemia in a Norwegian national cohort of extremely premature infants receiving very early full human milk feeding. *Pediatrics* **2005**, *115*, e269–e276. [CrossRef]
11. Liu, B.; Newburg, D.S. Human milk glycoproteins protect infants against human pathogens. *Breastfeed. Med.* **2013**, *8*, 354–362. [CrossRef] [PubMed]
12. Meinzen-Derr, J.; Poindexter, B.; Wrage, L.; Morrow, A.L.; Stoll, B.; Donovan, E.F. Role of human milk in extremely low birth weight infants' risk of necrotizing enterocolitis or death. *J. Perinatol.* **2009**, *29*, 57–62. [CrossRef]
13. Underwood, M.A. Human milk for the premature infant. *Pediatr. Clin. N. Am.* **2013**, *60*, 189–207. [CrossRef] [PubMed]
14. Rodriguez, N.A.; Meier, P.P.; Groer, M.W.; Zeller, J.M.; Engstrom, J.L.; Fogg, L. A pilot study to determine the safety and feasibility of oropharyngeal administration of own mother's colostrum to extremely low-birth-weight infants. *Adv. Neonatal Care* **2010**, *10*, 206–212. [CrossRef]
15. Zhang, Y.; Ji, F.; Hu, X.; Cao, Y.; Latour, J.M. Oropharyngeal Colostrum Administration in Very Low Birth Weight Infants: A Randomized Controlled Trial. *Pediatr. Crit. Care Med.* **2017**, *18*, 869–875. [CrossRef] [PubMed]
16. Rodriguez, N.A.; Meier, P.P.; Mw, G.; Zeller, J.M. Oropharyngeal administration of colostrum to extremely low birth weight infants: Theoretical perspectives. *J. Perinatol.* **2009**, *29*, 1–7. [CrossRef] [PubMed]
17. Lee, J.; Kim, H.S.; Jung, Y.H.; Choi, K.Y.; Shin, S.H.; Kim, E.K.; Choi, J.H. Oropharyngeal colostrum administration in extremely premature infants: An RCT. *Pediatrics* **2015**, *135*, e357–e366. [CrossRef] [PubMed]

18. Panchal, H.; Athalye-Jape, G.; Patole, S. Oropharyngeal Colostrum for Preterm Infants: A Systematic Review and Meta-Analysis. *Adv. Nutr.* **2019**, *10*, 1152–1162. [CrossRef]
19. Moreno-Fernandez, J.; Sanchez-Martinez, B.; Serrano-Lopez, L.; Martin-Alvarez, E.; Diaz-Castro, J.; Pena-Caballero, M.; Martin-Peregrina, F.; Alonso-Moya, M.; Maldonado-Lozano, J.; Ochoa, J.J.; et al. Enhancement of immune response mediated by oropharyngeal colostrum administration in preterm neonates. *Pediatr. Allergy Immunol.* **2019**, *30*, 234–241. [CrossRef]
20. de Vries, L.S.; Eken, P.; Dubowitz, L.M. The spectrum of leukomalacia using cranial ultrasound. *Behav. Brain Res.* **1992**, *49*, 1–6. [CrossRef]
21. Walsh, M.C.; Kliegman, R.M. Necrotizing enterocolitis: Treatment based on staging criteria. *Pediatr. Clin. N. Am.* **1986**, *33*, 179–201. [CrossRef]
22. Levy, M.M.; Fink, M.P.; Marshall, J.C.; Abraham, E.; Angus, D.; Cook, D.; Cohen, J.; Opal, S.M.; Vincent, J.L.; Ramsay, G. 2001 SCCM/ESICM/ACCP/ATS/SIS International Sepsis Definitions Conference. *Crit. Care Med.* **2003**, *31*, 1250–1256. [CrossRef] [PubMed]
23. Gephart, S.M.; Weller, M. Colostrum as oral immune therapy to promote neonatal health. *Adv. Neonatal Care* **2014**, *14*, 44–51. [CrossRef] [PubMed]
24. Sty, A.C.; Sangild, P.T.; Skovgaard, K.; Thymann, T.; Bjerre, M.; Chatterton, D.E.; Purup, S.; Boye, M.; Heegaard, P.M. Spray Dried, Pasteurised Bovine Colostrum Protects Against Gut Dysfunction and Inflammation in Preterm Pigs. *J. Pediatr. Gastroenterol. Nutr.* **2016**, *63*, 280–287. [CrossRef] [PubMed]
25. Rodriguez, N.A.; Groer, M.W.; Zeller, J.M.; Engstron, J.L.; Fogg, L.; Du, H.; Caplan, M. A Randomized Controlled Trial of the Oropharyngeal Administration of Mother's Colostrum to Extremely Low Birth Weight Infants in the First Days of Life. *Neonatal Intens. Care* **2011**, *24*, 31–35.
26. Nadeau-Vallee, M.; Chin, P.Y.; Belarbi, L.; Brien, M.E.; Pundir, S.; Berryer, M.H.; Beaudry-Richard, A.; Madaan, A.; Sharkey, D.J.; Lupien-Meilleur, A.; et al. Antenatal Suppression of IL-1 Protects against Inflammation-Induced Fetal Injury and Improves Neonatal and Developmental Outcomes in Mice. *J. Immunol.* **2017**, *198*, 2047–2062. [CrossRef]
27. Chiesa, C.; Pacifico, L.; Natale, F.; Hofer, N.; Osborn, J.F.; Resch, B. Fetal and early neonatal interleukin-6 response. *Cytokine* **2015**, *76*, 1–12. [CrossRef]
28. Schollin, J. Interleukin-8 in neonatal sepsis. *Acta Paediatr.* **2001**, *90*, 961–962. [CrossRef]
29. Machado, J.R.; Soave, D.F.; da Silva, M.V.; de Menezes, L.B.; Etchebehere, R.M.; Monteiro, M.L.; dos Reis, M.A.; Correa, R.R.; Celes, M.R. Neonatal sepsis and inflammatory mediators. *Mediat. Inflamm.* **2014**, *2014*, 269681. [CrossRef]
30. Labrousse, D.; Perret, M.; Hayez, D.; Da Silva, S.; Badiou, C.; Couzon, F.; Bes, M.; Chavanet, P.; Lina, G.; Vandenesch, F.; et al. Kineret®/IL-1ra Blocks the IL-1/IL-8 Inflammatory Cascade during Recombinant Panton Valentine Leukocidin-Triggered Pneumonia but Not during S. aureus Infection. *PLoS ONE* **2014**, *9*, e97546. [CrossRef]
31. Agarwal, S.; Karmaus, W.; Davis, S.; Gangur, V. Immune markers in breast milk and fetal and maternal body fluids: A systematic review of perinatal concentrations. *J. Hum. Lact* **2011**, *27*, 171–186. [CrossRef] [PubMed]
32. Ballard, O.; Morrow, A.L. Human Milk Composition: Nutrients and Bioactive Factors. *Pediatr. Clin. N. Am.* **2013**, *60*, 49–74. [CrossRef] [PubMed]
33. Rocha, G.; Proenca, E.; Guedes, A.; Carvalho, C.; Areias, A.; Ramos, J.P.; Rodrigues, T.; Guimaraes, H. Cord blood levels of IL-6, IL-8 and IL-10 may be early predictors of bronchopulmonary dysplasia in preterm newborns small for gestational age. *Dis. Markers* **2012**, *33*, 51–60. [CrossRef] [PubMed]
34. Buescher, E.S.; Malinowska, I. Soluble receptors and cytokine antagonists in human milk. *Pediatr. Res.* **1996**, *40*, 839–844. [CrossRef] [PubMed]
35. Castellote, C.; Casillas, R.; Ramirez-Santana, C.; Perez-Cano, F.J.; Castell, M.; Moretones, M.G.; Lopez-Sabater, M.C.; Franch, A. Premature delivery influences the immunological composition of colostrum and transitional and mature human milk. *J. Nutr.* **2011**, *141*, 1181–1187. [CrossRef]
36. Aghai, Z.H.; Saslow, J.G.; Mody, K.; Eydelman, R.; Bhat, V.; Stahl, G.; Pyon, K.; Bhandari, V. IFN-gamma and IP-10 in tracheal aspirates from premature infants: Relationship with bronchopulmonary dysplasia. *Pediatr. Pulmonol.* **2013**, *48*, 8–13. [CrossRef]

37. Harijith, A.; Choo-Wing, R.; Cataltepe, S.; Yasumatsu, R.; Aghai, Z.H.; Janer, J.; Andersson, S.; Homer, R.J.; Bhandari, V. A role for matrix metalloproteinase 9 in IFNgamma-mediated injury in developing lungs: Relevance to bronchopulmonary dysplasia. *Am. J. Respir. Cell Mol. Biol.* **2011**, *44*, 621–630. [CrossRef]
38. Smilowitz, J.T.; Lebrilla, C.B.; Mills, D.A.; German, J.B.; Freeman, S.L. Breast milk oligosaccharides: Structure-function relationships in the neonate. *Annu. Rev. Nutr.* **2014**, *34*, 143–169. [CrossRef]

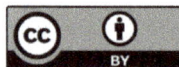

© 2020 by the authors. Licensee MDPI, Basel, Switzerland. This article is an open access article distributed under the terms and conditions of the Creative Commons Attribution (CC BY) license (http://creativecommons.org/licenses/by/4.0/).

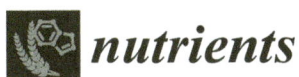 

Article

# Macronutrient Analysis of Target-Pooled Donor Breast Milk and Corresponding Growth in Very Low Birth Weight Infants

Ting Ting Fu [1,2,*], Paige E. Schroder [2] and Brenda B. Poindexter [1,2]

[1] Perinatal Institute, Division of Neonatology, Cincinnati Children's Hospital Medical Center, Cincinnati, OH 45229, USA
[2] Department of Pediatrics, University of Cincinnati College of Medicine, Cincinnati, OH 45267, USA
* Correspondence: tingting.fu@cchmc.org; Tel.: +1-513-636-8267

Received: 19 June 2019; Accepted: 9 August 2019; Published: 13 August 2019

**Abstract:** The macronutrient composition of target-pooled donor breast milk (DBM) (milk combined strategically to provide 20 kcal/oz) and growth patterns of preterm infants receiving it have not been characterized. Caloric target-pooled DBM samples were analyzed by near-infrared spectroscopy. Weekly growth velocities and anthropometric z-scores were calculated for the first 30 days and at 36 weeks corrected gestational age (CGA) for 69 very low birthweight (VLBW) infants receiving minimum one week of DBM. Samples contained mean 18.70 kcal/oz, 0.91 g/dL protein, 3.11 g/dL fat, 7.71 g/dL carbohydrate ($n$ = 96), less than labeled values by 2.43 kcal/oz and 0.11 g/dL protein ($p$ < 0.001). By week 3, growth reached 16.58 g/kg/day, 0.95 cm/week (length), and 1.01 cm/week (head circumference). Infants receiving <50% vs. >50% DBM had similar growth, but infants receiving >50% DBM were more likely to receive fortification >24 kcal/oz (83% vs. 51.9% in the <50% DBM group; $p$ = 0.005). From birth to 36 weeks CGA ($n$ = 60), there was a negative z-score change across all parameters with the greatest in length (−1.01). Thus, target-pooling does not meet recommended protein intake for VLBW infants. Infants fed target-pooled DBM still demonstrate a disproportionate negative change in length z-score over time.

**Keywords:** donor breast milk; human milk; milk analysis; very low birth weight; preterm; growth

## 1. Introduction

Neonatal practitioners commonly assume that human breast milk contains 20 kcal/oz, but the macronutrient content of human milk depends on many factors including gestational age [1]. Compared to preterm milk, term milk has less energy and protein, and in both populations, energy and protein content decreases over time as lactation progresses [2]. Because donor breast milk (DBM) commonly comes from mothers of term babies later in lactation, one major concern regarding the use of DBM in preterm infants is its nutritional adequacy, particularly its protein concentration, since higher protein intake and increased linear growth are associated with improved neurodevelopmental outcomes [3–5]. Pooled DBM has been shown to contain as low as 14.6 kcal/oz [6], and protein content in maternal preterm milk ranges from 1.2 to 1.7 g/dL in the first four weeks of lactation whereas the content in DBM is generally accepted as 0.9 g/dL [7]. For infants weighing less than 1 kg, the European Society for Pediatric Gastroenterology Hepatology and Nutrition (ESPGHAN) recommends an enteral intake of 4.0–4.5 g/kg/day of protein [8], which correlates to 2.7–3.0 g/dL assuming enteral fluid intake of 150 ml/kg/day. However, protein fortification for human milk is difficult, and standard multicomponent human milk fortifiers may still be insufficient as manufacturers of commercially available bovine-derived human milk fortifiers assume a baseline protein concentration of 1.4–1.6 g/dL in human milk [9,10].

Earlier studies comparing fortified DBM versus premature infant formula reported notably decreased growth velocities in the DBM group, particularly in weight and length [11,12]. However, more recent studies have shown similar growth can be achieved with adequate monitoring and fortification [13–15].

Target-pooling is a method that some milk banks employ to increase nutritional content by combining milk of multiple donors strategically, rather than randomly. One specific technique is to add skimmed fat from lower-calorie breast milk to higher-calorie breast milk to mimic hind milk and achieve a minimum of 20 kcal/oz. However, it is unclear how protein concentrations of DBM and subsequent infant growth are affected by caloric targeting. The objective of this study was to characterize the macronutrient composition and variability of caloric target-pooled DBM and the corresponding growth velocities of very low birth weight (VLBW) infants who receive it.

## 2. Materials and Methods

### 2.1. Patient Sample

This prospective observational study was performed at the neonatal intensive care unit (NICU) at TriHealth Good Samaritan Hospital in Cincinnati, Ohio, with milk analysis conducted at Cincinnati Children's Hospital Medical Center (CCHMC). The study was approved by the Institutional Review Board at both institutions with waiver of informed consent (CCHMC 2015-5191, TriHealth 15-085).

VLBW infants admitted to the NICU from December 2015 to April 2017 who received more than 1 week of DBM during the first 30 days of life as supplementation to maternal milk were eligible. Infants who transferred to another hospital or passed away in the first 30 days of life or did not follow the standardized feeding protocol (see below, Section 2.3) were excluded.

### 2.2. Milk Collection and Analysis

During the time period in which eligible infants were admitted, target-pooled DBM purchased from Mothers' Milk Bank of Ohio (MMBO, Columbus, Ohio) were screened for unique pools, and a representative bottle for each unique pool was marked. Caloric and protein content, as measured by MMBO and labeled on each bottle, was recorded. Per unit protocol, NICU milk technicians prepared feedings from refrigerator-thawed bottles by hand homogenizing and either pipetting or pouring into measured containers. From each marked bottle, a minimum of 1 ml of the remaining milk, more if allowed, was saved, and kept frozen for sample collection. For analysis, samples were heated to 37 °C, gently homogenized by hand, then homogenized for 30 seconds using a sonicator. Using a near-infrared (NIR) human milk analyzer (SpectraStar 2400, Unity Scientific, Brookfield, Connecticut), which was calibrated using a bias set of human breast milk obtained from MMBO, samples were then analyzed in 1–1.5 mL aliquots, triplicate if volume allowed.

### 2.3. Standardized VLBW Feeding Protocol

DBM is utilized for infants with birth weight </= 1500 g when maternal milk is not available for the first 30 days of life. Enteral feedings are initiated within 48 h of birth at 15 mL/kg/day for 3 days and subsequently advanced by 10 mL/kg/day every 12 h to a goal of 160 mL/kg/day. Fortification to 24 kcal/oz occurs at 75 mL/kg/day, usually day of life 7, using Similac (Abbott Nutrition, Columbus Ohio) human milk fortifier hydrolyzed protein concentrated liquid (HMF-HPCL). Additional fortification occurs as clinically indicated for poor growth using additional HMF-HPCL, Similac Special Care 30, Similac NeoSure, and/or Similac Liquid Protein Fortifier, per dietitian's discretion. In addition to enteral intake, parenteral nutrition provides 2.5 g/kg/day of protein starting on day of life 1, then 3.5 g/kg/day onward until intake is limited by fluid volume.

## 2.4. Enteral Intake Data

Enteral intake data were obtained from charted enteral feeding volumes and fortification status of donor and maternal milk for the first 30 days of life or until DBM was transitioned to formula. Percentage of DBM intake was calculated by dividing the volume of DBM by the total volume of human milk that the infant received during the studied time period. The last day on which DBM was given, whether the infant was still receiving DBM on day 30, and the highest caloric density of fortification of DBM were recorded. Utilizing the NICU's established milk tracking system (Women and Infants, Timeless Medical Systems, Charlottetown, Prince Edward Island, Canada), the source pool from each bottle of DBM that the infant received was identified.

## 2.5. Anthropometric Data

Weekly weight, length, and head circumference (HC), as recorded by clinical care, were collected until 4 weeks of age and also at 36 weeks corrected gestational age (CGA). Growth velocities, Olsen body mass index (BMI) [16], and Fenton z-scores [17] were calculated for each time point. Weight velocity was calculated using the two-point model. Per unit practice, length boards were used as needed to verify measurements that appeared abnormal. Outliers in length and HC (a gain of greater than 3 cm or a loss of greater than 2 cm) were excluded. For patients discharged prior to 36 weeks CGA, measurements at 35 weeks CGA were recorded if available. Small for gestational age (SGA) was defined as a birth weight below the 10th percentile, and appropriate for gestational age (AGA) was defined as birth weight between the 10th and 90th percentile.

## 2.6. Statistical Analysis

Analyses were performed using SAS Studio version 3.71. NIR results were compared to labeled values using paired t-test analysis. Subgroups comparisons of SGA vs. AGA status and DBM intake percentage (<50% vs. >50%) were analyzed using 2-tailed 2-sample t-tests and $\chi^2$ test. $P < 0.05$ was considered statistically significant. A sample size of 45 patients was estimated to detect a difference of 2.18 g/kg/day difference in weight (assuming full enteral feeding volume of 160 ml/kg/day with DBM fortified to 24 kcal/oz and baseline protein concentration 0.9 g/dL, yielding a projected protein intake of 3.87 g/kg/day, 0.63 g/kg/day less than ESPGHAN recommendations) with 80% power and alpha 0.05 and based on the largest randomized trial known at the time of study design describing growth in infants fed DBM [11].

## 3. Results

### 3.1. Study Infants

Of 235 infants screened, 85 met inclusion criteria (Figure 1). An additional 16 were excluded due to early discharge or modified feeding plans after completion of the standard feeding protocol. Thus, 69 had growth data available at 30 days, and 60 had measurements available at 36 weeks CGA. The summary of their characteristics can be found in Table 1. Of those 69 patients who had growth data, 65.9% were still receiving DBM as part or all of their feedings at 30 days old, and 5 additional patients were transitioned early from DBM to formula due to poor growth at 27–28 days. Further, 15.9% were SGA and 71.0% received increased fortification, which occurred on average at day 18.5.

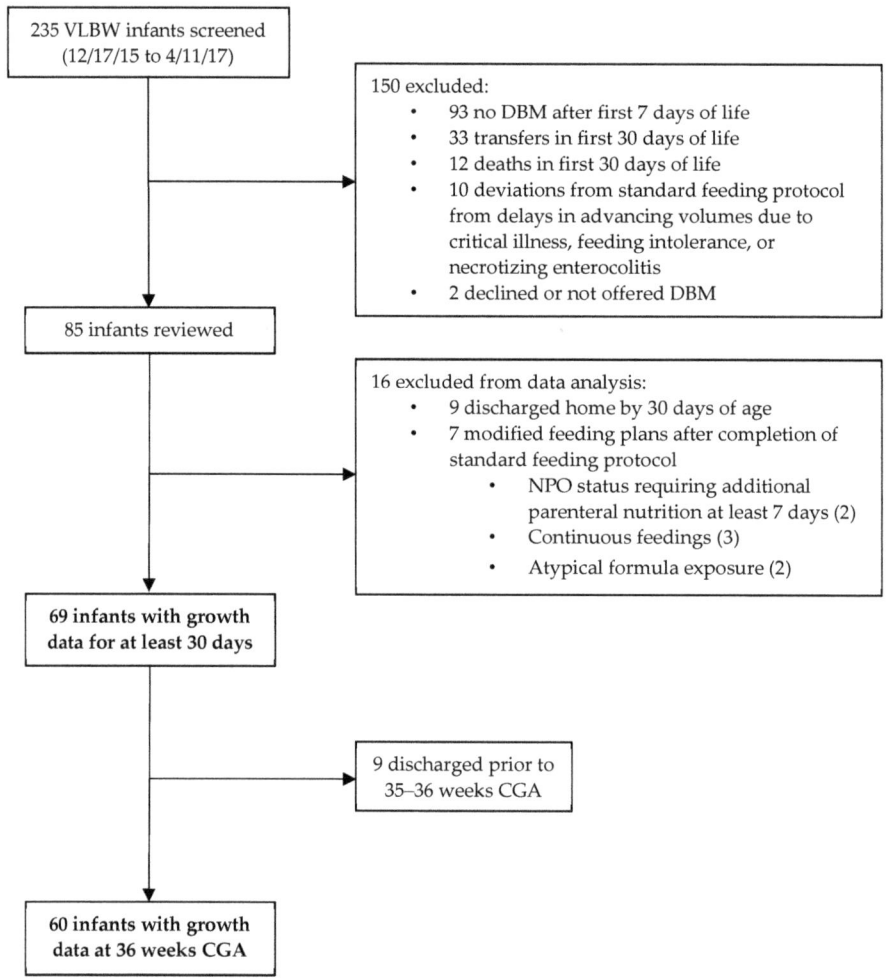

**Figure 1.** Flow diagram of study infants.

**Table 1.** Infant characteristics. Mean ± SD or $n$ (%).

|  | All Infants ($n = 85$) | Infants with 30 Days Growth Data ($n = 69$) | Infants Receiving <50% DBM ($n = 27$) | Infants Receiving >50% DBM ($n = 42$) | $p$-Value [1] |
|---|---|---|---|---|---|
| Male (%) | 47 (55.3%) | 38 (55.1%) | 17 (63.0%) | 21 (50%) | 0.291 |
| Gestational Age (weeks) | 29.4 ± 2.4 | 28.9 ± 2.0 | 29.6 ± 2.1 | 28.4 ± 1.8 | 0.011 |
| Birth Weight (g) | 1101.2 ± 266.5 | 1064.4 ± 260.0 | 1112.1 ± 264.5 | 1033.8 ± 255.5 | 0.225 |
| SGA (%) | 24 (28.2%) | 11 (15.9%) | 7 (25.9%) | 4 (9.5%) | 0.069 |
| Days on DBM | 26.5 ± 6.7 | 27.8 ± 5.4 | 24.9 ± 7.6 | 29.6 ± 1.7 | <0.001 |
| Infants on DBM at 30 days (%) | 56 (65.9%) [2] | 50 (72.5%) | 15 (55.6%) | 35 (83.3%) | 0.012 |
| Infants Needing >24 kcal/oz (%) | 59 (69.4%) | 49 (71.0%) | 14 (51.9%) | 35 (83.3%) | 0.005 |

[1] For DBM subgroups; [2] 5 patients were switched from DBM to preterm formula at 27–28 days due to poor growth.

## 3.2. Donor Milk Analysis

Samples from 96 unique pools were obtained. Review of enteral intake charting and milk tracking showed 146 unique pools of DBM were actually utilized during the study period. NIR analysis found mean contents of 18.70 ± 1.75 kcal/oz, 0.91 ± 0.19 g/dL protein, 3.11 ± 0.57 g/dL fat, and 7.71 ± 0.38 g/dL carbohydrate (Table 2). Mean coefficients of variation of triplicate or duplicate analysis were 1.61% for calories, 6.81% for protein, 2.68% for fat, and 1.81% for carbohydrate. Labeled nutritional information demonstrated mean calorie content of 21.13 ± 1.01 kcal/oz and mean protein content 1.02 ± 0.18 g/dL. On average, compared to labeled values, the samples had 2.43 kcal/oz less ($p < 0.001$) and 0.11 g/dL less protein ($p < 0.001$) (Table 3, Figure 2).

**Table 2.** Near-infrared (NIR) macronutrient analysis of donor breast milk (DBM) samples ($n = 96$).

|  | Calories (kcal/oz) | Protein (g/dL) | Fat (g/dL) | Carbohydrate (g/dL) |
|---|---|---|---|---|
| Minimum | 12.43 | 0.26 | 1.48 | 6.29 |
| Maximum | 22.27 | 1.36 | 4.51 | 8.48 |
| Mean | 18.70 | 0.91 | 3.11 | 7.71 |
| SD | 1.75 | 0.19 | 0.57 | 0.38 |
| Mean Coefficient of Variation | 1.61% | 6.81% | 2.68% | 1.81% |

**Table 3.** Comparison of labeled and NIR measured caloric and protein concentrations.

|  | Calories (kcal/oz) | | | Protein (g/dL) | | |
|---|---|---|---|---|---|---|
|  | Label | NIR | Difference | Label | NIR | Difference |
| Minimum | 19.51 | 12.43 | −8.22 | 0.62 | 0.26 | −0.62 |
| Maximum | 24.01 | 22.27 | 0.29 | 1.51 | 1.36 | 0.36 |
| Mean | 21.13 | 18.70 | −2.43 [1] | 1.02 | 0.91 | −0.11 [1] |
| SD | 1.01 | 1.75 | 1.66 | 0.18 | 0.19 | 0.21 |

[1] $p < 0.001$.

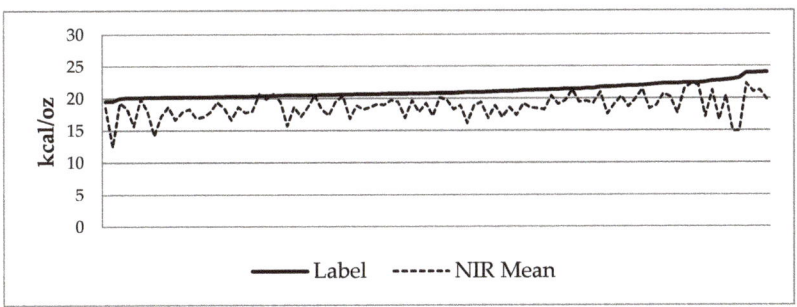

(a)

**Figure 2.** Cont.

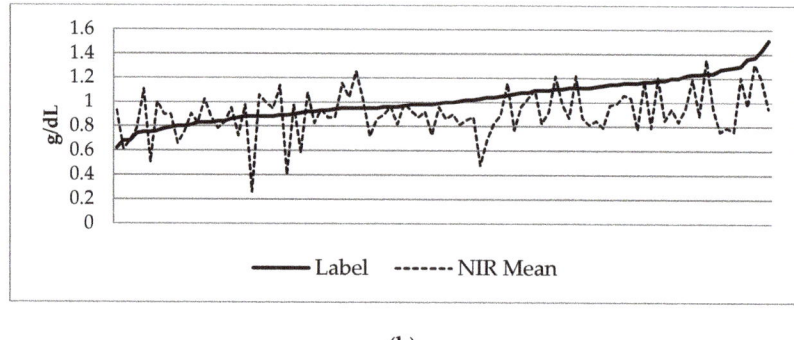

(b)

**Figure 2.** Labeled (solid line) vs. mean NIR analysis (dashed line) of (**a**) caloric and (**b**) protein content, ordered by increasing labeled values.

*3.3. Growth Analysis*

Mean weight velocity reached 16.58 g/kg/day by week 3, mean length velocity ranged from 0.95 to 1.03 cm/week during weeks 2-4, and mean HC velocity reached 1.01 cm/week by week 3 (Table 4). When comparing the subgroups of SGA and AGA infants, the mean velocities were statistically different for weight velocity in weeks 1 and 2 ($p = 0.001$, $p = 0.009$) (Table 4). There were no large-for-gestational-age infants. Infants whose enteral intake comprised of less than 50% DBM had similar growth velocities compared to those whose enteral intake was greater than 50% DBM with the exception of weight velocity at week 2 ($p = 0.024$) (Table 4). Further, 51.9% in the <50% DBM group and 83.3% in the >50% DBM group received fortification beyond 24 kcal/oz ($p = 0.005$).

**Table 4.** Weekly growth velocities including subgroups by small for gestational age (SGA) status and DBM intake. Mean ± SD.

|  | Overall ($n = 69$) | SGA ($n = 11$) | AGA ($n = 58$) | *p*-Value | <50% DBM ($n = 27$) | >50% DBM ($n = 42$) | *p*-Value |
|---|---|---|---|---|---|---|---|
| **Weight (g/kg/day)** | | | | | | | |
| Week 1 | 8.84 ± 6.81 | 15.07 ± 9.42 | 7.66 ± 5.56 | <0.001 | 8.50 ± 7.12 | 9.06 ± 6.68 | 0.742 |
| Week 2 | 12.95 ± 5.75 | 17.00 ± 6.96 | 12.18 ± 5.21 | <0.010 | 14.88 ± 6.08 | 11.71 ± 5.23 | 0.024 |
| Week 3 | 16.58 ± 5.13 | 18.45 ± 5.91 | 16.23 ± 4.95 | 0.189 | 17.21 ± 3.38 | 16.17 ± 6.01 | 0.415 |
| Week 4 | 16.11 ± 4.71 | 16.98 ± 3.71 | 15.94 ± 4.89 | 0.507 | 16.00 ± 3.50 | 16.18 ± 5.39 | 0.882 |
| **Length (cm/week)** | | | | | | | |
| Week 1 | 0.59 ± 0.85 | 0.60 ± 0.87 | 0.59 ± 0.86 | 0.982 | 0.45 ± 0.81 | 0.68 ± 0.88 | 0.299 |
| Week 2 | 0.97 ± 0.72 | 1.32 ± 0.72 | 0.91 ± 0.70 | 0.080 | 1.05 ± 0.65 | 0.92 ± 0.76 | 0.478 |
| Week 3 | 0.95 ± 0.78 | 0.70 ± 0.96 | 1.00 ± 0.74 | 0.244 | 0.94 ± 0.85 | 0.96 ± 0.75 | 0.914 |
| Week 4 | 1.03 ± 0.65 | 1.31 ± 0.45 | 0.97 ± 0.66 | 0.114 | 0.95 ± 0.67 | 1.08 ± 0.63 | 0.455 |
| **HC (cm/week)** | | | | | | | |
| Week 1 | 0.14 ± 0.77 | 0.39 ± 0.91 | 0.09 ± 0.74 | 0.235 | 0.06 ± 0.73 | 0.19 ± 0.80 | 0.490 |
| Week 2 | 0.67 ± 0.55 | 0.91 ± 0.58 | 0.63 ± 0.54 | 0.124 | 0.77 ± 0.58 | 0.61 ± 0.53 | 0.245 |
| Week 3 | 1.01 ± 0.54 | 1.20 ± 0.42 | 0.98 ± 0.56 | 0.216 | 0.96 ± 0.55 | 1.05 ± 0.53 | 0.525 |
| Week 4 | 1.01 ± 0.60 | 1.12 ± 0.59 | 0.99 ± 0.61 | 0.514 | 1.07 ± 0.59 | 0.97 ± 0.61 | 0.498 |

For the 60 infants who had growth measurements available at 36 weeks CGA, the Fenton z-score decreased for HC during weeks 1–2 and for both weight and length during all four weeks. From birth to 36 weeks CGA, there was a negative z-score change across all three parameters with the greatest change seen in length (−1.01) (Table 5, Figure 3). HC z-score improved to within 0.23 of birth, and a small increase (0.1) was noted in weight z-score between week 4 and 36 weeks CGA. Olsen BMI was the only measure to have a net increase in z-score over time. Further, 11/60 infants were SGA at birth; an additional 10 AGA infants became <10% for weight by 36 weeks CGA. There appeared to be a difference between the two DBM subgroups in both weight and length, though it was not statistically significant for any measurement (Figure 3), and with the exception of the change in BMI from week 4 to 36 weeks CGA, the weekly change in z-score and also net change from birth to 36 weeks CGA were not statistically different. After excluding the 11 SGA patients, again there was no statistically significant difference between the two DBM groups except between week 4 and 36 weeks CGA where the length z-score continued to decrease by −0.14 in the >50% DBM group but increased by 0.12 in the <50% DBM group ($p = 0.023$) (Figure 4).

Table 5. z-scores of anthropometric measurements each week and at 36 weeks corrected gestational age (CGA). Mean ± SD.

|  | Weight | HC | Length | BMI |
|---|---|---|---|---|
| Birth | −0.52 ± 0.89 | −0.45 ± 1.10 | −0.51 ± 1.06 | −0.30 ± 1.09 |
| Week 1 | −0.88 ± 0.81 | −1.30 ± 0.96 | −1.14 ± 1.06 | −0.41 ± 0.95 |
| Week 2 | −1.04 ± 0.77 | −1.45 ± 0.98 | −1.28 ± 1.02 | −0.43 ± 0.88 |
| Week 3 | −1.09 ± 0.79 | −1.41 ± 0.95 | −1.44 ± 1.05 | −0.24 ± 0.82 |
| Week 4 | −1.13 ± 0.83 | −1.28 ± 0.96 | −1.60 ± 1.00 | −0.09 ± 0.81 |
| 36 Weeks CGA | −1.03 ± 1.03 | −0.68 ± 0.90 | −1.64 ± 1.13 | 0.27 ± 0.85 |
| Net Change | −0.51 ± 0.47 | −0.23 ± 0.69 | −1.01 ± 0.57 | 0.60 ± 0.93 |

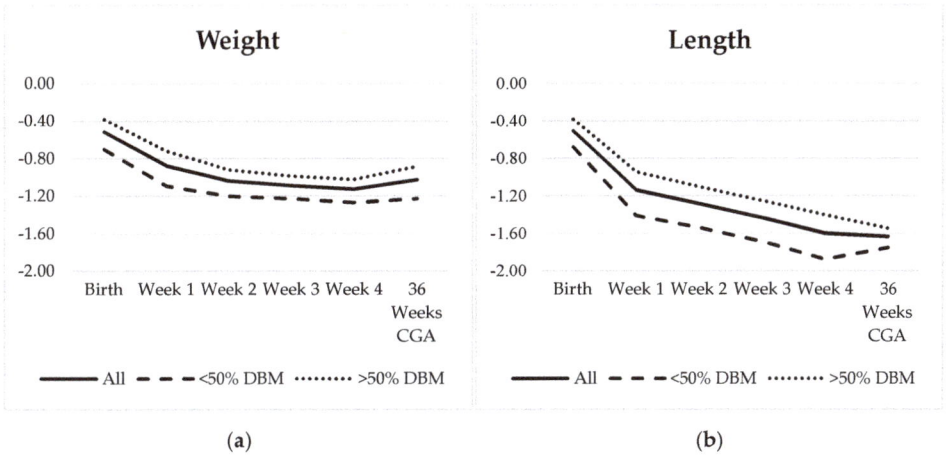

Figure 3. Cont.

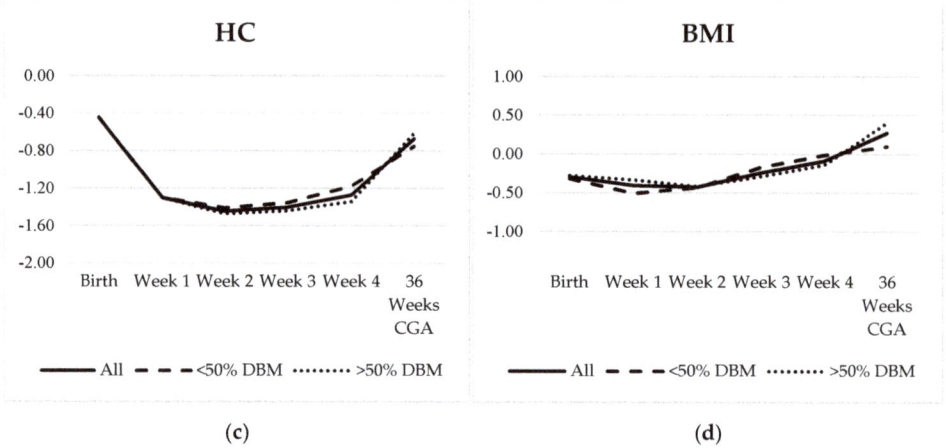

**Figure 3.** (**a**–**c**) Fenton z-score trajectories for weight, length, and head circumference (HC) and (**d**) Olsen z-score trajectory for body mass index (BMI) over time for all infants (solid line, $n = 60$), infants with <50% DBM intake (dashed line, $n = 25$), and infants with >50% DBM intake (dotted line, $n = 35$).

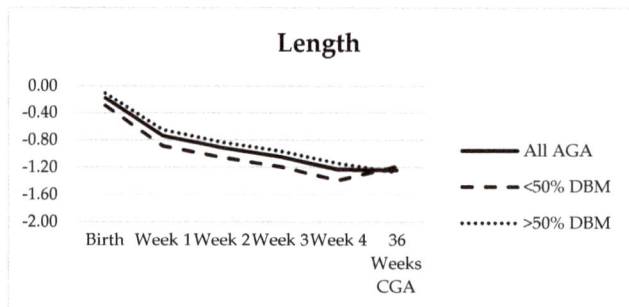

**Figure 4.** Fenton z-score trajectory for length in all appropriate-for-gestational-age (AGA) infants (solid line, $n = 49$) and subgroups of <50% DBM intake (dashed line, $n = 18$) and >50% DBM intake (dotted line, $n = 31$). Average rate of change from week 4 to 36 weeks CGA in the two subgroups were 0.12 and −0.14, respectively ($p = 0.023$).

## 4. Discussion

NIR analysis revealed that the target-pooled DBM samples contained similar calories (18.7 vs. 18.0–18.7 kcal/oz) and protein concentrations (0.91 vs. 0.88–1.0 g/dL) compared to other recent analyses of multi-donor random-pooled DBM [18,19]. However, in these studies, samples were measured pre-pasteurization. MMBO's labeled pre-pasteurization measurements showed the calorically targeted-pools contained mean 21.13 kcal/oz and 1.02 g/dL, reflective of their particular technique designed to mimic hind milk. As there are no dedicated regulations currently in place regarding pooling, the techniques utilized by other banks, which may include protein targeting, could result in different macronutrient ratios.

Furthermore, the measured concentrations for calories were, across the board, less than indicated on the corresponding labels (Figure 2), with one sample as low as 12.43 kcal/oz. Given that our NIR analyzer was calibrated utilizing milk and measurements provided by MMBO and that samples were collected after feeding preparations were completed for each shift, this suggests that nutrient loss likely occurred during preparation and handling. Handling from freezing and thawing of human milk has been shown to decrease caloric delivery [20], likely secondary to increased contact with plastic surfaces to which fat adheres, and the steps of feeding preparation, such as hand-homogenization and pouring versus using a transfer pipette, may also yield uneven distribution of macronutrients due to technician variation. The NIR-measured protein content was inconsistently matched with its label counterpart (Figure 2), potentially due to poor homogenization and compartmentalization. This carries implications in unequal delivery of nutrients between patients and also between feedings to individual patients, leading to unintended under- or over-nutrition. Developing consistent feeding preparation techniques to improve homogenization, minimize fat loss, and optimize nutrient delivery is an important focus for further research and quality improvement.

Growth parameters reached or approached goal velocities (15 g/kg/day for weight, 1 cm/week for length and HC) by weeks 3–4, but 71.0% of patients received additional fortification to maintain adequate growth (Tables 1 and 4). The clinical significance of the early weight velocity in SGA patients is unclear given the small subgroup size, though it could reflect a response to metabolic programming or a larger proportion of SGA infants in the <50% DBM group, though the latter was not statistically significant. The difference in weight velocity between the two DBM intake groups at week 2 and the narrowed gap at week 3 correlates, respectively, with infants approaching full enteral volumes with little or no parenteral nutrition and the point at which increased fortification occurred, supporting previous findings that acceptable growth velocities can be achieved on a DBM diet with appropriate fortification [14].

In addition, weekly Fenton z-scores suffered, and patients did not return to birth z-scores by 36 weeks CGA (Table 5, Figure 3). The greatest z-score change was seen in length, and the Olsen BMI z-score increased correspondingly. This suggests that monitoring z-scores in addition to growth velocities is necessary to determine whether weekly growth is adequate. Furthermore, despite the controlled caloric intake provided by target-pooled DBM, standard fortification to 24 kcal/oz alone does not provide adequate nutrition. Standard fortification of DBM increases the concentration from 0.9 g/dL to 2.42 g/dL, still below recommendations. Moreover, the switch to preterm formula at 30 days could not overcome the early growth faltering on DBM, highlighted by the 10/49 (20%) of AGA infants who developed postnatal growth failure (weight <10% at 36 weeks CGA). With studies associating poor linear growth and protein intake with worse neurodevelopmental outcomes [3,5], the persistent decreasing length z-score over time is particularly concerning. Thus, this population may benefit from earlier aggressive fortification of DBM with focused targeting of protein intake before growth faltering is demonstrated.

Though there appears to be a difference in weight and length at birth between the DBM subgroups, both groups actually had similar z-score trajectories over time. This is likely due to the increased percentage of infants who received additional fortification in the group that received >50% DBM. Colaizy et al. previously noted a net change in weight z-score from birth to discharge of −0.84 in infants who received >75% DBM [21]. In our >50% DBM subgroup, 32/35 patients received >75% DBM, and the net change in weight z-score was −0.49, an improvement possibly attributable to the target-pooling. Our net z-score changes for weight and length were also similar to findings of the DoMINO trial, the largest randomized controlled trial to date comparing DBM versus preterm formula as primary diet [13]. However, despite the improved growth potential that target-pooling may offer, the negative trends remain worrisome. Interestingly, over 95% of the study milk from the DoMINO trial was also purchased from MMBO. Providers may wish to inquire what pooling technique is utilized by the milk bank that provides their unit's donor milk, which may be different in content than the donor milk utilized in our study and the DoMINO study, thus limiting the generalizability of these findings.

Additionally, there was a gain in length z-score between week 4 and 36 weeks CGA for those who received <50% DBM and a decrease for those who received >50% DBM, though it was only statistically significant once the SGA infants were removed (Figure 4). Both of these groups transitioned to preterm formula as backup at 30 days, though many infants in the former likely continued to receive a larger percentage of maternal milk. Further investigation into the later feeding characteristics of these two cohorts and also comparison to infants who received almost exclusive maternal milk may provide additional insight.

One limitation of this study is the irregular sampling bias of DBM from leftover milk after feeding preparation, which may have affected our macronutrient analysis, but this poses new questions regarding human milk handling methods. Furthermore, while NIR human milk analyzers have been validated for precision in measuring protein and fat content, they are less accurate than mid-infrared analyzers [22,23]. A separate collaboration determined that the NIR analyzer used in this study may overestimate protein [24], suggesting that the protein content might be even lower than measured. Another limitation is the imprecision of length and head circumference measurements, and length boards had not been implemented as standard of care yet at the beginning of this study. We also sought to compare each infant's daily protein and caloric intake with weekly growth velocities. However, despite a protocol designed to identify all unique pools purchased by the NICU as shipments arrived, some shipments were missed, preventing us from capturing 50/146 (34%) of the unique pools that were utilized in these infants. Because bottles of DBM from the same pool may be dispersed among multiple patients, this unfortunately precluded us from calculating the enteral nutrient intake for the majority of the patients.

## 5. Conclusions

Target-pooling DBM to meet a caloric minimum alone does not meet recommended protein intake for VLBW infants. Infants fed calorically target-pooled DBM still demonstrate a disproportionate negative change in length z-score over time and would likely benefit from more aggressive and earlier fortification strategies that target protein as well. Whether target-pooled DBM offers improved growth compared to random-pooled DBM remains unknown.

**Author Contributions:** Conceptualization, T.T.F., B.B.P.; methodology, T.T.F.; formal analysis, T.T.F.; investigation, T.T.F., P.E.S.; data curation, T.T.F.; writing—original draft preparation, T.T.F.; writing—review and editing, T.T.F., B.B.P., P.E.S.; visualization, T.T.F.; supervision, T.T.F., B.B.P. All authors approved the final manuscript.

**Funding:** This research received no external funding.

**Conflicts of Interest:** The authors declare no conflict of interest.

## References

1. Tudehope, D.I. Human Milk and the Nutritional Needs of Preterm Infants. *J. Pediatr.* **2013**, *162*, S17–S25. [CrossRef] [PubMed]
2. Ballard, O.; Morrow, A.L. Human Milk Composition. *Pediatr. Clin. N. Am.* **2013**, *60*, 49–74. [CrossRef] [PubMed]
3. Ramel, S.E.; Demerath, E.W.; Gray, H.L.; Younge, N.; Boys, C.; Georgieff, M.K. The relationship of poor linear growth velocity with neonatal illness and two-year neurodevelopment in preterm infants. *Neonatology* **2012**, *102*, 19–24. [CrossRef] [PubMed]
4. Stephens, B.E.; Vohr, B.R. Protein Intake and Neurodevelopmental Outcomes. *Clin. Perinatol.* **2014**, *41*, 323–329. [CrossRef] [PubMed]
5. Stephens, B.E.; Walden, R.V.; Gargus, R.A.; Tucker, R.; McKinley, L.; Mance, M.; Nye, J.; Vohr, B.R. First-Week protein and energy intakes are associated with 18-month developmental outcomes in extremely low birth weight infants. *Pediatrics* **2009**, *123*, 1337–1343. [CrossRef] [PubMed]
6. Radmacher, P.G.; Lewis, S.L.; Adamkin, D.H. Individualizing fortification of human milk using real time human milk analysis. *J. Neonatal-Perinat. Med.* **2013**, *6*, 319–323. [CrossRef]
7. Ziegler, E.E. Human milk and human milk fortifiers. *World Rev. Nutr. Diet.* **2014**, *110*, 215–227. [CrossRef] [PubMed]
8. Agostoni, C.; Buonocore, G.; Carnielli, V.P.; De Curtis, M.; Darmaun, D.; Decsi, T.; Domellof, M.; Embleton, N.D.; Fusch, C.; Genzel-Boroviczeny, O.; et al. Enteral nutrient supply for preterm infants: Commentary from the European Society of Paediatric Gastroenterology, Hepatology and Nutrition Committee on Nutrition. *J. Pediatr. Gastroenterol. Nutr.* **2010**, *50*, 85–91. [CrossRef]

9. Abbott Nutrition. *Similac Human Milk Fortifier Hydrolyzed Protein Concentrated Liquid*; Abbott: Columbus, OH, USA, 2016.
10. Mead Johnson Nutrition. Enfamil Human Milk Fortifier Acidified Liquid. Available online: https://www.meadjohnson.com/pediatrics/us-en/product-information/products/newborns/enfamil-human-milk-fortifier-acidified-liquid (accessed on 19 October 2015).
11. Schanler, R.J. Randomized trial of donor human milk versus preterm formula as substitutes for mothers' own milk in the feeding of extremely premature infants. *Pediatrics* **2005**, *116*, 400–406. [CrossRef]
12. Cristofalo, E.A.; Schanler, R.J.; Blanco, C.L.; Sullivan, S.; Trawoeger, R.; Kiechl-Kohlendorfer, U.; Dudell, G.; Rechtman, D.J.; Lee, M.L.; Lucas, A.; et al. Randomized Trial of Exclusive Human Milk versus Preterm Formula Diets in Extremely Premature Infants. *J. Pediatr.* **2013**, *163*, 1592–1595. [CrossRef]
13. O'Connor, D.L.; Gibbins, S.; Kiss, A.; Bando, N.; Brennan-Donnan, J.; Ng, E.; Campbell, D.M.; Vaz, S.; Fusch, C.; Asztalos, E.; et al. Effect of supplemental donor human milk compared with preterm formula on neurodevelopment of very low-birth-weight infants at 18 months: A Randomized Clinical Trial. *JAMA* **2016**, *316*, 1897–1905. [CrossRef]
14. Hair, A.B.; Hawthorne, K.M.; Chetta, K.E.; Abrams, S.A. Human milk feeding supports adequate growth in infants ≤ 1250 grams birth weight. *BMC Res. Notes* **2013**, *6*, 459. [CrossRef] [PubMed]
15. Sisk, P.M.; Lambeth, T.M.; Rojas, M.A.; Lightbourne, T.; Barahona, M.; Anthony, E.; Auringer, S.T. Necrotizing Enterocolitis and Growth in Preterm Infants Fed Predominantly Maternal Milk, Pasteurized Donor Milk, or Preterm Formula: A Retrospective Study. *Am. J. Perinatol.* **2017**, *34*, 676–683. [CrossRef] [PubMed]
16. Olsen, I.E.; Lawson, M.L.; Ferguson, A.N.; Cantrell, R.; Grabich, S.C.; Zemel, B.S.; Clark, R.H. BMI Curves for Preterm Infants. *Pediatrics* **2015**, *135*, e572–e581. [CrossRef]
17. Fenton, T.R.; Kim, J.H. A systematic review and meta-analysis to revise the Fenton growth chart for preterm infants. *BMC Pediatr.* **2013**, *13*, 59. [CrossRef]
18. John, A.; Sun, R.; Maillart, L.; Schaefer, A.; Hamilton Spence, E.; Perrin, M.T. Macronutrient variability in human milk from donors to a milk bank: Implications for feeding preterm infants. *PLoS ONE* **2019**, *14*, e0210610. [CrossRef] [PubMed]
19. Piemontese, P.; Mallardi, D.; Liotto, N.; Tabasso, C.; Menis, C.; Perrone, M.; Roggero, P.; Mosca, F. Macronutrient content of pooled donor human milk before and after Holder pasteurization. *BMC Pediatr.* **2019**, *19*, 58. [CrossRef] [PubMed]
20. Vieira, A.A.; Soares, F.V.M.; Pimenta, H.P.; Abranches, A.D.; Moreira, M.E.L. Analysis of the influence of pasteurization, freezing/thawing, and offer processes on human milk's macronutrient concentrations. *Early Hum. Dev.* **2011**, *87*, 577–580. [CrossRef]
21. Colaizy, T.T.; Carlson, S.; Saftlas, A.F.; Morriss, F.H., Jr. Growth in VLBW infants fed predominantly fortified maternal and donor human milk diets: A retrospective cohort study. *BMC Pediatr.* **2012**, *12*, 124. [CrossRef]
22. Fusch, G.; Rochow, N.; Choi, A.; Fusch, S.; Poeschl, S.; Ubah, A.O.; Lee, S.-Y.; Raja, P.; Fusch, C. Rapid measurement of macronutrients in breast milk: How reliable are infrared milk analyzers? *Clin. Nutr.* **2015**, *34*, 465–476. [CrossRef]
23. Sauer, C.W.; Kim, J.H. Human milk macronutrient analysis using point-of-care near-infrared spectrophotometry. *J. Perinatol.* **2010**, *31*, 339–343. [CrossRef]
24. Fusch, G.; Kwan, C.; Rochow, N.; Fusch, C. Milk analysis using milk analyzers in a standardized setting (MAMAS) study: Preliminary results. *Monatsschrift Kinderheilkd.* **2016**, *164*, 233–390.

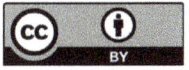

© 2019 by the authors. Licensee MDPI, Basel, Switzerland. This article is an open access article distributed under the terms and conditions of the Creative Commons Attribution (CC BY) license (http://creativecommons.org/licenses/by/4.0/).

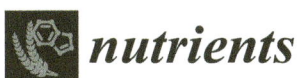 

Article

# Availability of Donor Milk for Very Preterm Infants Decreased the Risk of Necrotizing Enterocolitis without Adversely Impacting Growth or Rates of Breastfeeding

Débora Cañizo Vázquez [1], Sandra Salas García [2,*], Montserrat Izquierdo Renau [1] and Isabel Iglesias-Platas [1]

[1] Neonatology Department, Hospital Sant Joan de Déu, Universidad de Barcelona, BCNatal, 08950 Esplugues de Llobregat, Barcelona, Spain
[2] Neonatology Department, Hospital General Universitari Castelló, 12004 Castelló de la Plana, Spain
* Correspondence: sandrasalas33@gmail.com; Tel.: +34-689-951-982

Received: 11 July 2019; Accepted: 9 August 2019; Published: 14 August 2019

**Abstract:** Human milk contains non-nutritional factors that promote intestinal maturation and protect against infectious and inflammatory conditions. In the Neonatal Intensive Care Unit (NICU) setting, donor milk (DM) is recommended when availability of own mother's milk (OMM) is not enough. Our aim was to compare the incidence of necrotizing enterocolitis (NEC) and late-onset sepsis (LOS) in very preterm infants (VPI) after the introduction of DM. Growth and breastfeeding rates were examined as secondary outcomes. Single center, observational and retrospective cohort study comparing 227 VPI admitted to our neonatal unit before (Group 1, $n = 99$) and after (Group 2, $n = 128$) DM introduction. Enteral nutrition was started earlier after DM availability (2.6 ± 1.1 vs. 2.1 ± 1 days, $p = 0.001$). Incidence of NEC decreased in group 2 (9.1% vs. 3.4%, $p = 0.055$), especially in those born between 28 and 32 weeks (5.4 vs. 0.0%, $p = 0.044$). Surgical NEC was also less frequent. Suffering NEC was 4 times more likely in group 1 (multivariate analysis). Availability of DM did not impact breastfeeding rates or preterm growth. Our findings support the protective role of DM against NEC, particularly in non-extreme VPI, a group less frequently included in clinical guidelines and research studies on the use of DM.

**Keywords:** preterm infant; human milk; donor human milk; formula feeding; breastfeeding; necrotizing enterocolitis; growth

## 1. Introduction

The benefits of breastmilk for both mother and infant are well established [1,2]. Breast milk should be the first choice for feeding premature and low-birth weight newborns. Necrotizing enterocolitis (NEC) and late-onset sepsis (LOS) are infectious- inflammatory diseases of premature infants with a high rate of mortality, even today [3,4]. Breast milk has been shown to act as a preventative factor [5,6] and it is postulated that this is through several non-nutritional factors, such as immunoglobulins, growth factors and substances with antioxidant capacity [7,8]. Some of these compounds play a role in modulation of the immune system and in the pathophysiology of these and other diseases [7–11].

Establishing and maintaining an appropriate milk supply after preterm birth comes with its own challenges, including maternal illness, the need for artificial expression and stress surrounding separation from and worry about the well-being of the child [12]. International scientific societies recommend donor milk (DM) as the first alternative when the available quantity of own mother's milk (OMM) is not enough to cover the nutritional requirements of the premature infant [13]. It is unclear whether the advantages of pasteurized human milk can be similar to those of OMM.

Pasteurization does not alter caloric or macronutrient content, but there is controversy about how it does affect other biologically active components, such as IgA, lysozyme, lactoferrin, lymphocytes, lipase, alkaline phosphatase, cytokines (like IL10), growth factors and antioxidant capacity [8,14–16]. Several studies have shown a protective effect of DM against NEC [6,17] and an improvement in feeding tolerance [7,18] when comparing with formula feeding, and systematic reviews of published data find a decreased incidence of bronchopulmonary dysplasia (BPD) [19] and LOS [6]. Some even suggest better neurodevelopmental and cardiovascular outcomes with the use of DM [20,21].

Although growth of premature infants fed DM (especially if unfortified) might be slower when compared to formula-fed counterparts, no long-term nutritional compromise has been described [7]. Another concern that arose with the use of milk banks was that donor milk could threaten the motivation of the staff to provide support or the commitment of mothers to provide milk for their infants, but this does not seem to be the case [22].

The aim of this study was to compare the incidence of clinical complications (NEC and LOS) in very preterm infants (VPI) (≤32 weeks gestational age at birth) before and after the introduction of DM instead of artificial formula to supplement OMM when necessary. Rates of growth and breastfeeding in both groups were examined as secondary outcomes.

## 2. Materials and Methods

### 2.1. Study Design

Single center, observational retrospective cohort study of VPI admitted to a level III intensive care unit. The cohorts were defined by the use of premature artificial formula (Group 1) or donor milk (Group 2) for enteral feeding in the absence of enough OMM. Sample size was calculated to detect a reduction in the incidence of a composite outcome of NEC or LOS to a third (based on literature reports) of the basal figure of about 25% in our population of VPI. The estimated sample size was 82 patients per group for a confidence level of 95% with an 80% statistical power.

All subjects gave their informed consent for inclusion before they participated in the study. The study was conducted in accordance with the Declaration of Helsinki, and the protocol was approved by the local Ethics Committee (Fundació Sant Joan de Déu Ethics Committee; PIC-20-16).

### 2.2. Patients

Babies born at or before 32 completed weeks of gestational age were considered eligible. Inclusion criteria: Admission before 24 h of life and survival for longer than a week. Exclusion criteria: Major congenital malformations, chromosomal, genetic or metabolic abnormalities or the absence of clinical records. Group 1 comprised the 2 years before (2009–2010) and group 2 the 2 years after (2012–2013) the introduction of DM in our unit. The year of overlap (2011) was considered as an implementation period and not taken into consideration for the analysis. Clinical and growth variables as well as nutritional supplies were extracted from clinical charts.

### 2.3. Clinical Protocols

Nutritional management of VPI in our unit follows local written guidelines in accordance to international recommendations. In short and as previously described [23], parenteral nutrition (PN) is started immediately after birth through a central line for the provision of 2.5 g/kg of protein and 62 kcal/kg, with stepwise increases reaching 3.5–4 g/kg of protein and 100 kcal/kg depending on metabolic tolerance and progression of enteral feeding. Enteral nutrition is started as soon as possible depending on clinical condition of the patient. Own mother's milk is the first option. The difference between groups 1 and 2 was the supplementation with a preterm formula (Alprem®, Nestlé, Switzerland) or DM respectively, when the volume of enteral feeding prescribed was higher than the mother's milk supply. Donor milk is maintained if needed until one month of age if the baby is born under 28 weeks or 1000 g and during the first 3–7 days in newborns 28–32 weeks that are over 1 kg.

All human milk was fortified (Enfamil® Human Milk Fortifier Powder, Mead Johnson, Chicago, IL, USA) from an intake of 80–100 mL/kg/day.

There were no other changes in clinical protocols for any other areas of care in the unit during the study period.

*2.4. Study Variables*

Nutrition and growth: Volumes of enteral and parenteral nutrition administered were extracted from clinical charts. Macronutrients were calculated assuming standard compositions of preterm and term milk [24] or from manufacturer's information and considering the PN prescription. Nutritional supply was recorded daily for the first 14 days of life and again at 28 days and at 36 weeks postmenstrual age (PMA). Information on start of enteral feeding, achievement of full enteral nutrition and rates of OMM at 7, 14, 28 days of life, at full enteral nutrition and at discharge was also registered.

Weight was evaluated at admission, day 14 and day 28 of life and at 36 weeks PMA. We also collected data on minimum weight, days to maximum initial weight loss and days to regain birth weight. Length and head circumference (HC) data were available at birth and discharge. To allow for comparisons at different gestational ages, measurements of anthropometric parameters were transformed into z-scores for gestational age using local intrauterine growth standards [25,26].

Clinical variables: The main complications of prematurity were studied as clinical outcomes. A baby was considered to have NEC if fulfilling criteria compatible with Bell's stage 2 or higher [27]. Late-onset sepsis was defined as the presence of a positive culture of blood or a sterile fluid on or after the fourth day of life. Intraventricular hemorrhage was graded according to Papile et cols [28]. Patent ductus arteriosus (PDA) was diagnosed as the presence of clinical signs (heart murmur, hyperdynamic precordial impulse, full pulses, widened pulse pressure, and/or worsening of the respiratory status) with a ductal right-to-left shunt in the echocardiography. Bronchopulmonary dysplasia was defined as need for oxygen for more than 28 days. Retinopathy of prematurity (ROP) was staged according to the International Committee for classification of ROP [29] and considered as severe if requiring laser therapy.

*2.5. Statistical Analysis*

All data were analyzed with the SPSS® (Statistical Package for Social Sciences, IBM, Chicago, IL, USA) software, v17. Qualitative variables were expressed as frequencies or percentages and quantitative variables as means and standard deviations. Comparisons between Groups 1 and 2 were performed by chi-square and student $t$ tests as appropriate. Differences were considered significant if $p$-values were <0.05. Logistic regression models were used to analyze the risk of NEC in Groups 1 and 2 while adjusting for relevant covariates.

A secondary analysis for the groups ≤28 weeks and >28 weeks was performed on the basis of a higher risk of developing NEC among the extremely premature babies and because, as stated before, the protocol for administration of donor milk in our unit was different in the under and over 28 weeks groups (longer duration in the former).

## 3. Results

*3.1. Description of the Sample*

A total of 256 VPI were admitted to our unit during their first 24 h of life in the study period. Of them, 23 had exclusion criteria, leaving a total of 227 for analysis, 99 in Group 1 (before availability of DM) and 128 in Group 2 (after availability of DM) (Figure 1). Basal characteristics of the sample are summarized in Table 1. There were no differences between groups regarding gestational age, gender, multiparity, cesarean section, percentage of children with intrauterine growth restriction or severity of illness on admission as assessed by CRIB (Clinical Ric Index for Babies) score. Birth weight was slightly lower in Group 2, with no differences in z score (Table 1).

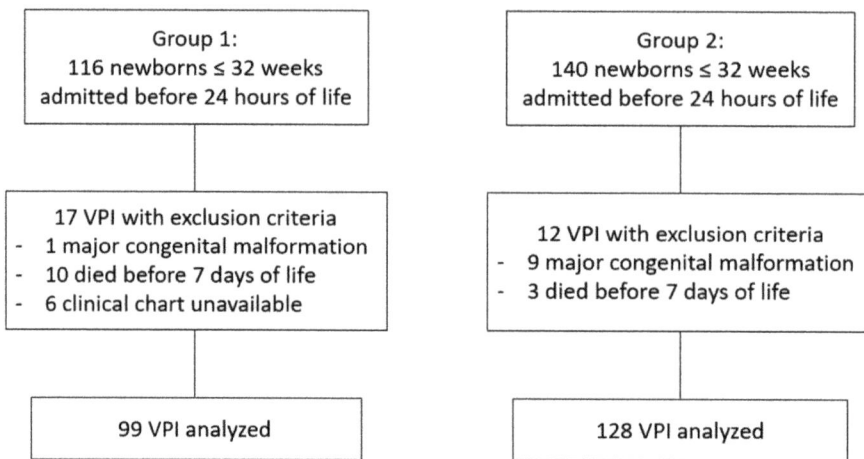

**Figure 1.** Flowchart of study participation.

*3.2. Enteral Nutrition Was Started Earlier after Availability of DM*

The start of enteral nutrition happened about half a day earlier in Group 2 (2.6 ± 1.1 vs. 2.1 ± 1.0 days, $p = 0.001$) and the percentage of fasted babies was lower on days of life 1 and 2 in Group 2. This did not impact age or milk volume at full enteral nutrition, days on parenteral nutrition or milk volumes fed during the 1st and 2nd weeks of life or at day 28 (Figure 2). There was a trend for a higher percentage of patients receiving only human milk on days 14 and 28 of life after the introduction of DM (65.2% vs. 76.9%, $p = 0.066$ and 62.9% vs. 75.2%, $p = 0.065$ respectively). This was significant for babies ≤ 28 weeks on day 14 (75.0% vs. 100.0%, $p = 0.004$). Nutrition during the second week of life and thereafter was homogenous between groups. During the first week we found small but significant differences in parenteral nutrition. Total fluid volume was higher in Group 1 (104.6 ± 11.0 vs. 96.3 ± 15.2, $p < 0.001$) and intravenous lipids (1.6 ± 0.7 vs. 1.9 ± 0.6, $p = 0.014$) were higher in Group 2. Total calories (78.4 ± 8.8 vs. 81.0 ± 9.1, $p = 0.035$) and protein (2.9 ± 0.4 vs. 3.0 ± 0.4, $p = 0.096$) were higher in Group 2.

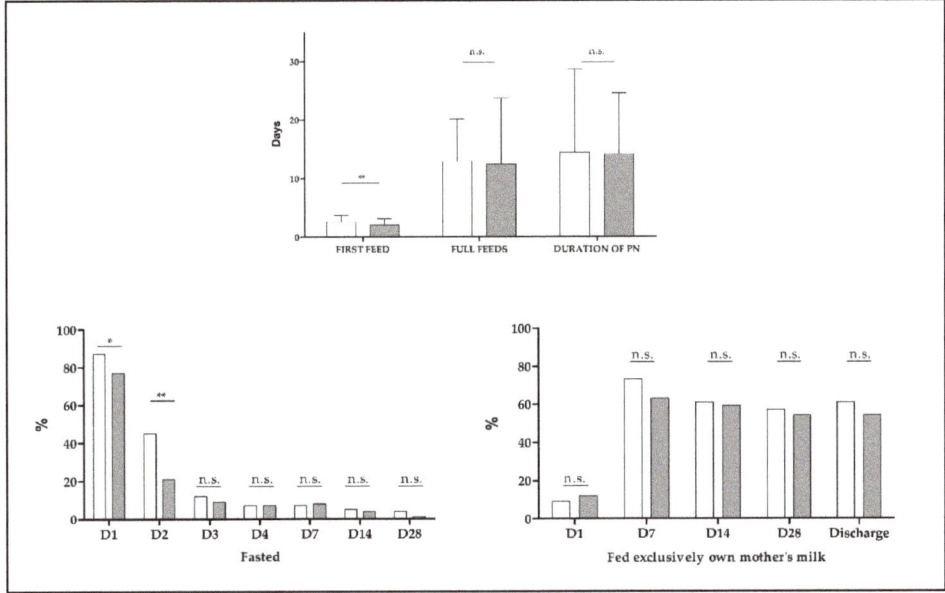

**Figure 2.** Summary of nutritional characteristics of very preterm infants (VPI) in G1 (white) and G2 (grey). * $p < 0.05$; ** $p < 0.001$; n.s.: non-significant ($p$-value > 0.05). G1: Group 1, G2: Group 2, D: Day of life, PN: Parenteral nutrition.

### 3.3. Breastfeeding Rates Did Not Change with the Introduction of Donor Milk

The percentage of children receiving their OMM was the same in both groups (Table 2). We have a rate of exclusive breastfeeding at discharge of 56.8% (60.6% in ≤28 weeks and 53.9% in >28 weeks).

### 3.4. Rates of Early Growth Were Better in Group 2

The percentage of weight loss immediately after birth was smaller in Group 2, due to differences in patients ≤28 weeks at birth (Table 2). There were no differences in age at minimum weight or days to recover birthweight. Fall in weight z-scores at 28 day of life (dol) was smaller in Group 2 than in Group 1, while no changes were seen at 36 weeks of PMA or discharge. In a multivariate analysis by linear regression, the group in which the patient was born was one of the determinants for fall in weight z-score at 28 dol after adjustment for confounders (Table S1). There were no differences between sexes in the growth and nutritional outcomes analyzed (data not shown).

### 3.5. The Incidence of Necrotizing Enterocolitis Decreased after the Introduction of DM

We found no differences between groups regarding ventilatory support, incidence of BPD, severe retinopathy or intraventricular hemorrhage. The rate of LOS was similar between groups and the same was true for duration of antibiotic treatment, days of central line and parenteral nutrition (Table 3). The incidence of NEC was slightly lower in Group 2 (9.1% vs. 3.4%, $p = 0.055$), especially in the group with a gestational age between 28 and 32 weeks at birth (5.4 vs. 0.0%, $p = 0.044$). Mortality was similar in both groups (4.0% vs. 5.5%, $p = 0.619$), but a history of NEC tended to be more frequent among very preterm babies that died in Group 1 (75.0% vs. 14.3%, $p = 0.088$). Surgical NEC was more frequent in G1 (5/99, 5.0% vs. 1/128, 0.8%), but this was not statistically significant ($p = 0.308$). An analysis of the risk of NEC in both groups including possible confounders showed that the odds of suffering NEC was 4 times higher before the introduction of DM (Table S2). There were no differences between boys and girls (data not shown).

Table 1. Comparison of basal characteristics of the patients from groups 1 and 2.

| | Whole Sample | | | Gestational Age ≤ 28 Weeks | | | Gestational Age > 28 Weeks | | |
|---|---|---|---|---|---|---|---|---|---|
| | Group 1 (n = 99) | Group 2 (n = 128) | p | Group 1 (n = 26) | Group 2 (n = 43) | p | Group 1 (n = 73) | Group 2 (n = 85) | p |
| | Mean ± SD | | | Mean ± SD | | | Mean ± SD | | |
| Gestational age (weeks) | 29.5 ± 2.3 | 29.1 ± 2.3 | 0.227 | 26.2 ± 1.3 | 26.3 ± 1.3 | 0.853 | 30.7 ± 1.1 | 30.5 ± 1.2 | 0.180 |
| Birth weight (g) | 1283 ± 393 | 1197 ± 370 | 0.095 | 844 ± 183 | 854 ± 210 | 0.759 | 1439 ± 323 | 1371 ± 306 | 0.499 |
| Birth weight z score | 0.11 ± 0.87 | −0.14 ± 0.93 | 0.204 | 0.05 ± 0.98 | −0.12 ± 1.05 | 0.516 | −0.00 ± 0.83 | −0.16 ± 0.87 | 0.261 |
| CRIB (Clinical Ric Index for Babies) score | 2.2 ± 3.0 | 2.8 ± 3.1 | 0.188 | 5.5 ± 3.8 | 5.1 ± 3.3 | 0.622 | 1.0 ± 1.4 | 1.6 ± 2.1 | 0.062 |
| | n (%) | | | n (%) | | | n (%) | | |
| Gender (boy) | 56 (56.6%) | 69 (53.9%) | 0.690 | 14 (53.8%) | 23 (53.5%) | 0.977 | 42 (57.5%) | 46 (54.1%) | 0.666 |
| Intrauterine growth restriction (IUGR) | 18 (18.2%) | 15 (11.7%) | 0.171 | 7 (26.9%) | 4 (9.3%) | 0.087 | 11 (15.2%) | 11 (12.9%) | 0.700 |
| Small for gestational age (SGA) | 7 (7.2%) | 10 (8.6%) | 0.706 | 3 (11.5%) | 4 (10.0%) | 1.000 | 4 (5.6%) | 6 (7.9%) | 0.747 |
| Multiple pregnancy | 39 (39.4%) | 47 (36.7%) | 0.771 | 8 (30.8%) | 12 (27.9%) | 0.800 | 31 (42.5%) | 35 (41.2%) | 0.870 |
| Cesarean section | 55 (55.6%) | 86 (67.2%) | 0.073 | 17 (65.4%) | 29 (67.4%) | 0.861 | 38 (52.1%) | 57 (67.1%) | 0.055 |
| Prenatal steroid course (2 doses) | 69 (69.7%) | 79 (61.7%) | 0.211 | 14 (53.8%) | 29 (67.4%) | 0.259 | 55 (75.3%) | 50 (58.8%) | 0.028 |

Table 2. Growth parameters of patients in Group 1 and 2.

| Mean ± SD | Whole Sample | | | Gestational Age ≤ 28 Weeks | | | Gestational Age > 28 Weeks | | |
|---|---|---|---|---|---|---|---|---|---|
| | Group 1 (n = 99) | Group 2 (n = 128) | p | Group 1 (n = 26) | Group 2 (n = 42) | p | Group 1 (n = 73) | Group 2 (n = 85) | p |
| Age at minimum weight (days) | 3.8 ± 1.6 | 3.9 ± 1.5 | 0.612 | 3.9 ± 1.8 | 4.2 ± 1.7 | 0.517 | 3.8 ± 1.6 | 3.8 ± 1.4 | 0.982 |
| % weight loss | 11.4 ± 5.1 | 9.2 ± 8.6 | 0.026 | 13.8 ± 6.0 | 7.8 ± 5.5 | <0.001 | 10.6 ± 4.5 | 10.0 ± 9.8 | 0.617 |
| Age at recovery of birth weight (days) | 11.1 ± 4.1 | 1.4 ± 5.1 | 0.287 | 11.5 ± 5.6 | 10.8 ± 6.9 | 0.663 | 11.0 ± 3.4 | 10.3 ± 3.9 | 0.230 |
| Fall in weight z-score from | | | | | | | | | |
| birth to 28 dol | −1.18 ± 0.41 | −0.96 ± 0.66 | 0.003 | −1.33 ± 0.59 | −0.91 ± 0.94 | 0.055 | −1.13 ± 0.32 | −0.98 ± 0.46 | 0.023 |
| birth to 36 weeks PMA | −1.69 ± 0.79 | −1.64 ± 0.70 | 0.652 | −2.31 ± 0.95 | −2.04 ± 0.76 | 0.217 | −1.43 ± 0.53 | −1.38 ± 0.51 | 0.588 |
| birth to discharge | −1.42 ± 0.77 | −1.42 ± 0.79 | 0.951 | −1.96 ± 1.04 | −1.86 ± 0.99 | 0.692 | −1.23 ± 0.55 | −1.21 ± 0.56 | 0.793 |

dol: Days of life, PMA: Postmenstrual age.

Table 3. Comparison of clinical outcomes between Group 1 and 2. Continuous variables are summarized as mean ± standard deviation and compared by Student's *t* tests. Categorical variables are expressed as number and percentage and compared by chi-square tests or Fisher's exact tests as appropriate.

| Clinical Outcomes During Admission | Whole Sample | | | Gestational Age ≤ 28 Weeks | | | Gestational Age > 28 Weeks | | |
|---|---|---|---|---|---|---|---|---|---|
| | Group 1 (n = 99) | Group 2 (n = 128) | p | Group 1 (n = 26) | Group 2 (n = 43) | p | Group 1 (n = 73) | Group 2 (n = 85) | p |
| Days on mechanical ventilation | 6.4 ± 15.4 | 5.6 ± 10.8 | 0.651 | 21.2 ± 24.7 | 13.2 ± 13.8 | 0.141 | 1.1 ± 2.4 | 1.7 ± 5.9 | 0.401 |
| Days on non-invasive respiratory support | 18.4 ± 21.6 | 21.3 ± 23.2 | 0.339 | 41.9 ± 26.3 | 42.3 ± 24.0 | 0.943 | 10.1 ± 11.1 | 10.7 ± 13.7 | 0.761 |
| Days on oxygen | 16.8 ± 33.0 | 16.3 ± 30.0 | 0.915 | 50.1 ± 49.0 | 42.6 ± 38.6 | 0.485 | 4.9 ± 10.4 | 3.0 ± 8.8 | 0.218 |
| Days on antibiotics | 10.8 ± 12.7 | 12.7 ± 12.9 | 0.267 | 24.4 ± 17.7 | 23.8 ± 14.4 | 0.884 | 6.0 ± 4.6 | 7.1 ± 7.2 | 0.253 |
| Days on central line | 14.4 ± 14.3 | 14.1 ± 10.5 | 0.864 | 25.0 ± 21.8 | 21.7 ± 12.2 | 0.420 | 9.4 ± 5.8 | 10.4 ± 5.0 | 0.247 |
| Days on parenteral nutrition | 13.5 ± 13.9 | 14.2 ± 9.7 | 0.658 | 25.8 ± 23.4 | 23.1 ± 12.8 | 0.542 | 10.3 ± 4.9 | 9.6 ± 4.7 | 0.308 |
| Patent ductus arteriosus | 44/99 (44.4%) | 57/128 (44.5%) | 0.990 | 21/26 (80.8%) | 31/43 (72.1%) | 0.418 | 23/73 (31.5%) | 26/59 (30.6%) | 0.901 |
| Surgical patent ductus arteriosus | 16/99 (16.2%) | 11/128 (8.6%) | 0.081 | 13/26 (50%) | 10/43 (23.3%) | 0.022 | 3/73 (4.1%) | 1/85 (1.2%) | 0.336 |
| Necrotizing enterocolitis | 9/99 (9.1%) | 4/128 (3.1%) | 0.055 | 5/26 (19.2%) | 4/43 (9.3%) | 0.282 | 4/73 (5.5%) | 0/85 (0%) | 0.044 |
| Surgical necrotizing enterocolitis | 5/9 (55.6%) | 1/4 (25%) | 0.308 | 1/26 (3.8%) | 1/43 (2.3%) | 1.000 | 0/73 | 0/85 | - |
| Late-onset sepsis | 18/99 (18.2%) | 27/128 (21.1%) | 0.585 | 14/26 (53.8%) | 22/43 (51.2%) | 0.829 | 4/73 (5.5%) | 5/73 (5.9%) | 0.913 |
| Bronchopulmonary dysplasia | 21/96 (21.9%) | 28/124 (22.6%) | 0.901 | 15/24 (62.5%) | 25/39 (64.1%) | 0.898 | 6/72 (8.3%) | 3/85 (3.5%) | 0.172 |
| Retinopathy of prematurity (any stage) | 27/87 (31%) | 43/113 (38.1%) | 0.302 | 19/23 (82.6%) | 26/40 (65.0%) | 0.136 | 8/64 (12.5%) | 17/56 (23.3%) | 0.103 |
| Severe retinopathy of prematurity | 5/81 (6.2%) | 6/112 (5.4%) | 0.809 | 5/23 (21.7%) | 6/39 (15.4%) | 0.732 | 0/58 (0%) | 0/73 (0%) | - |
| Severe intraventricular hemorrhage (grade III-IV) | 6/99 (6.1%) | 12/128 (9.4%) | 0.359 | 6/26 (23.1%) | 9/43 (20.9%) | 0.834 | 0/73 (0.0%) | 3/85 (3.5%) | 0.250 |
| Death | 4/99 (4%) | 7/128 (5.5%) | 0.619 | 3/26 (11.5%) | 6/43 (14.0%) | 1.000 | 1/73 (1.4%) | 1/85 (1.2%) | 1.000 |

## 4. Discussion

Enteral feeding with DM when own mother's milk is not available or is not enough has been associated with reduced mortality and a decrease in morbidity of VPI [6,18,19]. However, there is a concern about nutritional requirements of VPI fed with DM because artificial formula results in higher rates of weight gain and linear growth due to its greater amounts of nutrients. Preterm formulas are energy-enriched and variably protein and mineral-enriched when compared to mature human milk, and the nutrient content of donor milk may be further compromised by pasteurization [30]. Nevertheless, the role of an exclusive human milk diet is well recognized in the prevention of NEC and other severe complications like invasive infections. In a recent publication, this effect has been related to the presence of antioxidants in breast milk, and these could be impaired by DM processing [11].

Nowadays it remains unclear if DM has the same advantages as OMM and may have some disadvantages related to growth with respect to artificial formula. Our aim was to compare short-term outcomes of VPI admitted in our unit before and after the availability of DM, while also taking into account feeding and growth indicators.

Since the introduction of DM, there has been a reduction in both the percentage of VPI that are fasted in their first two days of life and in the age at initiation of enteral feeding, in line with other reports in the literature (16 h in Castellano Yañez et al., 12 h in our data) [31]. The results of an international survey published in 2012 [32] showed that when DM was available, the start of feedings was earlier and faster, maybe reflecting a better gastrointestinal tolerance to human milk when compared to artificial premature formula [18,30]. Despite this, we did not see a shortening in time on parenteral nutrition or at full enteral feedings. Our findings are similar to the data reported by Corpeleijn in 2016 [33] and might explain why, unlike others [6,34], we did not see a decrease in the incidence of LOS, which is consistent with other series [22,33,35].

There has been some degree of controversy regarding the impact of availability of DM on the rates of availability of own mother's milk, with either stability or increase being reported. In our unit, the introduction of banked milk did not change the percentage of exclusive breastfeeding at discharge, and this is in line with the observation in a slightly more mature population of preterms [31] as well as with the conclusion of a systematic review [36], which found no differences in exclusive administration of OMM on the first 28 days of life or at discharge. An Italian survey published in 2013 [13] describes that units where DM is available show higher rates of exclusive breastfeeding at discharge, although this might reflect baseline differences in the attitude towards human milk feeding. A multicentric Californian database analysis [37] observed an increase of about 10% in the rates of exclusive breastfeeding at discharge in infants under 1500 g admitted to Neonatal Intensive Care Units of mixed complexity after the introduction of DM; nevertheless, this increase was also seen in the same period of time among units that had no access to banked milk.

Milk produced by mothers that deliver preterm is richer in lipids, protein and calories [38] and is better suited for the needs of their infants regarding growth and neurodevelopment [39]. Even so, it is common practice in neonatal units to apply the same fortification protocol for OMM and DM, which is mainly supplied by mothers of term babies. This could be one of the reasons behind reported differences in growth in preterm babies fed OMM, DM and preterm formula [7,40]. A systematic review and metaanalysis [30], including 11 randomized controlled trials and 1809 patients concluded that preterms fed formula had faster rates of growth (weight, length and HC) when compared to the ones fed DM, whether exclusively or as a supplement of OMM. Interestingly, there were no differences in long term growth or neurodevelopment [30].

In our study, sequential weight, length and HC and their z-scores are similar between groups, contrary to previous reports [7,30,31,40]. What is more, the fall in weight z score at day 28 of life significantly decreased from group 1 to 2, although the difference was small (IC 95%: $-1.18 \pm 0.41$ vs. $-0.96 \pm 0.66$, $p = 0.003$) and disappeared by discharge time. Due to known differences in nutritional content between preterm and banked milk, this must be explained by other factors. Sisk et al. [41] also found preserved growth rates at discharge, but their classification of groups by predominant milk meant that babies in the DM group could be receiving up to 49% of their OMM. In our case, a detailed analysis exposes a slight but significant difference in early parenteral provision of nutrients, which has been shown to have an impact in growth during the first month [23].

Previous evidence points to a reduction of about 4% in the incidence and severity of NEC in VPI fed human milk [17,32,42], and this has been summarized recently [43]. It seems that the bigger the volume and the longer the duration of human milk feeding, the more impact in the occurrence of NEC [6]. Since the introduction of DM in our unit, we see a tendency to a decrease in the incidence of NEC, which is most prominent in babies born after 28 weeks of gestation, maybe because they are the ones that receive the most artificial formula (in the whole sample, 16.1% of babies born ≤ 28 weeks received some volume of formula on day 28 of life vs. 37.8% of those born at > 28 weeks, $p = 0.002$; this was 7.9% vs. 33.3%, respectively, in Group 2, $p = 0.003$). Mortality was similar before and after DM in our population as well as others [6,30], but we saw a history of NEC was more frequent in those who died in Group 1 when compared with Group 2. Surgical NEC was also less frequent in G2, although this was not statistically significant. The conclusion of a metanalysis on the impact of DM on the risk of surgical NEC was in line with this result [44]. Interestingly, if we add our numbers to the ones reported (although the metanalysis did not include observational studies), the incidence of surgical NEC would decrease from 5.2% in the group receiving formula to 1.8% in the group receiving DM, with a $p$-value of 0.002.

A recent metaanalysis [19] also describes a decrease in the incidence of BPD in DM fed versus formula fed preterm babies. Other multicentric studies [42] also found a decrease in days on mechanical ventilation or oxygen. Duration of invasive ventilation in extreme preterms (≤28 w) seemed shorter in Group 2, but the study was not powered to draw a conclusion. In any case, due to the before-after design of our study, this could merely reflect a global tendency to earlier extubation in neonatal care.

The presence of differences between sexes in the incidence of neonatal complications [45] and in growth responses to varied exposures [46] have been recently highlighted in the literature. As we mentioned, further analysis of our cohort showed that the same general conclusions apply to both sexes as well as to the whole population. When sex was introduced in the multivariate analysis, the final model did not vary and the contributing factors to NEC were gestational age, period of availability of donor milk and being SGA.

In this study, we contribute relevant information on morbidity, growth and breastfeeding outcomes of DM use in a third level neonatal unit. The single-center design should contribute to homogeneity on other aspects of care between groups. Although there is an increasing amount of literature about benefits of human milk when compared to artificial formulas, there is a high degree of variability in the methodology applied. There are differences in time windows analyzed (for example 10 days of life in Corpeleijn et al. [33]), the type of formula in the comparison group (4 standard term formula and 7 preterm formula in the 11 RCTs included in the 2018 Cochrane systematic review and metaanalysis [30]) or type of fortifier (human milk based vs. cow milk based [30]). Each center also has different criteria for the initiation, advancement and duration of DM feeding [47]. Our patients received DM under a pre-specified protocol, and we also include a detailed analysis of other growth and nutritional variables (like parenteral supply), which lacks in many other reports.

A remarkable finding of our study is that patients in the range from 28 to 32 weeks benefit more than those under 28 when using DM in terms of NEC-reduction under the conditions of our study. Most protocols of DM supplementation apply to patients born under 28 weeks GA. Even in our guidelines, patients under 28 are candidates for DM use for a longer period than those between 28 and 32 weeks. This makes us consider if this group (28–32 weeks GA) might be more sensitive to certain strategies for NEC prevention, including maybe, the use of DM, and if the results could improve with providing it for a longer time. Also, we did not find any differences in growth at discharge or in breastfeeding rates, which are two of the most reported undesired effects of using DM instead of formula for supplementation of OMM in the Neonatal Intensive Care Unit (NICU).

One of the limitations of our study is the available sample size. Also, the retrospective design does not allow for conclusions in causality. The pre- and post-period design rather than the analysis of actual intakes better reflects the impact of DM availability in a neonatal unit. Nevertheless, it should be taken into account that we have a moderately high rate of breastfeeding, so that more than half of the sample in both periods was receiving exclusively their OMM throughout admission, which might make it difficult to uncover any further differences between DM and formula. Another limitation is that the cause of preterm birth was not considered for the analysis. A higher risk of NEC has been described in some preterm subpopulations, like premature babies born after a period of intrauterine growth restriction (IUGR) [48] and they could benefit even more from the use of DM. Our study was not powered enough to detect differences in the effect of donor milk between different premature populations, which might be an area granting future attention.

## 5. Conclusions

Since the introduction of donor milk in our unit we have seen a reduction in NEC, particularly in the VPI between 28 and 32 weeks. We did not find significant differences in the incidence of other complications of prematurity or in rates of growth or breastfeeding.

Ours results support the evidence that donor milk feeding is safe and beneficial, not only for the most extreme premature babies, and that it can be implemented without impairment in nutritional outcomes while maintaining rates of breastfeeding.

**Supplementary Materials:** The following are available online at http://www.mdpi.com/2072-6643/11/8/1895/s1, Table S1: Multivariate analysis by linear regression of the determinants of fall in weight z-score at 28 day of life, Table S2: Multivariate analysis by logistic regression of the determinants of NEC.

**Author Contributions:** D.C.V. and S.S.G., reviewed the cases and collected the data, then collaborated in the data analysis. In addition, they reviewed the bibliography, prepared and wrote the first draft of this paper, and coordinated manuscript revisions and submission. M.I.R. and I.I.-P., planned and design the study, revised the methodology and led the statistical analysis. All the authors have seen and approved the final version.

**Funding:** This work is part of the project PI17/00107, from the National Plan of R+D+I and cofounded by the Instituto de Salud Carlos III (ISCIII)—General Assistant Direction for Evaluation and Promotion of Health Research and the European Regional Development Fund (ERDF).

**Acknowledgments:** We would like to thank all participants and their families as well as all the clinical staff in the Neonatal Unit.

**Conflicts of Interest:** The authors declare no conflict of interest.

## References

1. Morales, Y.; Schanler, R.J. Human Milk and Clinical Outcomes in VLBW Infants: How Compelling Is the Evidence of Benefit? *Semin. Perinatol.* **2007**, *31*, 83–88. [CrossRef] [PubMed]
2. Schanler, R.J.; Shulman, R.J.; Lau, C. Feeding Strategies for Premature Infants: Beneficial Outcomes of Feeding Fortified Human Milk Versus Preterm Formula. *Pediatrics* **1999**, *103*, 1150–1157. [CrossRef] [PubMed]
3. Frost, B.L.; Modi, B.P.; Jaksic, T.; Caplan, M.S. New Medical and surgical insights into neonatal necrotizing enterocolitis a review. *JAMA Pediatr.* **2017**, *171*, 83–88. [CrossRef] [PubMed]
4. Shane, A.L.; Sánchez, P.J.; Stoll, B.J. Neonatal sepsis. *Lancet* **2017**, *390*, 1770–1780. [CrossRef]
5. Cacho, N.T.; Parker, L.A.; Neu, J. Necrotizing Enterocolitis and Human Milk Feeding: A Systematic Review. *Clin. Perinatol.* **2017**, *44*, 49–67. [CrossRef] [PubMed]
6. Miller, J.; Tonkin, E.; Damarell, R.A.; McPhee, A.J.; Suganuma, M.; Suganuma, H.; Middleton, P.F.; Makrides, M.; Collins, C.T. A Systematic Review and Meta-Analysis of Human Milk Feeding and Morbidity in Very Low Birth Weight Infants. *Nutrients* **2018**, *10*, 707. [CrossRef]
7. Quigley, M.; Mcguire, W. Formula versus donor breast milk for feeding preterm or low birth weight infants. *Cochrane Libr.* **2014**, CD002971. [CrossRef]
8. Aksu, T.; Atalay, Y.; Türkyilmaz, C.; Gülbahar, Ö.; Hirfanoğlu, I.M.; Demirel, N.; Önal, E.; Ergenekon, E.; Koç, E. The effects of breast milk storage and freezing procedure on interleukine-10 levels and total antioxidant activity. *J. Matern. Neonatal Med.* **2015**, *28*, 1799–1802. [CrossRef]

9. Manti, S.; Lougaris, V.; Cuppari, C.; Tardino, L.; Dipasquale, V.; Arrigo, T.; Salpietro, C.; Leonardi, S. Breastfeeding and IL-10 levels in children affected by cow's milk protein allergy: A restrospective study. *Immunobiology* **2017**, *222*, 358–362. [CrossRef]
10. Arrigo, T.; Leonardi, S.; Cuppari, C.; Manti, S.; Lanzafame, A.; D'Angelo, G.; Gitto, E.; Marseglia, L.; Salpietro, C. Role of the diet as a link between oxidative stress and liver diseases. *World J. Gastroenterol.* **2015**, *21*, 384–395. [CrossRef]
11. Aceti, A.; Beghetti, I.; Martini, S.; Faldella, G.; Corvaglia, L. Oxidative stress and necrotizing enterocolitis: Pathogenetic mechanisms, opportunities for intervention, and role of human milk. *Oxid. Med. Cell. Longev.* **2018**, *2018*, 7397369. [CrossRef]
12. Asztalos, E.V. Supporting mothers of very preterm infants and breast milk production: A review of the role of galactogogues. *Nutrients* **2018**, *10*, 600. [CrossRef]
13. Arslanoglu, S.; Corpeleijn, W.; Moro, G.; Braegger, C.; Campoy, C.; Colomb, V.; Decsi, T.; Domellöf, M.; Fewtrell, M.; Hojsak, I.; et al. Donor human milk for preterm infants: Current evidence and research directions. *J. Pediatr. Gastroenterol. Nutr.* **2013**, *57*, 535–542. [CrossRef]
14. Goelz, R.; Hihn, E.; Hamprecht, K.; Dietz, K.; Jahn, G.; Poets, C.; Elmlinger, M. Effects of different CMV-heat-inactivation-methods on growth factors in human breast milk. *Pediatr. Res.* **2009**, *65*, 458–461. [CrossRef]
15. Daniels, B.; Schmidt, S.; King, T.; Israel-Ballard, K.; Mansen, K.A.; Coutsoudis, A. The effect of simulated flash-heat pasteurization on immune components of human milk. *Nutrients* **2017**, *9*, 178. [CrossRef]
16. Untalan, P.B.; Keeney, S.E.; Palkowetz, K.H.; Rivera, A.; Goldman, A.S. Heat Susceptibility of Interleukin-10 and Other Cytokines in Donor Human Milk. *Breastfeed. Med.* **2009**, *4*, 137–144. [CrossRef]
17. Cristofalo, E.A.; Schanler, R.J.; Blanco, C.L.; Sullivan, S.; Trawoeger, R.; Kiechl-Kohlendorfer, U.; Dudell, G.; Rechtman, D.J.; Lee, M.L.; Lucas, A.; et al. Randomized Trial of Exclusive Human Milk versus Preterm Formula Diets in Extremely Premature Infants. *J. Pediatr.* **2013**, *163*, 1592–1595. [CrossRef]
18. Bertino, E.; Giuliani, F.; Baricco, M.; Di Nicola, P.; Peila, C.; Vassia, C.; Chiale, F.; Pirra, A.; Cresi, F.; Martano, C.; et al. Benefits of donor milk in the feeding of preterm infants. *Early Hum. Dev.* **2013**, *89*, S3–S6. [CrossRef]
19. Villamor-Martínez, E.; Pierro, M.; Cavallaro, G.; Mosca, F.; Kramer, B.W.; Villamor, E. Donor human milk protects against bronchopulmonary dysplasia: A systematic review and meta-analysis. *Nutrients* **2018**, *10*, 238. [CrossRef]
20. Unger, S.; Gibbins, S.; Zupancic, J.; O'Connor, D.L. DoMINO: Donor milk for improved neurodevelopmental outcomes. *BMC Pediatr.* **2014**, *14*, 1–12. [CrossRef]
21. Zhou, J.; Shukla, V.V.; John, D.; Chen, C. Human Milk Feeding as a Protective Factor for Retinopathy of Prematurity: A Meta-analysis. *Pediatrics* **2015**, *136*, e1576–e1586. [CrossRef]
22. Larena Fernández, I.; Vara Callau, M.; Royo Pérez, D.; López Bernués, R.; Cortés Sierra, J.; Samper Villagrasa, M.P. Estudio de los efectos de la implantación de un banco de leche donada en los recién nacidos pretérmino en Aragón. *Enferm. Clin.* **2015**, *25*, 57–63. [CrossRef]
23. Izquierdo, M.; Martínez-Monseny, A.F.; Pociello, N.; Gonzalez, P.; Del Rio, R.; Iriondo, M.; Iglesias-Platas, I. Changes in Parenteral Nutrition during the First Week of Life Influence Early but Not Late Postnatal Growth in Very Low-Birth-Weight Infants. *Nutr. Clin. Pract.* **2016**, *31*, 666–672. [CrossRef]
24. Tudehope, D. Human milk and the nutritional needs of preterm infants. *J. Pediatr.* **2013**, *162*, S17–S25. [CrossRef]
25. Corbes de referència de pes, perímetre cranial i longitut en néixer de nounats d'embarassos únics, de bessons i de trigèmins a Catalunya.
26. García Muñoz, F.; García-Alix, A.; Figueras, J.; Saavedra, P. Nuevas curvas poblacionales de crecimiento en recién nacidos extremadamente prematuros espanoles. *An. Pediatr.* **2013**, *6*, 1–8.
27. Bell, M.; Ternberg, J.; Feigin, L. Neonatal necrotizing enterocolitis: Therapeutic decisions based upon clinical staging. *Ann. Surg.* **1978**, *187*, 1–7. [CrossRef]
28. Papile, L.; Burstein, J.; Burstein, R.; Koffler, H. Incidence and evolution of subependimal and intraventricular hemorrhage: A study of infants with birth weight less than 1500 gm. *J. Pediatr.* **1978**, *92*, 529–534. [CrossRef]
29. Patz, A. The new international classification of retinopathy of prematurity. *Arch. Ophthalmol.* **1984**, *74*, 160–161. [CrossRef]
30. Quigley, M.; Embleton, N.D.; Mcguire, W. Formula versus donor breast milk for feeding preterm or low birth weight infants. *Cochrane Database Syst. Rev.* **2018**, *6*, CD002971. [CrossRef]

31. Castellano Yáñez, C.; Castillo Barrio, B.; Muñoz Labián, M.D.C.; Ortiz Movilla, R.; García Lara, N.R.; Royuela Vicente, A.; Marín Gabriel, M.A. Providing very preterm infants with donor human milk led to faster breastfeeding rates but worse biometric gains. *Acta Paediatr. Int. J. Paediatr.* **2018**, *12*, 1–2. [CrossRef]
32. Klingenberg, C.; Embleton, N.D.; Jacobs, S.E.; O'Connell, L.A.F.; Kuschel, C.A. Enteral feeding practices in very preterm infants: An international survey. *Arch. Dis. Child. Fetal Neonatal Ed.* **2012**, *97*, 1–3. [CrossRef]
33. Corpeleijn, W.E.; De Waard, M.; Christmann, V.; Van Goudoever, J.B.; Jansen-Van Der Weide, M.C.; Kooi, E.M.W.; Koper, J.F.; Kouwenhoven, S.M.P.; Lafeber, H.N.; Mank, E.; et al. Effect of donor milk on severe infections and mortality in very low-birth-weight infants: The early nutrition study randomized clinical trial. *JAMA Pediatr.* **2016**, *170*, 654–661. [CrossRef]
34. Assad, M.; Elliott, M.J.; Abraham, J.H. Decreased cost and improved feeding tolerance in VLBW infants fed an exclusive human milk diet. *J. Perinatol.* **2015**, *36*, 216–220. [CrossRef]
35. De Silva, A.; Jones, P.W.; Spencer, S.A. Does human milk reduce infection rates in preterm infants? A systematic review. *Arch. Dis. Child. Fetal Neonatal Ed.* **2004**, *89*, 509–514. [CrossRef]
36. Williams, T.; Nair, H.; Simpson, J.; Embleton, N. Use of Donor Human Milk and Maternal Breastfeeding Rates. *J. Hum. Lact.* **2016**, *32*, 212–220. [CrossRef]
37. Kantorowska, A.; Gould, J.B.; Cohen, R.S.; Lee, H.C.; Wei, J.C.; Lawrence, R.A. Impact of Donor Milk Availability on Breast Milk Use and Necrotizing Enterocolitis Rates. *Pediatrics* **2016**, *137*, e20153123. [CrossRef]
38. Underwood, M.A. Human milk for premature infants. *Pediatr. Clin. N. Am.* **2013**, *60*, 189–207. [CrossRef]
39. Van Goudoever, J.B.; Vlaardingerbroek, H.; Van den Akker, C. Amino Acids and Proteins. *World Rev. Nutr. Diet.* **2014**, *110*, 49–63.
40. Brownell, E.A.; Matson, A.P.; Smith, K.C.; Moore, J.E.; Esposito, P.A.; Lussier, M.M.; Lerer, T.J.; Hagadorn, J.I. Dose-response Relationship between Donor Human Milk, Mother's Own Milk, Preterm Formula, and Neonatal Growth Outcomes. *J. Pediatr. Gastroenterol. Nutr.* **2018**, *67*, 90–96. [CrossRef]
41. Sisk, P.M.; Lambeth, T.M.; Rojas, M.A.; Lightbourne, T.; Barahona, M.; Anthony, E.; Auringer, S.T. Necrotizing Enterocolitis and Growth in Preterm Infants Fed Predominantly Maternal Milk, Pasteurized Donor Milk, or Preterm Formula: A Retrospective Study. *Am. J. Perinatol.* **2017**, *34*, 676–683.
42. Verd, S.; Porta, R.; Botet, F.; Gutiérrez, A.; Ginovart, G.; Barbero, A.H.; Ciurana, A.; Plata, I.I. Hospital Outcomes of Extremely Low Birth Weight Infants After Introduction of Donor Milk to Supplement Mother's Milk. *Breastfeed. Med.* **2015**, *10*, 150–155. [CrossRef]
43. Available online: https://www.amerihealthcaritaspa.com/pdf/provider/resources/clinical/policies/170401-donor-human-milk.pdf (accessed on 25 April 2019).
44. Silano, M.; Milani, G.P.; Fattore, G.; Agostoni, C. Donor human milk and risk of surgical necrotizing enterocolitis: A meta-analysis. *Clin. Nutr.* **2019**, *38*, 1061–1066. [CrossRef]
45. Binet, M.-E.; Bujold, E.; Lefebre, F.; Tremblay, Y.; Piedboeuf, B. Role of gender in morbidity and mortality of extremely premature neonates. *Am. J. Perinatol.* **2012**, *29*, 159–166. [CrossRef]
46. Alur, P. Sex Differences in Nutrition, Growth, and Metabolism in Preterm Infants. *Front. Pediatr.* **2019**, *7*, 1–9. [CrossRef]
47. Sáenz de Pipaón, M.; Closa, R.; Gormaz, M.; Lines, M.; Nabona, E.; Rodríguez-Martínez, G.; Uberos, J.; Zozaya, C.; Couce, M.L. Nutritional practices in very low birth weight infants: A national survey. *Nutr. Hosp.* **2017**, *34*, 1067–1072.
48. Barone, G.; Maggio, L.; Saracino, A.; Perri, A.; Romagnoli, C.; Zecca, E. How to feed small for gestational age newborn. *Ital. J. Pediatr.* **2013**, *39*, 1–5. [CrossRef]

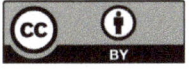

© 2019 by the authors. Licensee MDPI, Basel, Switzerland. This article is an open access article distributed under the terms and conditions of the Creative Commons Attribution (CC BY) license (http://creativecommons.org/licenses/by/4.0/).

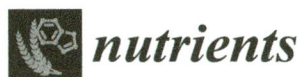 

Article

# Supplementation of Mother's Own Milk with Donor Milk in Infants with Gastroschisis or Intestinal Atresia: A Retrospective Study

Rebecca Hoban [1,2,3,*], Supriya Khatri [1], Aloka Patel [3] and Sharon L. Unger [1,2,4]

1. Department of Paediatrics, Division of Neonatology, Hospital for Sick Children, Toronto, ON M5G 1X8, Canada; supriya.khatri@sickkids.ca (S.K.); sharon.unger@sinaihealthsystem.ca (S.L.U.)
2. Faculty of Medicine, University of Toronto, Toronto, ON M5S 1A8, Canada
3. Department of Pediatrics, Division of Neonatology, Rush University Children's Hospital, Chicago, IL 60612, USA; Aloka_Patel@Rush.edu
4. Department of Paediatrics, Sinai Health, Toronto, ON M5G 1X5, Canada
* Correspondence: rebecca.hoban@sickkids.ca; Tel.: +1-416-813-6345; Fax: +1-416-813-5245

Received: 30 January 2020; Accepted: 20 February 2020; Published: 24 February 2020

**Abstract:** Background: Mother's own milk (MOM) improves in-hospital outcomes for preterm infants. If unavailable, donor milk (DM) is often substituted. It is unclear if DM vs. formula to supplement MOM is associated with improved in-hospital outcomes in term/late preterm surgical infants with gastroschisis or intestinal atresia. Methods: This retrospective study included infants born ≥33 weeks gestational age (GA) with a birth weight of >1500 g who were admitted to a quaternary neonatal intensive care unit (NICU). Using Chi square and Mann-Whitney u testing, we compared hospital outcomes (length of stay, parenteral nutrition and central line days) before and after a clinical practice change to offer DM instead of formula in this surgical population. Results: Baseline characteristics were similar between eras for the 140 infants (median GA 37 weeks). Fewer infants in DM era were receiving formula at discharge (50.0% vs. 31.4%, $p = 0.03$). In sub-analyses including only small bowel atresia and gastroschisis infants, the median length of stay (35 vs. 25, $p < 0.01$) and the central line days (28 vs. 20, $p < 0.01$) were lower in the DM era. Conclusion: In this retrospective study, offering DM instead of formula was associated with less formula feeding at discharge, and in infants with gastroschisis or small bowel atresia, shorter length of stay and central line days.

**Keywords:** human milk; donor milk; neonatal; gastroschisis; intestinal atresia

## 1. Introduction

Infants born with congenital malformations of the gastrointestinal (GI) tract, specifically those with gastroschisis or intestinal atresia, require surgical intervention early in life. Their abnormal GI tract necessitates prolonged parenteral nutritional (PN) [1,2] support prior to and after surgery, which puts these infants at risk of morbidities such as central line-associated sepsis and PN-induced cholestasis. In addition, once enteral feedings are initiated these infants commonly experience feeding intolerance and secondary morbidities such as necrotizing enterocolitis (NEC) [1,3] because of bowel exposure to inflammatory amniotic fluid and/or distension during fetal life [3]. All of these challenges, combined with the fact that these infants are often born late preterm [2], result in prolonged courses of PN and long hospital length of stays (LOS). Human milk (HM), which is most often mother's own milk (MOM), reduces the incidence of NEC in high-risk populations such as infants with preterm birth or gastroschisis [4–6]. Additionally, HM has been reported to shorten LOS, PN time and time to full enteral feeds in congenital GI malformations requiring surgery (gastroschisis, atresia) [7,8]. HM also reduces PN time and PN-associated liver disease in infants with short bowel syndrome [9,10] or intestinal failure, which may be a consequence of congenital GI malformations. Infants with congenital GI malformations are nothing by mouth (NPO, nil per os), are separated from their mothers after birth, and are often late preterm, requiring their mothers to initiate lactation exclusively with a breast pump, resulting in lactation challenges, risks of poor MOM supply [11–15] and lower rates of breastfeeding. If a supplement to MOM is required, the current standard of care in the term/late preterm population is the use of formula.

In other high-risk populations, namely very preterm (<32 weeks gestation) infants, pasteurized donor human milk (DM) is now commonly used if exclusive MOM is unavailable. Pasteurization and multiple freeze thaw cycles result in a product quite different than MOM in a myriad of ways, from bioactive to nutritional properties [16], but in the preterm population DM use avoids the risks of formula, specifically NEC [17]. Since DM is an expensive and limited resource, most Neonatal Intensive Care Units (NICUs) limit DM provision to very preterm infants, excluding most infants with congenital GI malformations. There are no trials of its efficacy in infants with congenital GI malformations, although it has been suggested that DM could have benefit in this population based on extrapolation from the preterm infant literature [12].

In 2013, the Hospital for Sick Children (HSC), in conjunction with the Rogers Hixon Ontario Human Milk Bank, changed its practice from only supplying DM to very preterm infants to also offer DM in-hospital to infants with congenital GI malformations in the first month post-surgery if MOM supply was inadequate. Given the limited literature, we sought to determine whether the use of DM for infants with congenital GI malformations who would not otherwise qualify for DM was associated with improved outcomes after this practice change. Primary outcomes included days of PN and central venous line (CL) as well as LOS. Secondary outcomes included comparing the use of MOM in both eras as a balancing measure, as offering DM could affect MOM provision [16]; comparing growth in both eras, as DM in the preterm population has been variably associated with poor growth [16,18]; and to compare risks of NEC (medical or surgical), culture positive sepsis and death in the pre-DM and DM eras.

## 2. Materials/Subjects and Methods

This was a retrospective single center study that included neonates admitted to an urban, quaternary outborn neonatal intensive care unit (NICU) in Toronto, Canada (the Hospital for Sick Children) prior to any surgical intervention who held a diagnosis of gastroschisis or congenital intestinal atresia.

*2.1. Sample*

Eligible infants had a birthweight (BW) >1500 g and/or gestational age (GA) at birth ≥33 weeks with a diagnosis of gastroschisis and/or congenital lower intestinal atresia (duodenal, jejunal, or ileal atresia or colonic/rectal atresia without a fistula). Included infants in this convenience sample were born between 1 July 2011 and 31 December 2012 (pre-DM era) and between 1 January 2014 and 31 May 2015 (DM era) to encompass approximately equal eras surrounding a practice change to use DM in late preterm or term surgical infants in early 2013. 2013 was excluded as a "wash-out" year to ensure complete separation between groups given long LOS and to allow for clinical uptake of the practice change. Of note, feeding initiation and advancement guidelines were slightly modified at our institution in early 2011 (prior to the study) and did not change for the duration of the study. Term and late preterm infants with congenital GI malformations would typically receive unfortified MOM or term formula; DM had protein powder added to approximate typical MOM protein levels. Infants would only receive bovine-based HM fortifiers for clinical concerns of poor growth once full enteral feeding tolerance was achieved. Infants were excluded if their initial admission to the NICU occurred after surgical intervention (i.e., transferred from another tertiary institution for second opinion or continued care). Other congenital gastrointestinal surgical conditions such as omphalocele, esophageal atresia, and anorectal malformation with fistula were not included unless co-existing with an included condition (such as both duodenal atresia and omphalocele). Lactation consultation and support was available to all mothers, as was a hospital grade double electric pumps for use in-hospital or to borrow without cost for home use. DM was offered after the practice change with parental consent when MOM supply was inadequate for the first post-operative month or until nearing discharge, whichever occurred sooner, with gradual weaning to formula occurring over a 48 h period.

*2.2. Design and Measures*

This study was approved by the institutional Research Ethics Board at the Hospital for Sick Children, and given its retrospective nature, was exempted from consent. Data were extracted from the electronic medical records for both eras after relevant medical record numbers were pulled from an internal NICU electronic database based on the study inclusion criteria of diagnosis, birthweight, gestational age and date of birth. Relevant electronic medical records were then hand searched to obtain and confirm each subject's relevant surgical primary (and secondary, if applicable) diagnosis, birth GA (completed weeks), sex, and birth anthropometrics (BW in grams, length and head circumference in cm). Outcomes collected included corrected GA at discharge, discharge anthropometrics (weight, length and head circumference), total days on PN, total days with a CL (peripherally inserted and/or surgically placed central catheter and/or umbilical venous catheter) during hospital stay (intermittent days summed if not continuous), hospital length of stay (LOS; days) and the dichotomous outcomes of any use of MOM, any use of DM and any use of formula during hospital stay and when this occurred (≤30 days of life vs. >30 days of life), MOM use in the 48 h prior to hospital discharge, death before discharge, NEC (if yes, medical or surgical) and culture positive blood steam infection. Data were de-identified upon chart extraction.

*2.3. Data Analysis*

Study data were collected and managed using REDCap electronic data capture tools [19] hosted at the Hospital for Sick Children and were analyzed using SPSS version 26 (IBM, Armonk, NY, USA). Descriptive statistics were used to summarize sample characteristics, and after testing for normalcy, pre-DM and DM infants were compared using t-testing, Mann-Whitney u testing or chi-square. Large diagnostic groups (i.e., gastroschisis and atresia) were studied as a whole as well as separately to assess for different signals, specifically focusing on small bowel atresias, which commonly exhibit prenatal bowel distension unlike large bowel atresias [2,15] and gastroschisis, in which the bowel may also exhibit distension in addition to being subjected to irritating amniotic fluid in the latter case. If an infant had both gastroschisis and intestinal atresia, gastroschisis was considered the primary diagnosis and dictated diagnostic grouping.

## 3. Results

*Characteristics of the Sample*

Infants ($n$ = 167) were initially identified in an electronic search using the inclusion criteria. After manually extracting all data from the electronic record, 27 were excluded due to a diagnosis of colonic/rectal atresia with a fistula, as these infants may not require neonatal surgery, leaving 140 infants for analysis. Characteristics of the sample separated by era (Table 1) are reported for the whole sample, the sample excluding large bowel atresia (i.e., including small bowel atresia and gastroschisis), and including only gastroschisis. As a whole, infants in the two eras did not differ by BW, GA, or sex. The mean (SD) birth GA fell into the late preterm/early term range [20,21]. The type of congenital gastrointestinal conditions differed between the eras, with the DM era having more infants with small bowel atresia and fewer with large bowel atresia.

**Table 1.** Characteristics of the sample.

| Median (IQR) or n (%) | Pre-DM Era | DM Era | p Value, Mann Whitney u Test or Chi-Square |
|---|---|---|---|
| **Whole Sample** | n = 70 | n = 70 | |
| Birthweight (grams) | 2790 (2388, 3310) | 2810 (2423, 3161) | 0.83 |
| Birth length (cm) | 47.5 (44.0, 50.0) n = 45 | 47.0 (45.0, 50.0) n = 65 | 0.87 |
| Birth HC (cm) | 32.8 (31.4, 33.5) | 33.0 (32.0, 34.0) n = 69 | 0.43 |
| Birth GA (weeks) | 37 (36, 38) | 37 (36, 38) | 0.80 |
| Male sex | 44 (62.9%) | 40 (57.1%) | 0.49 |
| Multiple GI malformations (i.e., gastroschisis + atresia) | 5 (7%) | 7 (10%) | 0.36 |
| Gastroschisis | 25 (35.7%) | 19 (27.1%) | |
| Small bowel atresia (duodenal, jejunal, ileal) | 22 (31.4%) | 39 (55.7%) | 0.01 * |
| Rectal/colonic atresia without fistula | 23 (32.9%) | 12 (17.1%) | |
| **Excluding Large Bowel (Rectal/Colonic) Atresia** | n = 47 | n = 58 | |
| Birthweight (grams) | 2690 (2300, 3070) | 2715 (2423, 3159) | 0.45 |
| Birth length (cm) | 46.8 (44.0, 50.0) n = 30 | 47.0 (45.0, 50.0) n = 53 | 0.36 |
| Birth HC (cm) | 32.5 (31.0, 33.0) | 33.0 (32.0, 34.0) n = 57 | 0.13 |
| Birth GA (weeks) | 36.3 (35.0, 38.0) | 37.0 (36.0, 38.0) | 0.07 |
| Male sex | 27 (57.4%) | 32 (55.2%) | 0.82 |
| Gastroschisis | 25 (53.2%) | 19 (32.8%) | 0.04 * |
| Small bowel atresia | 22 (46.8%) | 39 (67.2%) | |
| **Only Gastroschisis** | n = 25 | n = 19 | |
| Birthweight (grams) | 2480 (2205, 2918) | 2640 (2430, 3080) | 0.15 |
| Birth length (cm) | 45.0 (42.9, 48.8) n = 16 | 45.0 (43.0, 49.0) | 0.94 |
| Birth HC (cm) | 32.0 (31.0, 33.0) | 33.0 (32.0, 34.0) | 0.03 * |
| Birth GA (weeks) | 36.0 (35.0, 37.0) | 37.0 (36.0, 37.0) | 0.02 * |
| Male sex | 15 (60.0%) | 10 (52.6%) | 0.63 |

IQR: intraquartile range; DM: donor milk; HC: head circumference; GA: gestational age in completed weeks; GI: gastrointestinal. * $p < 0.05$.

Table 2 delineates the type of enteral feedings received during hospitalization. Feeding categories were non-exclusive, with many infants receiving multiple types of feeds (MOM, DM, or formula) during their hospitalization. As DM was weaned prior to discharge to the planned at-home feeding regimen, no infants received DM in the 48 h prior to discharge. In the first 30 days, for the whole cohort, infants received similar amounts of HM overall, with percentage of MOM in the pre-DM era exactly equal to MOM + DM in the DM era. DM use was relatively infrequent in the DM era (5.7% in the DM group), with a vast majority of infants receiving MOM (88.6% in the DM group) in the first 30 days in both eras. Formula use in the DM era was still common, likely reflecting infants with short length of stay who were supplemented with formula instead of DM (which is not available after discharge) when planning for prompt discharge.

It was noted that fewer infants received formula in the 48 h prior to discharge in the DM era, a drop of nearly 20% for the cohort as a whole ($p = 0.03$), suggesting that the aforementioned use of formula in the first 30 days was only intermittent as a supplement or a bridge to MOM, not to replace MOM.

In-hospital outcomes (Table 3) did not differ between eras for the group as a whole. When large bowel atresias were excluded, hospital LOS and CL days were 10 and 8 days shorter, respectively, in the DM era. Although not reaching statistical significance ($p = 0.10$), infants in the DM era were discharged at 1.2 weeks younger corrected GA (41.1 vs. 42.3 weeks). When the infants at highest risk of feeding intolerance (gastroschisis) were analyzed separately, statistical significance was lost, likely due to low numbers (total n of 44.) Trends remained, however, with LOS 15 days shorter ($p = 0.10$) and central line days 11 days shorter ($p = 0.07$) in the DM era. NEC was rare overall (4 in pre-DM and 2 in DM era) and did not differ between eras in any analysis.

Table 2. Enteral feeding during hospitalization.

| n (%) | Pre-DM Era | DM Era | p Value, Chi-Square |
|---|---|---|---|
| Whole Sample | n = 70 | n = 70 | |
| Received during the first 30 days of life | | | |
| MOM | 66 (94.3%) | 62 (88.6%) | 0.23 |
| DM | 0 | 4 (5.7%) | 0.04 * |
| Formula | 37 (52.9%) | 34 (48.6%) | 0.61 |
| Received in the 48 h prior to discharge | | | |
| MOM | 50 (71.4%) | 56 (80.0%) | 0.24 |
| Formula | 35 (50.0%) | 22 (31.4%) | 0.03 * |
| Excluding Large Bowel (Rectal/Colonic) Atresia | n = 47 | n = 58 | |
| Received during the first 30 days of life | | | |
| MOM | 45 (95.7%) | 51 (87.9%) | 0.16 |
| DM | 0 | 4 (6.9%) | 0.07 |
| Formula | 22 (46.8%) | 28 (48.2%) | 0.88 |
| Received in the 48 h prior to discharge | | | |
| MOM | 32 (68.1%) | 47 (81.0%) | 0.13 |
| Formula | 24 (51.1%) | 19 (32.8%) | 0.06 |
| Only Gastroschisis | n = 25 | n = 19 | |
| Received during the first 30 days of life | | | |
| MOM | 25 (100%) | 15 (78.9%) | 0.02 * |
| DM | 0 | 1 (5.3%) | 0.25 |
| Formula | 14 (56.0%) | 13 (68.4%) | 0.40 |
| Received in the 48 h prior to discharge | | | |
| MOM | 15 (60.0%) | 14 (73.7%) | 0.34 |
| Formula | 15 (60.0%) | 10 (52.6%) | 0.63 |

DM: donor milk; MOM: mother's own milk. * $p < 0.05$.

Table 3. Outcomes.

| Median (IQR) or n (%) | Pre-DM Era | DM Era | p Value, Mann Whitney—u Test or Chi-Square |
|---|---|---|---|
| Whole Sample | n = 70 | n = 70 | |
| Hospital LOS (days) | 28.0 (17.8, 54.3) | 25.0 (16.75, 45.0) | 0.26 |
| PN days | 11.0 (6.0, 23.0) | 14.0 (8.0, 24.3) | 0.38 |
| Central line days | 21.0 (6.0, 44.5) | 18.0 (10.8, 29.3) | 0.34 |
| NEC | 4 (1 medical, 3 surgical) (5.7%) | 2 (surgical) (2.9%) | 0.40 |
| Culture positive bloodstream infection | 6 (11.4%) | 8 (8.6%) | 0.57 |
| Death prior to discharge | 1 (1.4%) | 1 (1.4%) | 1.00 |
| Discharge weight (grams) | 3169 (2734, 3532) | 3056 (2625, 3560) n = 69 | 0.31 |
| Discharge HC (cm) | 33.5 (32.6, 34.9) n = 52 | 33.3 (32.5, 34.7) n = 36 | 0.57 |
| Discharge CGA (weeks) | 41.1 (40.1, 44.7) | 41.1 (39.6, 44.2) | 0.29 |
| Excluding Large Bowel (Rectal/Colonic) Atresia | n = 47 | n = 58 | |
| Hospital LOS (days) | 35.0 (22.0, 76.0) | 25.0 (18.0, 43.5) | 0.01 * |
| PN days | 14.5 (8.8, 26.8) | 14.5 (9.0, 24.3) | 0.82 |
| Central line days | 28.0 (15.0, 71.0) | 20.0 (12.5, 29.3) | 0.01 * |
| NEC | 4 (1 medical, 3 surgical) (8.5%) | 2 (both surgical) (3.4%) | 0.27 |
| Culture positive bloodstream infection | 8 (17%) | 4 (6.9%) | 0.11 |
| Death prior to discharge | 0 | 1 (1.7%) | 0.37 |
| Discharge weight (grams) | 3135 (2705, 3670) | 3125 (2668, 3680) | 0.54 |
| Discharge HC (cm) | 33.8 (32.2, 34.6) n = 34 | 34.0 (32.5, 35.0) n = 27 | 0.77 |
| Discharge GA (weeks) | 42.3 (40.1, 47.9) | 41.1 (39.6, 44.6) | 0.10 |
| Only gastroschisis | n = 25 | n = 19 | |
| Hospital LOS (days) | 44.0 (34.5, 77.0) | 29.0 (26.0, 52.0) | 0.10 |
| PN days | 15.0 (10.0, 29.0) | 21.0 (12.0, 34.0) | 0.64 |
| Central line days | 36.0 (26.0, 73.5) | 25.0 (21.0, 45.0) | 0.07 |
| NEC | 3 (1 medical, 2 surgical) (12.0%) | 1 surgical (5.3%) | 0.44 |
| Culture positive bloodstream infection | 4 (16%) | 1 (5.3%) | 0.27 |
| Death prior to discharge | 0 | 0 | |
| Discharge weight (grams) | 3100 (2698, 3625) | 2810 (2625, 3865) | 0.74 |
| Discharge HC (cm) | 33.0 (32.0, 34.5) n = 18 | 33.3 (32.5, 35.0) n = 8 | 0.34 |
| Discharge CGA (weeks) | 43.0 (40.3, 50.0) | 41.3 (40.6, 44.9) | 0.33 |

IQR: intraquartile range; DM: donor milk; LOS: length of stay; PN: parenteral nutrition; NEC: necrotizing enterocolitis; HC: head circumference; CGA: corrected gestational age. * $p < 0.05$.

## 4. Discussion

This retrospective study suggests that there is a potential benefit in offering post-operative DM to reduce the LOS and central line days in a subset of the late preterm/term congenital GI malformation population with gastroschisis and small bowel atresias Although not reaching statistical significance, infants in the DM era were discharged at 1.2 weeks younger corrected GA, a clinically significant value not likely explained by the birth GA that was only a few days older in the DM era ($p = 0.07$, 37 vs. 36.3 weeks). No obvious benefit was seen when infants with colonic/rectal atresias were included. The results are scientifically plausible—dysmotility and feeding intolerance frequently feature in these "high-risk" diagnoses (small bowel atresias and gastroschisis), in which the bowel may experience prolonged periods of distension and/or amniotic fluid exposure prenatally [3]. In contrast, infants with large bowel atresias typically present with distension post-natally and often have rapid return of bowel function after receiving a diverting colostomy [15], reflected in the cohort's longer LOS when infants with large bowel atresias were removed from the analyses (Table 3).

It is unclear for the small bowel atresia and gastroschisis infants if the DM itself is beneficial, as the number receiving DM was small, or if it was the lower rates of formula feeding with accompanying higher rates of MOM feeding around the time of discharge that might have facilitated a decreased LOS, or a combination of the two. Although studies are limited, previous authors have found that offering DM can be associated with higher rates of MOM provision [22,23]. In a retrospective study of 163 infants, Shinnick et al. reported that an exclusively HM diet in a neonatal surgical population consisting mostly of infants with gastroschisis and intestinal atresia was associated with decreased LOS, PN days, and days to full enteral feeds; a mixed diet consisting of partial HM/partial formula did not show similar benefits [7]. The authors report that "very few" of the infants received DM in this cohort, whose mean GA fell into the late preterm range and included infants >1250 g, but no further information was reported. Gulack et al. reported in a retrospective study that the use of HM, defined as MOM or DM, vs. formula resulted in shorter hospital LOS in infants with gastroschisis, but data was not available to differentiate between MOM vs. DM. Given the study time frame of 1997–2012, when DM use was less common even in preterm populations, it is likely that the majority of this HM was MOM, not DM [24]. Kohler et al. reported shorter time to full feeds with exclusive HM vs. mixed diet or exclusive formula in a retrospective gastroschisis study in a similar time frame to Gulack; DM use was not reported [6].

In keeping with our findings of lower rates of formula feeding at NICU discharge in the DM era, previous studies have linked HM, but not DM specifically, to improved outcomes in the gastroschisis and small bowel atresia population [5–8]. Growth factors such as epidermal growth factor in HM may promote small bowel epithelial growth [25] and gut barrier protection [16]; HM fed infants demonstrate decreased intestinal permeability, which can protect against pathogens in a fragile gut [26]. The milk microbiome can also modulate epithelial cells and promotes a healthy gut microbial environment [16], and bioactive components such as lactoferrin, immunoglobulins and oligosaccharides have anti-inflammatory and prebiotic properties that could promote improved feeding tolerance. Although these components and others are postulated to mediate the myriad of benefits of HM and specifically MOM in the neonatal population, DM has an altered composition. Many, but not all, growth factors and bioactive components are reduced while all living cells are eradicated with pasteurization and processing [27], which likely explains why DM has not been shown to improve morbidities like sepsis in the same way that MOM does [25]. The benefits associated with the DM era in our study could simply be due to less exposure to formula, which can increase intestinal permeability and inflammation. This formula avoidance is postulated to partially explain the reduction in NEC in preterm infants with DM use [16,28], and could also explain the findings of Kohler et al. and Shinnick et al., who reported that exclusive HM diets had better outcomes than even infants fed a majority HM, but some formula, in the congenital GI malformation population [5–7]. However, the dose of MOM vs. DM may be important given the aforementioned differences, and researchers should not combine

MOM and DM together as "HM" [16]. It is important to study differences in DM outcomes according to the dose of MOM fed.

The strengths of our study were the utilization of a high volume single center with consistent feeding protocols between eras in a relatively short time frame. Access to records that differentiated between MOM and DM was a particular strength of our study that addresses a common limitation of previous research in this area. This is the first study we are aware of specifically assessing DM to supplement MOM in the congenital GI malformation surgical population. Limitations include a retrospective study with a relatively small n, although in keeping with other cohorts given diagnostic rarity [6,7]. The low NEC rates in both eras limited our ability to detect any differences with DM. Although there were no other significant practice changes implemented in our NICU between the two eras, it is possible that other confounding factors may have been responsible for the differences seen between the eras. Finally, our data included the type of feed, but not the proportion of each type of feed, so we were unable to determine doses of MOM or DM versus formula or exclusivity of MOM.

Our study provides the first evidence of potential benefit of offering post-operative DM when MOM is limited in supply in the congenital GI malformation population, specifically for infants with gastroschisis and small bowel atresia. More studies of DM in this population are warranted, and could include additional congenital GI conditions with motility challenges such as omphalocele and Hirschprung's disease. Although DM is a costly product, it has been shown to be cost effective in the very preterm population based on reductions in NEC [29]. In addition, if offering DM is associated with increased rates of MOM feeding, then this practice could have significant short and long-term secondary benefits. A randomized controlled trial of DM vs. formula to supplement inadequate MOM in this population would provide further evidence and may help address important questions such as how long to continue DM post-operatively, when to introduce formula if needed, and the cost-effectiveness of DM. Finally, centers with low baseline rates of MOM feedings may see larger outcome differences with the use of DM compared to our cohort, in which MOM use is relatively prevalent.

## 5. Conclusions

In conclusion, a practice change to offer DM was associated with shorter LOS and central line days in a late preterm and term population with gastroschisis and small bowel atresia, providing the first evidence for the potential use of a limited resource in this high-risk surgical population when MOM volumes are insufficient. More studies are needed to confirm our findings at other centers as well as to delineate the duration of DM therapy and its cost effectiveness.

**Author Contributions:** R.H. designed the study, performed the analysis, and contributed to interpretation of the data and drafting the article. S.K. performed the data extraction and data entry and contributed to interpretation of the data and drafting and editing the article. A.P. and S.L.U. contributed to interpretation of the data and drafting and editing the article. All authors have read and agreed to the published version of the manuscript

**Funding:** This research received no external funding.

**Conflicts of Interest:** The authors declare no conflict of interests.

## Abbreviations

| | |
|---|---|
| BW | birth weight |
| DM | donor human milk |
| GA | gestational age |
| LOS | length of stay |
| MOM | mother's own milk |
| NEC | necrotizing enterocolitis |
| PN | parenteral nutrition |

## References

1. Singh, S.J.; Fraser, A.; Leditschke, J.F.; Spence, K.; Kimble, R.; Dalby-Payne, J.; Baskaranathan, S.; Barr, P.; Halliday, R.; Badawi, N.; et al. Gastroschisis: Determinants of neonatal outcome. *Pediatr. Surg. Int.* **2003**, *19*, 260–265. [CrossRef]
2. Gamba, P.; Midrio, P. Abdominal wall defects: Prenatal diagnosis, newborn management, and long-termoutcomes. *Semin. Pediatr. Surg.* **2014**, *23*, 283–290. [CrossRef]
3. Jayanthi, S.; Seymour, P.; Puntis, J.W.; Stringer, M.D. Necrotizing enterocolitis after gastroschisis repair: A preventable complication? *J. Pediatr. Surg.* **1998**, *33*, 705–707. [CrossRef]
4. Morrison, J.J.; Klein, N.; Chitty, L.S.; Kocjan, G.; Walshe, D.; Goulding, M.; Geary, M.P.; Pierro, A.; Rodeck, C.H. Intra-amniotic inflammation in human gastroschisis: Possible aetiology of postnatal bowel dysfunction. *BJOG* **1998**, *105*, 1200–1204. [CrossRef] [PubMed]
5. Gulack, B.C.; Laughon, M.M.; Clark, R.H.; Burgess, T.; Robinson, S.; Muhammad, A.; Zhang, A.; Davis, A.; Morton, R.; Chu, V.H.; et al. Enteral Feeding with Human Milk Decreases Time to Discharge in Infants following Gastroschisis Repair. *J. Pediatr.* **2016**, *170*, 85–89. [CrossRef] [PubMed]
6. Kohler, J.A.S.; Perkins, A.M.; Bass, W.T. Human milk versus formula after gastroschisis repair: Effects on time to full feeds and time to discharge. *J. Perinatol.* **2013**, *33*, 627–630. [CrossRef]
7. Shinnick, J.K.; Wang, E.; Hulbert, C.; McCracken, C.; Sarson, G.Y.; Piazza, A.; Karpen, H.; Durham, M.M. Effects of a Breast Milk Diet on Enteral Feeding Outcomes of Neonates with Gastrointestinal Disorders. *Breastfeed Med.* **2016**, *11*, 286–292. [CrossRef]
8. Storm, A.P.; Bowker, R.M.; Klonoski, S.C.; Iantorno, S.E.; Shah, A.N.; Pillai, S.; Bell, J.; Patel, A.L. Mother's own milk dose is associated with decreased time from initiation of feedings to discharge and length of stay in infants with gastroschisis. *J. Perinatol.* **2020**. [CrossRef]
9. Kulkarni, S.; Mercado, V.; Rios, M.; Arboleda, R.; Gomara, R.; Muinos, W.; Reeves-Garcia, J.; Hernandez, E. Breast milk is better than formula milk in preventing parenteral nutrition-associated liver disease in infants receiving prolonged parenteral nutrition. *J. Pediatr. Gastroenterol. Nutr.* **2013**, *57*, 383–388. [CrossRef]
10. Andorsky, D.J.; Lund, D.P.; Lillehei, C.W.; Jaksic, T.; Dicanzio, J.; Richardson, D.S.; Collier, S.B.; Lo, C.; Duggan, C. Nutritional and other postoperative management of neonates with short bowel syndrome correlates with clinical outcomes. *J. Pediatr.* **2001**, *139*, 27–33. [CrossRef]
11. Meier, P.P.; Patel, A.L.; Hoban, R.; Engstrom, J.L. Which breast pump for which mother: An evidence-based approach to individualizing breast pump technology. *J. Perinatol.* **2016**, *36*, 493–499. [CrossRef] [PubMed]
12. Salvatori, G.; Foligno, S.; Occasi, F.; Pannone, V.; Valentini, G.B.; Dall'Oglio, I.; Bagolan, P.; Dotta, A. Human milk and breastfeeding in surgical infants. *Breastfeed Med.* **2014**, *9*, 491–493. [CrossRef] [PubMed]
13. Demirci, J.; Caplan, E.; Brozanski, B.; Bogen, D. Winging it: Maternal perspectives and experiences of breastfeeding newborns with complex congenital surgical anomalies. *J. Perinatol.* **2018**, *38*, 708–717. [CrossRef] [PubMed]
14. Crippa, B.L.; Colombo, L.; Morniroli, D.; Consonni, D.; Bettinelli, M.E.; Spreafico, I.; Vercesi, G.; Sannino, P.; Mauri, P.A.; Zanotta, L.; et al. Do a Few Weeks Matter? Late Preterm Infants and Breastfeeding Issues. *Nutrients* **2019**, *11*, 312. [CrossRef] [PubMed]
15. Dalla Vecchia, L.K.; Grosfeld, J.L.; West, K.W.; Rescorla, F.J.; Scherer, L.R.; Engum, S.A. Intestinal atresia and stenosis: A 25-year experience with 277 cases. *Arch. Surg.* **1998**, *133*, 490–497. [CrossRef] [PubMed]
16. Meier, P.; Patel, A.; Esquerra-Zwiers, A. Donor Human Milk Update: Evidence, Mechanisms, and Priorities for Research and Practice. *J. Pediatr.* **2017**, *180*, 15–21. [CrossRef]
17. Patel, A.L.; Kim, J.H. Human milk and necrotizing enterocolitis. *Semin. Pediatr. Surg.* **2018**, *27*, 34–38. [CrossRef]
18. Hoban, R.; Schoeny, M.E.; Esquerra-Zwiers, A.; Kaenkumchorn, T.K.; Casini, G.; Tobin, G.; Siegel, A.H.; Patra, K.; Hamilton, M.; Wicks, J.; et al. Impact of Donor Milk on Short- and Long-Term Growth of Very Low Birth Weight Infants. *Nutrients* **2019**, *11*, 241. [CrossRef]
19. Harris, P.A.; Taylor, R.; Thielke, R.; Payne, J.; Gonzalez, N.; Conde, J.G. Research electronic data capture (REDCap)—a metadata-driven methodology and workflow process for providing translational research informatics support. *J. Biomed. Inform.* **2009**, *42*, 377–381. [CrossRef]
20. ACOG Committee Opinion No 579: Definition of term pregnancy. *Obstet. Gynecol.* **2013**, *122*, 1139–1140. [CrossRef]

21. Engle, W.A.; Tomashek, K.M.; Wallman, C. Committee on Fetus and Newborn, American Academy of Pediatrics "Late-preterm" infants: A population at risk. *Pediatrics* **2007**, *120*, 1390–1401. [CrossRef] [PubMed]
22. Kantorowska, A.; Wei, J.C.; Cohen, R.S.; Lawrence, R.A.; Gould, J.B.; Lee, H.C. Impact of Donor Milk Availability on Breast Milk Use and Necrotizing Enterocolitis Rates. *Pediatrics* **2016**, *137*, 1–8. [CrossRef] [PubMed]
23. Williams, T.; Nair, H.; Simpson, J.; Embleton, N. Use of Donor Human Milk and Maternal Breastfeeding Rates: A Systematic Review. *J. Hum. Lact.* **2016**, *32*, 212–220. [CrossRef] [PubMed]
24. Updegrove, K.H. Donor human milk banking: Growth, challenges, and the role of HMBANA. *Breastfeed Med.* **2013**, *8*, 435–437. [CrossRef]
25. Cummins, A.G.; Thompson, F.M. Effect of breast milk and weaning on epithelial growth of the small intestine in humans. *Gut* **2002**, *51*, 748–754. [CrossRef]
26. Taylor, S.N.; Basile, L.A.; Ebeling, M.; Wagner, C.L. Intestinal permeability in preterm infants by feeding type: mother's milk versus formula. *Breastfeed Med.* **2009**, *4*, 11–15. [CrossRef]
27. Pitino, M.A.; Unger, S.; Doyen, A.; Pouliot, Y.; Aufreiter, S.; Stone, D.; Kiss, A.; O'Connor, D. High Hydrostatic Pressure Processing Better Preserves the Nutrient and Bioactive Compound Composition of Human Donor Milk. *J. Nutr.* **2019**, *149*, 497–504. [CrossRef]
28. Quigley, M.; Embleton, N.D.; McGuire, W. Formula versus donor breast milk for feeding preterm or low birth weight infants. *Cochrane Database Syst. Rev.* **2018**, *6*, CD002971. [CrossRef]
29. Buckle, A.; Taylor, C. Cost and Cost-Effectiveness of Donor Human Milk to Prevent Necrotizing Enterocolitis: Systematic Review. *Breastfeed Med.* **2017**, *12*, 528–536. [CrossRef]

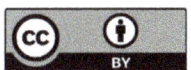

© 2020 by the authors. Licensee MDPI, Basel, Switzerland. This article is an open access article distributed under the terms and conditions of the Creative Commons Attribution (CC BY) license (http://creativecommons.org/licenses/by/4.0/).

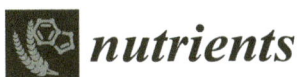 

Article

# Parent and Provider Perspectives on the Imprecise Label of "Human Milk Fortifier" in the NICU

Jennifer Canvasser [1,*], Amy B. Hair [2], Jae H. Kim [3] and Sarah N. Taylor [4]

1. NEC Society, PO Box 72271, Davis, CA 95617, USA
2. Baylor College of Medicine, Texas Children's Hospital, Houston, TX 77030, USA; abhair@texaschildrens.org
3. Cincinnati Children's Hospital Medical Center, University of Cincinnati College of Medicine, Cincinnati, OH 45229, USA; jae.kim@cchmc.org
4. Yale School of Medicine, New Haven, CT 06520, USA; sarah.n.taylor@yale.edu
* Correspondence: jennifer@necsociety.org

Received: 3 February 2020; Accepted: 4 March 2020; Published: 9 March 2020

**Abstract:** In the critical care of preterm infants, feeding is complex and potentially harmful to an immature gastrointestinal system. Parents have expressed the desire to be fully informed about what is being fed to their child, as this places them in the best position to nurture their child's health. In the parent-engaged setting of the Necrotizing Enterocolitis Symposium, NICU parents expressed concern and confusion about how cow's milk product and donor human milk product both carry the label "Human Milk Fortifier" (HMF). Accordingly, two online surveys were developed to characterize how the label HMF is used and interpreted in the NICU by parents and providers. Of 774 United States participants, only 21.9% of providers reported consistently describing the source of HMF to parents, and only 20.6% of parents whose child received an HMF product report knowing the source. Parents expressed that they were "not given information" regarding HMF, while both parents and healthcare providers expressed that "the label (HMF) is misleading". This study documents the ambiguity around the label HMF as well as the need for more specific language and clearer communication.

**Keywords:** necrotizing enterocolitis; human milk fortifier; patient empowerment; breast milk; neonatal nutrition; prematurity; communication; product labeling; donor milk; NICU parent

## 1. Introduction

For new parents, feeding their baby is one of the most primal and meaningful experiences of their lives. When a baby is born prematurely or with a medical condition requiring intensive care, this basic responsibility is taken from new parents and entrusted to professionals. Parents are forced to quickly adapt to parenting in the intensive care setting, where many of their original plans are derailed and they are met with a new and often unexpected reality.

In the critical care of preterm infants, feeding is complex and potentially harmful to an immature gastrointestinal system. Parents are informed of many neonatal intensive care unit (NICU) nutrition and feeding practices, some of which actively rely on maternal production of milk for the infant. For example, parents commonly receive education regarding the lifesaving potential of mother's own milk and pasteurized human donor milk for preterm and medically fragile infants, which can help protect against necrotizing enterocolitis (NEC), sepsis, and death [1–3]. Strategies to optimize the production of mother's own milk, as well as the rationale for parental consent if pasteurized donor milk is necessary, are often prioritized in parental education.

Human milk alone typically cannot meet the nutritional needs of infants born before 34 weeks' postmenstrual age (PMA) [4,5]. Accordingly, most NICUs in the United States provide these infants with a Human Milk Fortifier (HMF) that aims to increase the nutritional and caloric density of a mother's own milk or pasteurized human donor milk. There are two main types of HMF available for use in NICUs based in the United States: one is derived from cow's milk and the other is derived from pasteurized donor human milk. The term, HMF, does not reflect which type of fortifier is being used. During the NEC Symposium at the University of Michigan (2–5 June 2019, Ann Arbor, MI, USA), the patient-family advocates in attendance described the label HMF as ambiguous, vague, and misleading. These patient-family advocates, whose babies received intensive care, expressed that they felt uninformed when they learned that their babies' breast milk was being fortified with an HMF product that they misunderstood. These comments led to the development of this survey study examining parental and healthcare provider perceptions of HMF, as well as their understanding of the constituents and purpose of HMF.

## 2. Materials and Methods

### 2.1. Survey Development

This study was reviewed by the Yale University Institutional Regulatory Board (IRB) (New Haven, CT, USA) and was determined to be exempt from IRB approval. Two online surveys were developed for (1) parents and (2) providers in order to characterize how the label "Human Milk Fortifier" (Supplementary Materials) is used and interpreted in the NICU, as well as to establish potential alternative label choices. Each survey contained an introductory paragraph that described the purpose, the eligibility criteria, and how participation in the survey was voluntary. The respondent's completion of the survey served as documentation of consent to participate in the study.

The survey questions included both multiple choice and open-ended text fields, which were developed by parents whose children have been affected by NEC, in partnership with neonatologists affiliated with the NEC Society (www.necsociety.org). The survey questions stemmed from the lived experience of parents in the NICU. NICU parents selected 19 adjectives from a list of some of the most common human feelings which could be used to describe potential emotions associated with various infant feeding types. Prior to dissemination, both surveys were distributed to an expert panel of parents and scientists from the NEC Society for face validity and question optimization.

The first survey was developed for NICU parents > 18 years old from the United States. These questions were adapted to address parents whose infant(s) received care in an NICU, including those parents whose infant(s) have been affected by NEC or have died. Optional demographic information included parent age, education level, and race/ethnicity categories.

The second survey was directed to healthcare providers in the NICU, including nurses, physicians, nurse practitioners, physician assistants, lactation consultants, dietitians, and other members of the clinical care team in the NICU. Providers had the option to include years of experience and race/ethnicity categories.

### 2.2. Survey Distribution

The two surveys were created and distributed through the online-based survey platform Qualtrics© (Seattle, Washington, USA). Links to the survey were disseminated via the NEC Society's listserv, social media pages, and blog. The NICU Parent Network also circulated links to the survey on their listserv and social media pages. The provider survey was emailed to contacts at 11 United States level III/IV academic NICU centers who were requested to distribute the survey to all NICU clinical staff. The surveys were available to respondents from 15 August 2019, through to 23 September 2019.

### 2.3. Analysis

These surveys were exploratory and, therefore, no sample size calculations were performed. Survey data was compiled into summary statistics including the proportion of respondents providing each answer. Test answers were coded for themes using Dedoose Version 7.0.23, web application for managing, analyzing, and presenting qualitative and mixed method research data (2016). Los Angeles,

California, USA: SocioCultural Research Consultants, LLC. Relative risk (RR) with 95% confidence intervals (CI) were calculated by Chi-squared analysis.

## 3. Results

### 3.1. Parent Survey

#### 3.1.1. Demographics

The parent survey had 395 respondents in the United States. Demographics are presented in Table 1. The parent respondents who opted to answer the demographic questions were primarily white, college-educated, 30–39 years of age, with a child born between 2011 and 2019 who received NICU care.

Table 1. Parent demographics.

|  | Parent Cohort % (n) |
|---|---|
| Age (years): | N = 345 |
| Under 18 | 0.5% (2) |
| 18–29 | 20% (68) |
| 30–39 | 57% (195) |
| 40–50 | 21% (74) |
| 50 Years or above | 1.5% (6) |
| Race/Ethnicity: | N = 358 |
| White | 85% (305) |
| Hispanic or Latino | 7% (24) |
| Black | 3% (11) |
| Asian/Asian Indian | 3% (12) |
| Other | 2% (6) |
| Formal Education: | N = 344 |
| High School Degree | 20% (69) |
| College Graduate | 45% (156) |
| Post-Graduate Degree | 30% (101) |
| Other | 5% (18) |
| Year Child was Born: | N = 395 |
| 2010 and Below | 14% (54) |
| 2011–2013 | 16% (62) |
| 2014–2016 | 25% (101) |
| 2017–2019 | 45% (177) |
| Child Gestational Age at Birth: | N = 395 |
| 22–24 weeks | 17% (65) |
| 25–28 weeks | 35% (137) |
| 29–33 weeks | 29% (115) |
| 34–36 weeks | 12% (49) |
| 37–42 weeks | 7% (29) |

#### 3.1.2. Feeding Type

Among the 395 parent respondents, 90.6% reported that their child received their mother's own milk in the NICU, 71.1% reported that their child received HMF, and 44.5% remember being told that human milk helps to reduce the risk of NEC.

Regarding formula feeding, 48.6% of parents reported that their child received formula in the NICU, and of those 192 parent respondents, 68% reported that they were asked to give consent prior to their child receiving formula.

3.1.3. Necrotizing Enterocolitis

In this survey, 49.9% of parent respondents reported that their child was diagnosed with NEC in the NICU. Of these, 30.5% had a child who died, with 96.7% of these cases due to NEC or complications related to NEC.

3.1.4. Adjectives Describing Mother's Own Milk or Fortification

Parents were asked to choose up to five adjectives in response to the questions "How did you feel about your baby receiving mother's milk?" and "Reflecting back to your time in the NICU with your baby, how did you feel about fortification then?" The percentage of parent respondents who chose each adjective for each question is shown in Figure 1.

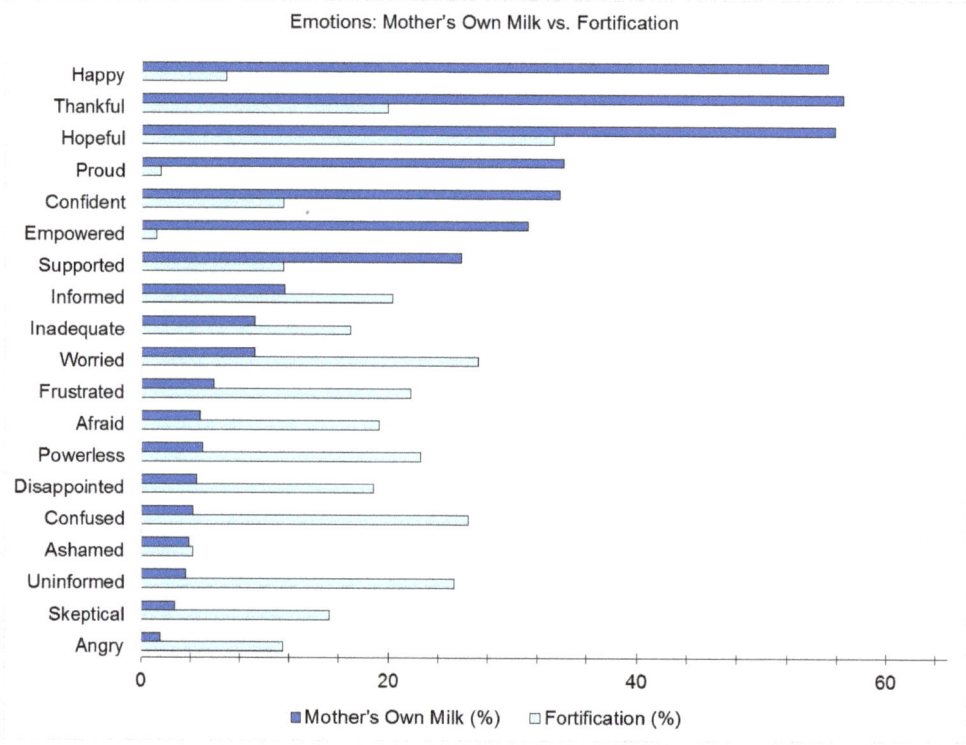

**Figure 1.** The percentage of respondents choosing each listed adjective in response to the questions "How did you feel about your baby receiving mother's milk?" and "Reflecting back to your time in the NICU with your baby, how did you feel about fortification then?".

## 3.2. Provider Survey

Demographics

The provider survey had 379 respondents in the United States. Provider demographics are provided in Table 2. Provider respondents were primarily white nurses and physicians who have provided NICU care for over 10 years.

Table 2. Provider demographics.

|  | Provider Cohort |
|---|---|
|  | N = 379 |
|  | % (n) |
| **Position:** |  |
| Nurse | 52% (196) |
| Physician | 28% (108) |
| Neonatal Nurse Practitioner | 8% (29) |
| Registered Dietitian | 6% (21) |
| Fellow/Resident | 4% (15) |
| Physician Assistant | 1% (5) |
| Lactation Consultant | 1% (5) |
| **Length of Providing NICU Care:** |  |
| More Than 20 Years | 27% (101) |
| 10–19 years | 31% (117) |
| 5–9 years | 25% (96) |
| 1–4 years | 15% (58) |
| Less Than a Year | 2% (7) |
| **Race/Ethnicity:** |  |
| White | 80% (305) |
| Asian/Asian Indian | 8.5% (32) |
| Hispanic or Latino | 5% (18) |
| Black | 3% (11) |
| Other | 3.5% (13) |

## 3.3. Human Milk Fortifier Information and Labeling

Of the 281 parent respondents who answered that their child received HMF, 60.1% reported that they were told about HMF prior to their child receiving it and 82.6% of those parents reported being told why their child was receiving HMF. However, only 20.6% report knowing the source of their child's HMF. Reflecting back to their time in the NICU, only 8.8% of parent respondents interpreted the product as potentially meaning a cow's milk-based product. In fact, many parents (n = 48%) did not know that HMF could be derived from cow's milk or pasteurized human donor milk until they participated in this survey study: provider report of communication with parents regarding HMF.

Of the 379 provider respondents, 21.9% answered that they consistently inform parents as to whether their child's HMF is cow's milk- or human milk-based, 23.3% answered that they sometimes inform parents, and 54.8% stated that they do not inform parents of this information.

Parent and provider responses as to what the term "HMF" means to them are shown in Table 3, and recommendations to improve clarity are provided in Table 4. Regarding fortifiers derived from cow's milk, 73% of parent respondents and 54% of provider respondents thought that bovine fortifiers should include the label "Cow's Milk" to improve clarity.

Table 3. Parent and provider responses regarding the term "human milk fortifier".

| %(n) Choosing the Response * | Parent Survey:"In the NICU, What Did HMF Mean to You?" | Parent Survey:"Today, What Words Describe HMF?" | %(n) Choosing the Response * | Provider Survey:"What Does the Label HMF Mean to You?" |
|---|---|---|---|---|
| Cow's milk-based product | 10% (35) | 22% (75) | Cow's milk-based product | 52% (194) |
| Human milk-based product | 21% (71) | 49% (171) | Human milk-based product | 35% (133) |
| Vitamins and minerals | 27% (93) | 19% (67) | Concentrated formula | 12% (45) |
| Additional calorie source | 64% (221) | 44% (151) | Supplement in addition to human milk | 39% (146) |
| Not sure | 13% (44) | 14% (48) | Additive to human milk | 83% (313) |
| Other | 7% (24) | 4% (13) | Other | 2% (8) |

* Able to choose more than one response.

Table 4. Parent and provider recommendations for the best way to describe Human Milk Fortifier (HMF).

| Response | Parent (n = 344) | Provider (n = 377) |
|---|---|---|
| **For cow's milk-based fortifier** | | |
| Cow's milk-based fortifier | 73% (251) | 54% (203) |
| Concentrated formula | 20% (70) | 8% (31) |
| Human milk fortifier | 4% (13) | 27% (100) |
| Other* | 3% (10) | 11% (43) |
| **For human milk-based fortifier** | | |
| Human milk-based fortifier | 53% (183) | 59% (224) |
| Donor milk fortifier | 24% (83) | 19% (70) |
| Human milk fortifier | 20% (67) | 17% (66) |
| Other* | 3% (10) | 5% (19) |

* Other suggestions for "cow's milk-based fortifier" from parents included "bovine milk fortifier", "non-human milk fortifier", and "fortifier". Other suggestions for "cow's milk-based fortifier" from providers included "cow's milk-based human milk fortifier", "nutrient-enriched fortifier for human milk", "fortifier that contains broken-down cow's milk proteins as well as many other nutrients", "bovine-based", "cow's milk-based fortifier for human milk", "bovine-derived fortifier", "formula-based fortifier", "cow's milk-derived fortifier", "dairy-based fortifier", "supplement for growth", "milk fortifier", "an additive to your breast milk that comes from cow's milk", "cow's milk-based human milk fortifier", "fortifier for your milk that is cow's milk-based", "fortifier to human milk containing hydrolyzed cow's milk protein", and "fortifier". Other suggestions for "human milk-based fortifier" from parents included "donor breast milk", "donor milk-based fortifier", "breast milk-based fortifier", and "human donor milk fortifier". Other suggestions for "human milk-based fortifier" from providers included "donor human milk-based fortifier", "donor human milk-based fortifier for human milk", "purchase-pooled human milk-based fortifier", "human milk-derived fortifier", "human milk-based human milk fortifier", "human milk-derived fortifier", "concentrated human milk", "donor milk-based fortifier", "human milk-derived human milk fortifier", "an additive to your breast milk that comes from donated human milk", and "fortifier for your milk that is made from pasteurized donor human milk".

In an analysis of provider characteristics and their relationship with providing parental information regarding fortifier sources, providers with greater experience (at least 10 years) were not significantly more likely to inform parents when compared to providers with less experience (RR 1.01, 95% CI 0.86–1.18). However, when comparing provider role in the NICU, nurses were less likely to inform parents about the source of HMF compared to other providers (RR 1.63, 95% CI 1.35–1.96).

Qualitative Survey Data

Throughout the open-ended text field in the parent survey, phrases including "the label is misleading" and "it should be clear" were mentioned in the context of HMF labeling. The most common theme expressed by parents was that they were "not given information", with 21 parent respondents providing open-ended text that included this theme. Excerpts from parent comments that best represent these themes include:

*"I wish I would have been told that the fortifier was cow's-milk based. The name is way too confusing."*

*"It should be very clear whether the fortifier is derived from cow's-milk formula or breast milk. A label with "human milk" should only mean it's FROM humans."*

*"While in the NICU with my baby, I had to ask what HMF stood for and I only really understood what it was once we were home and I could see the bottle and read the ingredient label."*

*"Until today, I had no understanding of what "fortifier" meant when nurses used that term. It's disappointing how uninformed parents are in the NICU during such a vulnerable time."*

The theme of "the label is misleading" was mentioned by providers in the open-ended text field, as shown by the following example:

*"The labeling of our cow's milk-based fortifiers is misleading because it still has the label "human milk."*

## 4. Discussion

To our knowledge, this is the first study to formally document how the label HMF is used and interpreted by parents and providers in the NICU. In this survey study, we found that while most parents (n = 82.6%) were told why their child was receiving HMF, few parents (n = 20.6%) reported knowing the source of their child's HMF. Reflecting back to their time in the NICU, only 8.8% of parent respondents interpreted the product as potentially meaning a cow's milk-based product. In fact, until they participated in this survey study, many parents (n = 48%) did not know that HMF could be derived from cow's milk or pasteurized human donor milk. Only 21.9% of providers reported consistently describing the source of HMF to parents. The lack of a transfer of information from provider to parent was also evident in the qualitative open-ended text responses, where parents expressed a feeling of being misinformed and needing clarity, with the most common theme being "not informed".

Most providers acknowledged that HMF can be derived from cow's milk or human milk, and yet provider awareness did not translate into parental knowledge in this study. While nurses were significantly less likely to inform parents of the derivation of their child's HMF, the study results cannot determine the basis for this lack of transfer of information. This study raises the possibility that providers have this information but do not find it pertinent to share it with parents. It is also possible that some providers may find it challenging to clearly articulate the differences between fortifiers to parents, or perhaps they do not characterize their professional role as having to inform parents of this type of information. Nevertheless, parents rely on the bedside team as a vital source of information. Clearly, there are a plethora of issues for NICU providers to determine if, how, and when to share with NICU parents. Providers may fear that sharing more information with parents will only further overwhelm them. On the contrary, NICU parents are empowered when information is presented with empathy as early as possible [6]. Gadepalli and colleagues found that informed parents are more satisfied with care, even when their infant's outcome is poor, because it allows them to better engage and contribute as a member of their child's care team. Indeed, there are opportunities for education and further research focused on communication between NICU providers and parents, which go beyond the labeling of HMF products.

Given that both NICU parents and providers find the label HMF to be ambiguous and misleading, there is an urgent need for an alternative, more precise product name. This study demonstrates that the label HMF thwarts an NICU parent's ability to be fully informed and a provider's ability to deliver clear information to families. Accordingly, it is vital for providers to not only fully understand the products that they are prescribing to their patients, but also to have the capacity to clearly articulate to NICU parents the basic components and purpose of the products they are prescribing.

Clarity in labeling is not only a priority for parents and providers, but also for the U.S. Food and Drug Administration. Under Section 403 (a) (1) of the Federal Food, Drug, and Cosmetic Act (FD&C Act) (21 U.S.C. 343 (a) (1)), food labeling, including that concerning infant formula and human milk fortifiers, must be truthful and not misleading. This guidance specifically addresses function claims such as the benefit of the formula/fortifier, but significant emphasis is placed on removing any "misleading" information. The results of this study support the argument that the current label HMF is misleading.

Gooding and colleagues emphasized the importance of open and honest communication between parents and providers in the NICU as it fosters family-centered care (FCC). FCC takes a holistic approach to optimizing infant outcomes by actively engaging the parents. In FCC, providers recognize their role is to care for patients in the context of their family and community. Accordingly, providers engage parents in decision-making and serve as a mentor as parents learn how to care for their medically fragile infant. Importantly, FCC can help to improve parental mental health, increase parent–infant bonding, decrease the NICU length of stay, and improve developmental outcomes [7]. Given the gravity of clear communication between NICU parents and providers, a more transparent product label for HMF should be of high priority.

Communication between parents and providers may potentially affect how an NICU parent engages in their child's care. Pineda et al. stressed that when NICU parents tune in and provide hands-on care for their baby, they actually help to optimize their infant's brain development and long-term outcomes. Nurturing interactions between the parent and infant in the NICU may also strengthen parent–child attachment, which can further support a child's long-term healthy development [8]. When providers support parents in understanding what is being fed to their child, they may help to foster the parents' engagement and active participation. NICU parents who are empowered with information may be better able to contribute and engage in a meaningful way. Parents seek to know precisely what is being fed to their baby, which can help them serve as informed and engaged members of their child's care team. Yet, the label HMF is imprecise.

This study has multiple limitations that warrant mention. Convenience sampling was used, as a random sample of NICU parents and providers was not available. Since the NEC Society developed the surveys, it is not surprising that 49.9% of parent respondents had a child that was affected by NEC. Additionally, the self-selected parents and providers who participated may bias the sample towards individuals who have stronger perspectives about the label HMF. Parents and providers may also have recall bias due to the retrospective nature of the study. Furthermore, parents and providers of diverse backgrounds were underrepresented.

## 5. Conclusions

This study demonstrates the need to clarify the term and concept of HMF" to parents and specify the source of the product. It may b/e beneficial to explore formal label changes to these commercial products.

**Supplementary Materials:** The Human Milk Fortifier (HMF) label survey questions for parents as well as for providers are available as supplementary materials online at http://www.mdpi.com/2072-6643/12/3/720/s1.

**Author Contributions:** Conceptualization, J.C., A.B.H., J.H.K., and S.N.T.; methodology, J.C., A.B.H., J.H.K., and S.N.T.; formal analysis, J.C., A.B.H., and S.N.T.; data curation, J.C., A.B.H., and S.N.T.; interpretation of data, J.C., A.B.H., J.H.K., and S.N.T.; writing—Original draft preparation, J.C.; writing—Review and editing, J.C., A.B.H., J.H.K., and S.N.T. All authors have read and agreed to the published version of the manuscript.

**Funding:** This research received no external funding.

**Acknowledgments:** We thank Erin Umberger, M.Arch. for designing this study's graphical abstract. The NEC Society is grateful to the Patient-Centered Outcomes Research Institute (PCORI) for the Engagement Award in support of the 2019 NEC Symposium. We thank the NICU Parent Network for distributing the survey links to their members and community. We acknowledge the parents and providers who not only responded but also shared the survey with others. Special thanks to clinical staff of Yale New Haven Hospital NICU, Nationwide Children's Hospital NICU, C.S. Mott Children's Hospital Pediatric Surgery and NICU, Washington University NICU, Texas

Children's Hospital NICU, Cincinnati Children's Hospital NICU, Riley Hospital NICU, Beth Israel Deaconess Medical Center NICU, University of Iowa Stead Family Children's Hospital NICU, Children's Healthcare of Atlanta NICU, and UC Davis Children's Hospital NICU.

**Conflicts of Interest:** J.C. has no conflicts of interest to declare. A.H. receives research grants from Prolacta Bioscience and Fresenius Kabi for two unrelated studies. J.H.K. received unrelated research grants from Fresenius Kabi and Mallinckrodt, is a consultant for Medela, Astarte Medical, and Fujifilm, and has shares in Nicolette and Astarte Medical. S.T. serves as principal investigator at Yale for unrelated research funded by Mallinckrodt Pharmaceuticals, Pfizer, Inc., and Prolacta Biosciences, and S.T. is a consultant for Alcresta Therapeutics.

## References

1. Meinzen-Derr, J.; Poindexter, B.; Wrage, L.; Morrow, A.L.; Stoll, B.; Donovan, E.F. Role of human milk in extremely low birth weight infants' risk of necrotizing enterocolitis or death. *J. Perinatol.* **2009**, *29*, 57–62. [CrossRef] [PubMed]
2. Miller, J.; Tonkin, E.; Damarell, R.; McPhee, A.; Suganuma, M.; Suganuma, H.; Middleton, P.; Makrides, M.; Collins, C. A Systematic Review and Meta-Analysis of Human Milk Feeding and Morbidity in Very Low Birth Weight Infants. *Nutrients* **2018**, *10*, 707. [CrossRef] [PubMed]
3. Quigley, M.; Embleton, N.D.; McGuire, W. Formula versus donor breast milk for feeding preterm or low birth weight infants. *Cochrane Database Syst. Rev.* **2014**, *4*. [CrossRef] [PubMed]
4. Brown, J.V.; Embleton, N.D.; Harding, J.E.; McGuire, W. Multi-nutrient fortification of human milk for preterm infants. *Cochrane Database Syst. Rev.* **2016**, *5*. [CrossRef] [PubMed]
5. Atkinson, S.A.; Bryan, M.H.; Anderson, G.H. Human milk feeding in premature infants: Protein, fat, and carbohydrate balances in the first two weeks of life. *J. Pediatrics* **1981**, *99*, 617–624. [CrossRef]
6. Gadepalli, S.K.; Canvasser, J.; Eskenazi, Y.; Quinn, M.; Kim, J.H.; Gephart, S.M. Roles and Experiences of Parents in Necrotizing Enterocolitis: An International Survey of Parental Perspectives of Communication in the NICU. *Adv. Neonatal Care* **2017**, *17*, 489–498. [CrossRef] [PubMed]
7. Gooding, J.S.; Cooper, L.G.; Blaine, A.I.; Franck, L.S.; Howse, J.L.; Berns, S.D. Family Support and Family-Centered Care in the Neonatal Intensive Care Unit: Origins, Advances, Impact. *Semin. Perinatol.* **2011**, *35*, 20–28. [CrossRef] [PubMed]
8. Pineda, R.; Bender, J.; Hall, B.; Shabosky, L.; Annecca, A.; Smith, J. Parent participation in the neonatal intensive care unit: Predictors and relationships to neurobehavior and developmental outcomes. *Early Hum. Dev.* **2018**, *117*, 32–38. [CrossRef] [PubMed]

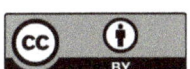

© 2020 by the authors. Licensee MDPI, Basel, Switzerland. This article is an open access article distributed under the terms and conditions of the Creative Commons Attribution (CC BY) license (http://creativecommons.org/licenses/by/4.0/).

MDPI
St. Alban-Anlage 66
4052 Basel
Switzerland
Tel. +41 61 683 77 34
Fax +41 61 302 89 18
www.mdpi.com

*Nutrients* Editorial Office
E-mail: nutrients@mdpi.com
www.mdpi.com/journal/nutrients

www.ingramcontent.com/pod-product-compliance
Lightning Source LLC
LaVergne TN
LVHW070418100526
838202LV00014B/1481